Jackie Rafferty
Jan Steyaert
David Colombi
Editors

Human Services in the Information Age

Pre-publication
REVIEWS,
COMMENTARIES,
EVALUATIONS . . .

"This work joins an important set of volumes in the human services. . . . The collection of papers in this particular volume document artful progress made in computer applications across a broad scope of human services, including disability, deviance, ethics and privacy, learning and a variety of direct client services. Anyone interested in the current state of the development of human service information systems of all types needs to read this volume.

Walter F. LaMendola, PhD
Consultant

More pre-publication
REVIEWS, COMMENTARIES, EVALUATIONS . . .

"In our ever more integrating world of the information age, sharing experiences and views across national development projects becomes vital, and this is exactly what this book does, and it does it well. This need makes conferences like HUSITA and books like this one extremely important.

Not only does it reflect the important presentations of the previous HUSITA conference, but provides us with expansive and topical world-wide information about the progress of information technology in the human services. It is worth noticing that this sector is not only a customer of the IT industry, but a major player in the development and innovative use of this technology. . . .

As a person responsible for the arrangements of the next HUSITA conference, taking place in June 1996, I feel that this book is coming into the market just in time. It gives a solid ground for the discussions that will continue in that international gathering. I hope this book will find many readers in all parts of our global community.

Victor Savtschenko, M.A.
Senior Planning Officer, IT in the Human Services STAKES, Finland's National Research and Development Centre for Welfare and Health

"The spread of IT across all areas of the human services is well-represented in this book. The editors have succeeded in putting together a rich picking of more than 30 short papers from the HUSITA 3 conference to give the reader an up-to-date and international compendium of how care professionals are using IT to improve their services.

Fred Yates, PhD
Research Psychologist,
Centre for Alcohol
and Drug Studies
Plummer Court,
Carliol Place,
Newcastle-upon-Tyne,
UK

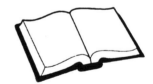

More advance
REVIEWS, COMMENTARIES, EVALUATIONS . . .

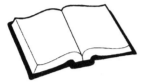

. . . The book is another milestone in bringing together the imaginative and creative skills of human service practitioners who are harnessing technology for human purposes. Indeed it really represents a view of Information Services in the Human Age.

Professor Norman J. Smith
Dean, Faculty of Social Work
The University of Queensland

"**T**his edited collection of papers gives us a glimpse of innovation in human service practice and thinking, using information technology in a creative way. The book balances a number of different but highly relevant themes and represents work from a number of countries. It is a timely publication for it successfully brings together the diversity of what has been achieved in line with its title as well as widening the frontiers open to imaginative work to achieve the editors underlying aim, the empowerment of all people through information generation and control.

The Haworth Press, Inc.

Human Services
in the Information Age

Human Services in the Information Age

Jackie Rafferty
Jan Steyaert
David Colombi
Editors

The Haworth Press, Inc.,
New York • London

Human Services in the Information Age has also been published as *Computers in Human Services*, Volume 12, Numbers 1/2/3/4 1995.

The Haworth Press, Inc., 10 Alice Street, Binghamton, NY 13904-1580 USA

Library of Congress Cataloging-in-Publication Data

Human services in the information age / Jackie Rafferty, Jan Steyaert, David Colombi, editors.
    p. cm.
Originally published as v. 12, nos. 1-4 of Computers in human services.
Includes bibliographical references.
ISBN 1-56024-768-1 (alk. paper)
    1. Human services–Data processing. I. Rafferty, Jackie. II. Steyaert, Jan. III. Colombi, David, 1945- .
HV41.H717 1996   96-4783
361'.00285–dc20   CIP

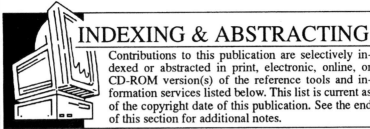

INDEXING & ABSTRACTING

Contributions to this publication are selectively indexed or abstracted in print, electronic, online, or CD-ROM version(s) of the reference tools and information services listed below. This list is current as of the copyright date of this publication. See the end of this section for additional notes.

- *Abstracts of Research in Pastoral Care & Counseling*, Loyola College, 7135 Minstrel Way, Suite 101, Columbia, MD 21045

- *ACM Guide to Computer Literature*, Association for Computing Machinery, 1515 Broadway, New York, NY 10036

- *Applied Social Sciences Index & Abstracts (ASSIA) (Online: ASSI via Data-Star)*, Bowker- Saur Limited, Maypole House, Maypole Road, East Grinstead, West Sussex RH19 1HH, England

- *caredata CD: the social and community care database*, National Institute for Social Work, 5 Tavistock Place, London WC1H 9SS, England

- *CNPIEC Reference Guide: Chinese National Directory of Foreign Periodicals*, P.O. Box 88, Beijing, People's Republic of China

- *Computer Abstracts*, MCB University Press, 60/62 Toller Lane, Bradford, West Yorkshire BD8 9BY, England

- *Computer Literature Index*, Applied Computer Research, Inc., P.O. Box 82266, Phoenix, AZ 85071-2266

- *Computing Reviews*, Association for Computing Machinery, 1515 Broadway, 17th Floor, New York, NY 10036

- *Current Contents: Clinical Medicine/Life Sciences (CC: CM/LS) (weekly Table of Contents Service)*, and *Social Science Citation Index*. Articles also searchable through *Social SciSearch*, ISI's online database and in ISI's *Research Alert* current awareness service. Institute for Scientific Information, 3501 Market Street, Philadelphia, PA 19104-3302

- *Engineering Information (PAGE ONE)*, Bibliographic Services Department, Castle Point on the Hudson, Hoboken, NJ 07030

- *Information Science Abstracts*, Plenum Publishing Company, 233 Spring Street, New York, NY 10013-1578

(continued)

- *INSPEC Information Services*, Institution of Electrical Engineers, Michael Faraday House, Six Hills Way, Stevenage, Herts SG1 2AY, England
- *INTERNET ACCESS (& additional networks) Bulletin Board for Libraries ("BUBL"), coverage of information resources on INTERNET, JANET, and other networks.*
  - JANET X.29: UK.AC.BATH.BUBL or 00006012101300
  - TELNET: BUBL.BATH.AC.UK or 138.38.32.45 login 'bubl'
  - Gopher: BUBL.BATH.AC.UK (138.32.32.45). Port 7070
  - World Wide Web: http://www.bubl.bath.ac.uk./BUBL/ home.html
  - NISSWAIS telnetniss.ac.uk (for the NISS gateway) The Andersonian Library, Curran Building, 101 St. James Road, Glasgow G4 ONS, Scotland
- *Library & Information Science Abstracts (LISA)*, Bowker-Saur Limited, Maypole House, Maypole Road, East Grinstead, West Sussex RH19 1HH, England
- *Microcomputer Abstracts,* Learned Publications, 143 Old Marlton Pike, Medford, NJ 08055
- *Periodica Islamica*, Berita Publishing, 22 Jalan Liku, 59100 Kuala Lumpur, Malaysia
- *Psychological Abstracts (PsycINFO)*, American Psychological Association, P.O. Box 91600, Washington, DC 20090-1600
- *Referativnyi Zhurnal (Abstracts Journal of the Institute of Scientific Information of the Republic of Russia)*, The Institute of Scientific Information, Baltijskaja ul., 14, Moscow A-219, Republic of Russia
- *Sage Public Administration Abstracts*, Sage Publications, Inc., 2455 Teller Road, Newbury Park, CA 91320
- *Social Planning/Policy & Development Abstracts (SOPODA)*, Sociological Abstracts, Inc., P.O. Box 22206, San Diego, CA 92192-0206
- *Social Work Abstracts*, National Association of Social Workers, 750 First Street NW, 8th Floor, Washington, DC 20002
- *Sociological Abstracts (SA)*, Sociological Abstracts, Inc., P.O. Box 22206, San Diego, CA 92192-0206
- *Urban Affairs Abstracts*, National League of Cities, 1301 Pennsylvania Avenue NW, Washington, DC 20004

SPECIAL BIBLIOGRAPHIC NOTES

related to special journal issues (separates)
and indexing/abstracting

☐ indexing/abstracting services in this list will also cover material in any "separate" that is co-published simultaneously with Haworth's special thematic journal issue or DocuSerial. Indexing/abstracting usually covers material at the article/chapter level.

☐ monographic co-editions are intended for either non-subscribers or libraries which intend to purchase a second copy for their circulating collections.

☐ monographic co-editions are reported to all jobbers/wholesalers/approval plans. The source journal is listed as the "series" to assist the prevention of duplicate purchasing in the same manner utilized for books-in-series.

☐ to facilitate user/access services all indexing/abstracting services are encouraged to utilize the co-indexing entry note indicated at the bottom of the first page of each article/chapter/contribution.

☐ this is intended to assist a library user of any reference tool (whether print, electronic, online, or CD-ROM) to locate the monographic version if the library has purchased this version but not a subscription to the source journal.

☐ individual articles/chapters in any Haworth publication are also available through the Haworth Document Delivery Services (HDDS).

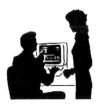

Human Services
in the Information Age

CONTENTS

REFLECTIONS

ABOUT THE EDITORS

Jackie Rafferty is a Senior Research Fellow at the Centre for Human Service Technology, University of Southampton. She is a member of the ENITH (European Network for Information Technology and Human Services) Executive and is one of the Editors of the journal *New Technology in the Human Services.* She researches the ethical and community use of the information technology and develops computer assisted learning for social work education.

Jan Steyaert is Consultant at Causa, the innovation centre of the Institute of Higher Professional Education, Faculty of Health Care and Social Work in Eindhoven, The Netherlands. He is coordinating information projects in Care and Welfare. He is also secretary of ENITH.

David Colombi is the Information Manager of West Sussex Probation Service in the UK. A shorter version of his doctoral thesis was published in 1994 as *The Probation Service and Information Technology* by the Avebury Press. He produces *Protocol Software* programs for probation and social work practice.

Colombi, Rafferty and Steyaert previously edited *Human Service and Information Technology: A European Perspective* (1993).

The three editors are currently working on a comparative analysis of information technology use in human services across 20 countries. This new publication is to be published at the HUSITA 4 conference in June 1996.

Foreword

In March 1991, I first came across Arthur Jansen, at that time employed by the provincial government of Limburg. It was on that occasion that I first heard the name HUSITA. He mentioned that the province had the idea to host an international conference on the application of information technology in human services. He knew LIOSE (Foundation for policy and management of welfare agencies) as an organisation that was capable of managing the organisation of such an event. At first, I was hesitant to commit LIOSE. This hesitation was the result of a limited knowledge on what it implied to organise an international conference about a subject I was hardly familiar with. Not withstanding this hesitation, we decided to go ahead, knowing that sufficient substantial knowledge would be available within the HUSITA network. When I met one of the spiders in this network–Bryan Glastonbury–I became convinced we probably could organise a good conference because he was chair of ENITH at the time (European Network for Information Technology in Human Services) and had good relations with the organisers of the previous HUSITA conferences. Another motivation resulted from both the provincial and state government having interest in holding the conference in the Netherlands. The Dutch government has for several years now had an active policy to raise the quality of service provision for citizens by applying information technology. Browsing through the numerous Dutch contributions to this volume, this certainly has had its effect.

To be fully prepared for the task awaiting us, I visited HUSITA 2 in New Brunswick, 1992. From that moment onwards, the preparation of HUSITA 3 really began to grow. We established important contacts and managed to get an idea of what lay ahead of us. The motivation of Marcos Leiderman, the organiser of HUSITA 2, was a great inspiration to us. We founded the HUSITA foundation and got started.

Theo Willemsen is Chair of HUSITA foundation.

[Haworth co-indexing entry note]: "Foreword." Willemsen, Theo. Co-published simultaneously in *Computers in Human Services* (The Haworth Press, Inc.) Vol. 12, No. 1/2, 1995, pp. xv-xvi; and: *Human Services in the Information Age* (ed: Jackie Rafferty, Jan Steyaert, and David Colombi) The Haworth Press, Inc., 1995, pp. xv-xvi. Single or multiple copies of this article are available from The Haworth Document Delivery Service [1-800-342-9678, 9:00 a.m. - 5:00 p.m. (EST)].

xv

I will not bother you with all further details of those preparations for the conference. Suffice it to say that a group has been working which set itself professional standards and was prepared for some hard work.

Point of departure was that the conference had to contribute to the improvement of *the quality of life and services* and that we would try hard to enable participants from Eastern European and third world countries to participate in the conference. These aims were established during a preliminary expert meeting in Valkenburg (the Netherlands) in January 1992 in which experts from 15 countries participated. The accessibility of HUSITA was increased by the foundation of a special fund to empower participants with limited resources.

Reflecting, I can state without any hesitation that the conference has been a successful one. More than 400 participants from 56 countries gathered in Maastricht, a good quantitative result. Although most of these participants came from Europe and North America, persons from Eastern Europe, Africa, the Middle East, Asia and Australia also were present. From the evaluation, it shows that participants rated the quality of the conference as high, especially because of the opportunities to establish and enlarge networks. Also, the city of Maastricht and its environment created an excellent surrounding in which work and leisure were perfectly to be combined.

The Haworth Press is to be applauded for taking the initiative for this book. It prolongs a tradition of good publications on the use of information technology in the human services. In their preface, the editors explain how HUSITA 3 is part of the established tradition of conferences and publications on this subject. They also provide an overview of the contents of this book. They have succeeded in making a good selection of papers presented during the conference. This book thereby becomes a valuable document. It can become an important contribution to the further improvement of the quality of life and services. The contents can therefore be a starting point for the HUSITA 4 conference in June 1996, Finland. I wish the organisers of HUSITA 4 a lot of success and the readers of this book a lot of inspiration.

See you in Finland. Electronic communication may become the item of the coming years, but nothing surpasses personal communication.

Theo Willemsen

Preface

During the last decade, a recurrent theme in the literature on the use of information technology in Human Services has been the slow progress of incorporating the new technologies into the activities of human service agencies. Since 1987, three international conferences, organised under the title of HUSITA (Human Service Information Technology Applications), have brought together people working in the human services to share and discuss ideas and developments. If these conferences have taught us one thing, it is that across the world, many agencies and people are taking up the challenge to use information technology to improve the quality, efficiency, and effectiveness of their service provision.

The 1987 HUSITA conference in Birmingham, UK and the 1992 HU-SITA 2 conference in New Jersey, USA laid the ground for the highly successful 1993 HUSITA 3 conference in Maastricht in the province of Limburg in the Netherlands. The conference had the theme of *Information Technology and the Quality of Life and Services*. Over 400 participants from 56 countries gathered for a week to present experiences and research findings, to share information, and to discuss important developments. The editors of this book have the luxury of not having been involved in organising the conference, so we can comment on how well it was organised without having real inside knowledge of how much hard work was involved. It can be and is an opportunity to record our thanks to all those who undertook the work in such a professional and dedicated manner and express our appreciation for the generous and warm hospitality of our Dutch hosts.

This book contains a selection of the papers presented at the HUSITA 3 conference, albeit many have been updated to take into account more recent developments. The conference was the occasion for the launch of two other significant publications. The first was a pre-conference selection

[Haworth co-indexing entry note]: "Preface." Rafferty, Jackie, Jan Steyaert, and David Colombi. Co-published simultaneously in *Computers in Human Services* (The Haworth Press, Inc.) Vol. 12, No. 1/2, 1995, pp. xvii-xxiii; and: *Human Services in the Information Age* (ed: Jackie Rafferty, Jan Steyaert, and David Colombi) The Haworth Press, Inc., 1995, pp. xvii-xxiii. Single or multiple copies of this article are available from The Haworth Document Delivery Service [1-800-342-9678, 9:00 a.m. - 5:00 p.m. (EST)].

of conference papers which were edited by Bryan Glastonbury (1993) and published by Van Gorcum as *Human Welfare and Technology*. The second was *Human Service and Information Technology: A European Perspective* (Colombi, Rafferty and Steyaert, 1993) which was published by ENITH and provided an overview of developments in Europe with contributions from fourteen countries. This publication was part of the contribution of ENITH (European Network for Information Technology in Human Services) to the HUSITA 3 conference.

In selecting from over sixty papers available for publication in the current volume, the editors have striven for a balance between the diverse themes presented at the conference as well as a representative geographical spread. The literature has, perhaps inevitably, been dominated by contributions from Western Europe and from North America, although from the start the HUSITA movement has been concerned with issues of empowerment within and between societies. The HUSITA conferences included presentations from Africa, Asia, the Middle East, Australia, North and South America, and East and West Europe. We are fortunate in having valuable and innovative contributions to this book from India, Israel, and from Eastern Europe in the form of the Czech Republic and Rumania.

However, there is still far to go in achieving a better balance worldwide and that remains a continuing challenge for HUSITA. It is of course part of a much wider issue of how technology transfer to the developing world is managed and priced and how developments are nurtured so that the true potential of information technology to contribute to the developing world can be realised. The present reality is a wide gap between the information rich and the information poor reflecting existing divisions between rich and poor in societies. Information and knowledge have the capacity to be shared and endlessly reproduced. This means they have inherently democratic properties which become accessible as the technology becomes increasingly available and affordable. We shall return to this theme in later discussion of the Internet which can be identified as perhaps one of the most powerful anarchic, democratic, and empowering forces against a prevailing trend of technology and media control by governments and multi-national corporations. Still within a geographic perspective, there are the relatively new phenomena of developments in rural contexts within societies, which are the subject matter of two absorbing papers in this book. Both are at the forefront of technological developments. The first is concerned with meeting information and communication needs of rural communities in Scotland and the second is about the development of communications camps in Finland.

Another important dimension is the issue of disability. Five papers are included which address disability issues and very different developments in India, Germany, Britain, the USA and Israel. These reflect human experiences as well as technological aspects. In two of the papers, the authors write about their own experiences of being helped to overcome their disabilities through information technology. Rather than treating disability as a separate issue, these papers are integrated into the wider thematic structure of the book. Reference to "disability" is itself an issue, with the term "physically challenged" gaining increasing recognition as a more appropriate term, particularly in North America. Throughout the book, the editors have sought to avoid use of discriminatory references whilst at the same time reflecting and respecting the approaches and thinking in different countries. At present the term "disability" is too firmly established in common usage to be rejected without violation to the work of authors–several of whom refer to non-physical disabilities as well. We can however note this as an issue and reflect on how far the issue of language is tied to the very different stages within countries in terms of establishing rights for people who are disabled.

The structure of the book is led by the theme of the conference and by the subject matter of the papers selected. Our aim was to select the best and most relevant papers rather than ones that fitted to a pre-ordained structure. Many of these fell into natural groupings such as those to do with "Social Work Education" or with "Widening Communications," which are clear growth areas in use of the technology. Many papers were to do with the adoption and development of systems within agencies. The primary division here was between those on the one hand that had to do directly with "Assessment and Provision of Services" to clients and on the other hand, those that had to do with "Information Systems for Agencies and Practitioners" at an organisational level. Another group of papers that addressed particular themes (such as race equality, health and safety, and privacy protection) that cut across these categories and which could be included under the heading of our opening section, "The Quality of Life." This left a small group of wide-ranging papers for the final section of "Reflections" written from more global or wide-ranging perspectives about the development and implications of use of technology in the human services.

Each of these sections has its own introduction which sets the individual papers in a wider context and comments on the contribution that each makes. Through this process, certain themes develop and are explored. With such a wide range of papers and subject matter, it is difficult, if not impossible, to summarise the themes into a coherent whole without distorting and diminishing the work of the authors. We can however seek to place some of the themes in the broad context of developments which can be charted through the history of the HUSITA movement and which leads on to the next HUSITA conference in Lapland in 1996. This book stands in succession to earlier conference books that between them provide a history of developments in this area. Even before the first HUSITA conference, *The Human Edge–Information Technology and Helping People* edited by Geiss and Viswanathan (1986) set the tone as a remarkable book following a conference held in Maryland, USA in 1984. This identified many of the themes, vision, hopes, and concerns that are still, despite all the technological changes, relevant to us ten years later. The link with HUSITA was made tangible by provision of *The Human Edge* to attendees at the first HUSITA conference in 1987 which was the first major international gathering of professionals working in this area. Two books of HUSITA conference papers followed: (1) *Information Technology and the Human Services* edited by Glastonbury, LaMendola and Toole (1988), and (2) *A Casebook of Computer Applications in the Social and Human Services* edited by LaMendola, Glastonbury and Toole (1989). These together with publication of other conference papers in the journal *Computers in Human Services* represented a major publishing endeavour. These papers marked in great detail the then state of development of the technology and reflected the sense of hope and excitement from the HUSITA conference for the future, tempered with concerns about issues of empowerment, privacy and control.

The second HUSITA conference in 1991 was followed by publication of *Technology in People Services* edited by Leiderman, Monnickendam, Guzzeta and Struminger (1993). Again a wide-ranging spread of papers marked progress that had been made, but it was also a period of some frustration as it became increasingly clear that developments were going to be slower than many of us wished. Applying expert system approaches within the imprecision of social work contexts was clearly a complex, time consuming and often frustrating task. Too many people were working on development areas that were inadequately resourced for the potential of the work to be fully realised. Some seemingly promising technologies were being outmoded just as they were starting to be seriously developed. In the later category emerging use of interactive video-disks as a teaching tool was being outmoded by the development of CD-ROM based multimedia systems. At a political level, issues of empowerment became more urgent and immediate through powerfully articulated expression within the conference. The latter was a positive factor as was progress recorded in many areas of development and important initiatives in the area of networking and extending this beyond being primarily a North American phenomenon. Although the conference was an undoubtable success, many of us came away uncertain and less sure about future directions after the heady excitement of the first HUSITA experience.

In this context a number of themes can be identified from HUSITA 3 and from this book. The first is the value of people from a wide range of cultures and backgrounds meeting together to listen to each other, to learn from each other, and to share experiences, ideas, and plans. The conference reinforced the value of the "HUSITA experience" which Schoech in the foreword to *Technology in People Services* (ibid.) described as a continuum of networking activities involving face-to-face meeting, literature, and electronic networking.

The second theme seemed to be the transition from a focus primarily on experimental innovative activities into continuing innovation balanced by more systematic application of established methodologies on a wider scale. More of the developments seemed to be happening not just within individual agencies and institutions but as part of a regional, national or international programme of development across a specific area of service provision. We see this clearly in papers included here on Dutch work on supporting integrated home care and their experiences with client databanks, on work in the Moravian Region of the Czech Republic on unemployment assistance, and on the Finnish experience of planning services for elderly people. At an international level, the work on rural communications in Scotland (referred to earlier) is part of a European project. This trend represents a growing confidence and respectability about the work, as the case for use of information technology to support and develop services moves into the heart of agency functioning and into the heart of social work education.

While it is rash to make any predictions about the future of information technology itself, there is in some ways a greater clarity now than there was at the start of the decade. The immediate future seems to be about graphical environments (particularly Windows), about CD-ROMs, about multimedia systems, and about electronic networking through the Internet and the World Wide Web. Use of the Windows environment and multimedia has brought with it new standards of presentation and quality, but also development tools that make those standards achievable. Never have the tools to develop applications that are relevant to enhancing practice in the human services and the technical means to share them been so available. It is encouraging to be able to report here on new initiatives that are making good use of those possibilities. However there still remain important barriers about learning to use the applications, having time and resources to develop and maintain information systems, and barriers to learning to explore and use the wealth of information that is increasingly accessible.

In this context, the section on *Widening Communications* includes valuable information on the development of access to electronic networks throughout the world. This is a fundamental issue for all of us struggling to make sense of the rich and confusing diversity of information. What is important here is not just the electronic networks, on-line databases, and bulletin boards, but the people networks established through HUSITA that can be maintained through electronic networks. The exponential growth in use of the Internet has major implications for how societies communicate internally and internationally in ways that can make McCluhan's concept of the global village begin to seem real. In an era of increasing control by multi-national corporations of television and other media, the Internet is an anarchic and uncontrolled genie that may prove impossible to put back in its magic lamp.

Whatever the future of the Internet and the Information Superhighway, the concept of low-cost, fast communications is here to stay and may become as much a part of our natural cultural environment as language itself.

As noted earlier, we live in a world of information insiders and information outsiders separated by barriers of wealth, power, privilege, race, geography, and nationality. Ultimately the success of all our work will depend on the extent to which we have recreated and moulded this extraordinary technology to serve and meet human needs. We must redress the balance of power away from the powerful and towards those in need of better services and a better quality of life. The HUSITA movement has an honourable record of good intentions and of some achievement in enabling the voices of those in need to be heard and met. It is however the end to which we must all continually strive if we are not to look back on this as an era of crucial opportunities lost through lack of vision and courage.

Jackie Rafferty
Jan Steyaert
David Colombi

REFERENCES

Colombi D.P., Rafferty J. and Steyaert J. (Eds.) (1993) *Human Service and Information Technology: A European Perspective.* Published by ENITH (available from the Centre for Human Service Technology, University of Southampton, Southampton, Hampshire, UK.)
Geiss G.R. & Viswanathan N. (1986) *The Human Edge-Information Technology and Helping People.* New York: Haworth.
Glastonbury B. (Ed.) (1993) *Human Welfare and Technology.* Assen, Netherlands: Van Gorcum.

Glastonbury B., LaMendola W. & Toole S. (1988) *Information Technology and the Human Services.* Chichester England: John Wiley and Sons.

LaMendola W., Glastonbury B. and Toole S. (1989) *A Casebook of Computer Applications in the Social and Human Services.* New York: Haworth.

Leiderman M., Monnickendam M., Guzzeta C. and Struminger L. (Eds.) (1993) *Technology in People Services.* New York: Haworth.

THE QUALITY OF LIFE

Introduction

Jackie Rafferty

The five papers in this section were chosen to reflect the main theme of the Husita 3 Conference, *Information Technology and the Quality of Life and Services.* The conference was notable for the number of participants from the less wealthy nations as well as service users, academics and professionals. Three of the five papers are from authors who combine a number of these roles. Their papers are a timely reminder that the sharing across frontiers of information, expertise, and experience on the use of technology in the human services is not an "academic exercise" but one that has the potential to reach millions of people and to enhance or deny their quality of life.

Joseph Varghese, Geoff Busby and Richard Reinoehl are academics and professionals who write from their own experiences of empowerment and disability through technology. Varghese in the first paper discredits the notion that technology and human services are a minority interest by pointing to the scope of technology to aid the estimated 100 million disabled people in India alone. Busby, in "Facilitating Citizenship," uses his

Jackie Rafferty is Senior Research Fellow at the Centre for Human Service Technology, University of Southampton, UK.

[Haworth co-indexing entry note]: "Introduction." Rafferty, Jackie. Co-published simultaneously in *Computers in Human Services* (The Haworth Press, Inc.) Vol. 12, No. 1/2, 1995, pp. 1-4; and: *Human Services in the Information Age* (ed: Jackie Rafferty, Jan Steyaert, and David Colombi) The Haworth Press, Inc., 1995, pp. 1-4. Single or multiple copies of this article are available from The Haworth Document Delivery Service [1-800-342-9678, 9:00 a.m. - 5:00 p.m. (EST)].

1

personal perspective and experience on disability and technology to challenge current preoccupations of governments with individualism. He suggests that a greater sense of community is required if people with disabilities are going to achieve the full rights of citizenship through technology. "The Computer Dilemma: Harming the Helpers," by Reinoehl et al., takes us down a related path, which is too often neglected. The authors share with us the preventative measures required to stop computer users from becoming disabled with soft tissue and joint dysfunction. The papers by Kish Bhatti-Sinclair and Erik Van Hove share a European focus and show the impact that data protection and security, or the lack of it, in information systems is having on individuals and different communities. Bhatti-Sinclair gives a fascinating insight into the use of information technology to track cross-border movement across Europe. She argues that the use of such systems is adversely affecting black people disproportionately. Finally, Van Hove concentrates on data protection legislation across Europe and the danger the legislation poses for the provision of research information to social policy makers and the potentially damaging effect this could have on people's lives.

Bryan Glastonbury in his prologue to *Human Welfare and Technology* (1993) writes:

.. that the aim of the participants (of HUSITA) remains to explain and push forward the part IT can play in strengthening the lives of the global community, not in a detached bureaucratic or 'number-crunching' way but in a way which is simultaneously helpful and without threat, life enhancing and not life controlling . . .

These five papers detail the potential for life enhancement but warn of the dangers and challenges that still need to be faced if the aim of HUSITA is to be realized.

Dr. Joseph Varghese in his paper "Independence to the Blind and Handicapped in Asia Through Modern Assistive Devices," links the need to improve the education and rehabilitation of disabled people in Asia to enable independence to the need for both global and local communities to take responsibility to achieve this. As a qualified social worker with a Doctorate in Special Education and also a person who lost his sight at the age of six, Varghese speaks both from the heart and the head as he describes the work of Ability Aids India International. He makes what is essentially a plea to the wealthy nations to share their expertise and assistive technologies in a way which will enable Asia to short-cut the developmental process. Disabled people could then profit from the work done elsewhere.

Geoff Busby is a professional in the computer industry and in his paper puts forward a very personal perspective on the importance of technology empowering both himself, as a person with cerebral palsy, and others to achieve full citizenship. Busby's paper links to the first by Varhgese as he challenges the stereotypes that people have about disability that is based on the western world view. Busby asks us to look to the lesser developed countries to find alternative concepts and values. He suggests a synthesis of both is needed for people who find themselves excluded from the mainstream of life. Busby and Varghese place the ethical agenda firmly in the centre. As Busby puts it, "Can the world ethically reject the opportunity to facilitate the complete citizenship of disabled people and their carers?"

The next paper presents another side of the coin as Reinoehl et al. write about the potential damage that computers can cause human service workers. It provides a detailed account of how "as we move towards a future of increased computer use, we also move toward a future of increased risk for computer related disabilities . . . " Reinoehl describes the problem areas in detail and addresses the treatments and ergonomic issues which can help. He argues that these problems are not individual physiological problems but systemic with ramifications throughout an organization. This is one of those subjects where "the can't happen to me syndrome" applies. It is not often a book of this nature contains a paper full of practical advice and the editors suggest every reader should take account of this issue as it may save you many painful years ahead.

Kish Bhatti-Sinclair's paper broadens the theme away from individuals to communities again as she discusses "Race Equality and Information Technology in Europe," through the focus of how IT systems impact on black people. She relates the rise of racism in Europe to the uncertain status of many non-nationals who do not have full rights of citizenship, the majority of whom are black. She also looks at the often clandestine nature of committees and groups responsible for European Policies on Immigration and IT. Her conclusion offers some avenues which would allow for greater equity and suggests that "the lack of established procedures and computerization has led in many instances to the discretionary interpretation of rules and regulations by officials. For black people discretion usually equals discriminatory behavior . . . "

We end this chapter with another cautionary tale which highlights a potential problem, initially, for the social research community of the privacy protection laws in Europe. One of the areas where human services takes some pride is in its concern for the privacy of individuals. This is most evidenced by the approach to confidentiality and data protection in human service training, education and practice. Yet as Erik Van Hove points out in his paper "The Legislation on Privacy Protection and Social Research,"

... The introduction of powerful information technology in scientific research and progress in emancipation of citizens raises the problem of controlling that flow of information in the research context as well as in other spheres of action. The research community has a tradition of open communication which can easily come into conflict with the need to be careful with personal information ...

Van Hove takes the reader through a definition of the "notion of privacy" as it affects individuals and the "attention to privacy protection" before laying out the main principles of the legislation and looking at a comparison among four European countries. He then outlines the objectives of the European Parliament to harmonize the rules concerning privacy protection in the twelve countries of the European Community and the consequences these will have on social research. Van Hove concludes by setting out a guide to good practice which would protect the individual whilst ensuring the possibility of continuing social research.

Five very different papers but with common themes involving the rights of individuals and the responsibilities of communities, whether the community is a small Indian village or the European Community. Glastonbury and LaMendola argue that human service professionals form an important part of the "ethics industry" (1993). These papers show us ways in which we have to act outside the traditional human service arenas if we are to meet the challenge of ensuring that technology empowers people.

REFERENCES

Glastonbury, B., (Ed.), *Human Welfare and Technology,* Van Gorcum, Assen, 1993. ISBN. 90-232-2831-6.
Glastonbury, B., and LaMendola, W., *The Integrity of Intelligence-A Bill of Rights for the Information Age,* St. Martin's Press, New York. pp 163-170.

Independence to the Blind
and Handicapped in Asia
Through Modern Assistive Devices

Joseph E. Varghese

SUMMARY. It is estimated that there are around 100 million disabled people in India alone. This is more than three times the population of Canada. The disabled in India and Asia are not in possession of many devices with which they may combat their disabilities. Some do have access to low-level technological devices. Very few have access to medium-tech devices. Only a handful have access to high-tech items. Production, distribution and promotion of assistive devices for the handicapped can only be achieved through the active co-operation of trans-national agencies. This is the need of the handicapped in Asia today. *[Article copies available from The Haworth Document Delivery Service: 1-800-342-9678.]*

INTRODUCTION

Asia is the largest continent on earth. More than 60% of the world's population live there and the continent cradled some of the major civilisations and religions of history. The people are friendly, hospitable and able.

Joseph E. Varghese, PhD, is Founder-President of The Christian Institute of Technology, Founder-Managing Director of The National Christian Service and The Ability Aids India International, Trivandrum, as well as being Founder-President of The Kerala Federation of the Blind and The International Institute of Ability Advancement, Inc., of New York. Dr. Varghese's Doctorate is in Special Education and Counselling from Wayne State University, Detroit. Dr. Varghese is also a certified social worker and rehabilitation counsellor.

[Haworth co-indexing entry note]: "Independence to the Blind and Handicapped in Asia Through Modern Assistive Devices." Varghese, Joseph E. Co-published simultaneously in *Computers in Human Services* (The Haworth Press, Inc.) Vol. 12, No. 1/2, 1995, pp. 5-12; and: *Human Services in the Information Age* (ed: Jackie Rafferty, Jan Steyaert, and David Colombi) The Haworth Press, Inc., 1995, pp. 5-12. Single or multiple copies of this article are available from The Haworth Document Delivery Service [1-800-342-9678, 9:00 a.m. - 5:00 p.m. (EST)].

5

They have the spirit to combat adversities, the strength to face realities and the audacity to reshape their destiny. Of course, they have conflicts, illiteracy, superstitions and poverty as constant and age-old companions to combat. In order to achieve any success they have to work hard and long.

With the exception of Japan, all countries in Asia are underdeveloped or developing. I do not forget the tremendous progress being achieved by Hong Kong and Singapore but these are city states. At the same time some of the countries in Asia are very backward economically and have yet to be introduced to modern life styles. When they are struggling to advance their living conditions of the general population, how can they think about improving the lot of their disabled brethren?

ESCO estimates that 10-15% of the world population is disabled. That means one out of every 8 or 10 persons is disabled. If the acute social and economic disadvantage of a person is also taken into consideration, the number of disabled persons might be much more. For example, malnourished children, though fully physically normal in infancy, may grow as mentally underdeveloped adults through no fault of their own. Similarly, untreated childhood diseases may result in disabilities later on.

India has the second largest population in the world today numbering nearly 900 million according to statistics just released. If such is the case, the total disabled population in India must number at least 135 million. That means the handicapped population of India comes to more than half the population of the United States of America, i.e., nearly 5 times the population of Canada and more than the combined populations of several countries in Europe. The problem, indeed, is colossal. A big problem demands a big solution.

The slow progress of education, technology and industrial development that Europe and America have experienced need not necessarily be repeated in Asia. Technology and industrial development can bypass and overstep centuries of slow development in any country. Examples are too numerous to narrate, just look at the tremendous progress achieved by Japan and pockets of development achieved by other countries.

India, for example, in nearly 40 years has come to the rocket, satellite and electronic age from the age of "bullock-cart." I am drawing this analogy to show that the disabled in Asian countries do not have to wait for centuries to get abreast of their western brethren.

WHAT ACTUALLY ARE ASSISTIVE DEVICES?

When human beings wanted to move people and cargo fast, they invented the wheel. When they wanted to cross large bodies of water, they invented boats. When they wanted to go from place to place still faster, they invented the aeroplane. When they wanted records kept, they made paper. Then they went to voice recording and filming. Now we have compact discs, video tapes and personal computers. A pencil, a pen, a coffee-maker, a shaver–all are assistive devices: Imagine a world without any of these consumer items. Now consider the world of the millions of disabled persons in the developing countries? Most of them do not have the means to keep any records or read a document. They do not have even a cane to guide them, let alone wheelchairs and electronic devices. We need to think about them and do need to do something for them. What shall we do? We have to harness modern technology on their behalf.

PERSONAL BACKGROUND

Let me backtrack a little bit, to give you brief background information about myself. I am 60 years old. I was born and raised in a village in Kerala, the southern-most part of India. When I lost my sight in 1938 at the age of 6, nobody in my family knew if I could continue my education. I was admitted to a school for the blind and I was taught Braille, which opened vistas of knowledge unavailable to me till then.

The only assistive devices I had seen during my school and college years were a Braille slate, a Stainsbury Braille writer and a reel-to-reel tape recorder. I had to wait more than two years, after leaving college, to purchase my first Braille watch from Switzerland. I purchased the watch only after laborious correspondence to obtain the foreign exchange and import license. I saw a cassette recorder only when I went to the United States of America for further education in the early 1970s. I learned to travel alone with a cane and got introduced to many sophisticated aids and appliances there. When I became adept with the technological wonders, blindness became to me just a physical nuisance, and nothing more.

EDUCATION AND REHABILITATION FOR ASIA

Visually handicapped students in America (I suspect in Europe as well) are familiar with reading machines, personal computers, travel-aids, Braille printers and many other gadgets that make their education and life much easier. These special aids and appliances help them to overcome their disabilities. The cases of locomotor-handicapped and hearing-handicapped persons are no different. Efficient electric wheelchairs, hearing aids and hand-controlled cars are common. The word-processor and the micro-computer have come of age on the college campus.

Unless we improve the education and rehabilitation of the disabled persons in Asia, we cannot think of their employment or independence. If we think of residential education for the handicapped, the disabled population in this continent will remain uneducated for the next 1000 years or more. An intense effort has to be undertaken akin to being on a war-footing to rehabilitate the disabled of Asia all at once. If we look towards the governments to get this done, that might take another 1000 years. Governments have to worry about many other things. Education and rehabilitation of the handicapped come low on their agenda.

The people have to take responsibility for their disabled brothers and sisters on a community basis. Non-governmental organisations and local governments have to be inspired, encouraged and helped to do the job. Let me illustrate by giving an example. If the Government of India were to educate, rehabilitate and employ the handicapped people of India, it would take for them trillions of rupees, millions of personnel and centuries to get the job done. On the other hand, if the local private organisations would come forward to help the local handicapped individuals, the job could be done more easily and quickly. For example: A few million rupees would get the job done in Trivandrum in three to five years. Similarly, each village, town and city must be motivated to educate and rehabilitate their own disabled population.

ABILITY AIDS INDIA INTERNATIONAL

The Ability Aids India International, of which I am Managing Director, wants to do something in this respect. We would like to manufacture essential special aids and appliances for the visually, hearing, locomotor and other handicapped persons. We would like to research and develop more special aids using indigenous materials and using modern technology. We have already produced prototypes of wheelchairs, tricycles and such other basic items for the physically handicapped. We have also started selling braillette boxes to teach Braille to the blind. We are planning to produce canes, crutches and other items of low technology. We would then like to produce medium technology items.

We, of course, have plans to enter the high technology field as well. There are modern research facilities nearby. The Electronics Research and Development Centre (ER&DC) is an Indian Government autonomous institution doing commendable research in electronics and allied disciplines. We have also the Institute of Human Resources Development for Electronics

(IHRDE), Electronics Regional Testing Laboratories (ERTL), Government Engineering College and many other institutions of higher learning and research. AAII has a good understanding and working relationships with them.

TECHNOLOGY TRANSFER

We are quite capable of doing research, designing, modifying, inventing and adapting all kinds of assistive devices for all categories of the handicapped. Engineers, technicians, skilled and unskilled workers are in plentiful supply in Kerala, where we are situated. Salaries are unbelievably low compared to the western countries. We would like to enter into collaboration with manufacturers of assistive devices from anywhere in the world. We do not intend to "reinvent the wheel." We want to take full advantage of scientific advancement and technological development on behalf of the disabled. We also would like to receive assistance in this regard. We need technological know-how, expert training and financial help. We, at the Ability Aids India International are ready, willing and able to go any distance and anywhere on behalf of the handicapped of Asia, in procuring their full freedom and independence for the 21st century.

ASSISTIVE DEVICES

The disabled of Asian countries need education. Not necessarily formal education but access to cassette recorders and cassette players that will enable them to listen to books and periodicals. We are planning to produce a four-track half-speed cassette player, the type that is used in the United States. We estimate that the player would cost less than $30 (in US currency) per unit if it is mass produced and the price will be much less in the course of time. We are also planning to enter into a contract with the Electronics Research and Development Centre (ER&DC) for transfer of technology for the right to produce the first electric wheelchair in India. We estimate the price to be less than $1500 (in US currency) per unit. Our present problems are the right kind of motor and batteries. Once we sort these things out, the price per unit may come down.

Two more items that may be of interest are an electronic chalk-board and an audio-visual telephone switchboard. We have identified more than forty other items, including talking watches and meters, audio-visual traffic signals, visual alarms (for the deaf), etc. These and other gadgets will open employment opportunities for the handicapped as never before in India and other Asian countries.

OPPORTUNITIES FOR TECHNOLOGY TRANSFER

The Government of India has recently liberalised economic and industrial policies, making it possible for foreign entrepreneurs and investors to come to India. Foreign exchange regulations are favourable as never before. AAII will guarantee the international intellectual property rights of any patent holder. We are looking for collaboration with manufacturers of special aids and appliances for the visually handicapped, the locomotor and physically handicapped, the hearing handicapped and other print-handicapped groups. We also would like to invite funding agencies to come forward to assist us in making essential assistive devices available for the ordinary handicapped persons in India at a price they could afford. We are confident we can prevail upon non-governmental organisations and local governments to come to the aid of handicapped individuals in procuring these devices.

PLAN FOR ACTION

AAII has a very well prepared plan of action. We aim to promote research, development, production and distribution of low, medium and high-tech aids and appliances for the disabled in Asian countries. We would like to promote the use of assistive devices among the handicapped through effective demonstrations, exhibitions and public education to individuals, groups, governments and non-governmental organisations on all aspects of special education and rehabilitation.

We will also be operating a comprehensive rehabilitation complex offering motivation and evaluation services, orientation and mobility, skill development services, rehabilitation engineering and technology services, production, servicing and distribution of assistive devices and several other innovative programs. We will also be providing help with employment and self-help projects to the disabled and disadvantaged persons, aiding in their full integration into the mainstream of society.

EXAMPLES OF PEOPLE WHO ARE RECEIVING SERVICES

Before concluding, let me draw before you the picture of two or three clients whom we have the privilege of serving:

A successful mechanical engineer accidentally falls from the second floor of a building. His spinal-cord is broken and instantaneously made immobile. We found him confined to his bed in his village home. He is now trained as a computer operator. He whizzes around in his wheelchair radiating exuberance all around.

We found a young woman talented and educated who due to polio and scoliosis was being suffocated by her bending body. The doctors told us that she might die of self-asphyxiation in a few years. Corrective surgeries were performed which cost more than eighty thousand rupees (approximately $3000). But imagine the joy of setting a "captive free"!

A young teenager goes to the hospital for the treatment for an ordinary disease and comes out totally blind due to the wrong medication being administered by the doctors. We would like to see her rehabilitated, leading an independent life following a useful career of her choice.

CONCLUSION

In conclusion, I would like to state a few things: The world has become very small. The cultural chasms are not as wide as before. The television has brought the world to our living rooms. Scientific and technological advances benefit humanity much more than ever before at a phenomenal speed. Yesterday's essentials have become today's necessities, even in the remote corners of the globe. The human family is one. We know that in our heads. Do we feel it in our hearts?

The disabled are part of the human family. A chain is only as strong as its weakest link. The weaker links of humanity have to be made strong. We need concerted, considered and concrete action.

Rehabilitation of the disabled is not the responsibility of one community or country alone any more. We cannot neglect or ignore, the needs of 15% of the human population. They have to be integrated educationally, culturally, economically and socially. They ought to be given the opportunity to lead their lives with dignity. They must earn a living rather than subsist on the mercy of others.

Assistive devices are absolutely essential for the independence of the blind and handicapped persons particularly in Asia and generally in the whole world. In order to maximise employment opportunities for disabled people we need to give them the full advantages and benefit of the scientific and technological advancements available to the non-handicapped. If some products could be produced cheaper and better in Asia than in a developed country, we must take steps to do just that. The benefit would go directly to the disabled, who happen to be on the bottom part of the economic totempole.

In order to make the blind and handicapped of Asia independent and self-sufficient, educationally, economically and socially, it takes the considerate and concerted efforts of all concerned in the human services community.

May the messages delivered and the spirit emanating from HUSITA-3 awaken the human conscience, inspire the human spirit and enhance the applied technology in liberating the handicapped people the world over.

Facilitating Citizenship

Geoff Busby

SUMMARY. Approximately 1 in 10 of the world's population is made up of people with disabilities. Such disabilities, even in the western world, has the effect of denying full citizenship in the terms of freedom of choice to do what you want, when you want and how. To some degree technology can help facilitate this citizenship. My paper attempts to describe this technology and moreover questions whether more could be done if there were to be a change in the sense of values in the more developed nations. *[Article copies available from The Haworth Document Delivery Service: 1-800-342-9678.]*

Most readers will be expecting a totally technical paper, in fact I would rather describe it as a technico/socio one. Most of the anecdotal references are subjective, but having been a person with Cerebral Palsy all my life and having spent the last eighteen years involving myself in technical

Geoff Busby, is Chief Executive (External Developments), GEC Computer Services, Ltd., Essex, UK. Geoff Busby is 50 years old and has the condition of cerebral palsy. Since 1975 he has been involved in the technology pertaining to disability and has led many projects in this area. He has travelled extensively, including visits to Iraq, Tokyo, USA and most of Europe. He is married with two sons.

Address correspondence to: Geoff Busby, MBE, D.Univ, MA, FBCS, C.Eng, Chief Executive (External Developments), c/o GEC Computer Services Ltd, Hanningfield Road, Chelmsford, Essex CM2 8HN, UK.

The author would like to thank GEC Computer Services Ltd, who have seconded me to the projects concerned with IT and disability, on which I have been working for the past eight years and Concept 2000 for sponsoring me to carry out all my European work.

[Haworth co-indexing entry note]: "Facilitating Citizenship." Busby, Geoff. Co-published simultaneously in *Computers in Human Services* (The Haworth Press, Inc.) Vol. 12, No. 1/2, 1995, pp. 13-20; and: *Human Services in the Information Age* (ed: Jackie Rafferty, Jan Steyaert, and David Colombi) The Haworth Press, Inc., 1995, pp. 13-20. Single or multiple copies of this article are available from The Haworth Document Delivery Service [1-800-342-9678, 9:00 a.m. - 5:00 p.m. (EST)].

13

solutions to disability, leading me into the sociopolitical arena, perhaps the subjectivity is not so serious as it may seem. I hope, indeed, that my life's experiences have afforded me greater insight into disability, thus enabling me to express opinions and disseminate information which a non-disabled person would not be able to do with the same degree of authority.

My disability is such that I am a wheelchair user with non-effective use of my hands and have a speech defect, which makes communication difficult with strangers. My public presentations are therefore given by the technique of using overhead foils of my text to support delegates who may not understand my speech.

We learn as much from sorrow as from joy, as much from illness as from health, from handicap as from advantage–indeed perhaps more

Pearl S. Buck

Inherent in my title is the suggestion of people with disabilities not being offered a choice of full citizenship. The Oxford English Dictionary defines citizenship as a person who has full rights in a county or commonwealth by birth or naturalization. This definition was obviously written before the European Economic Community was founded, otherwise it would have surely included "community." Rights could be said to equate freedom of choice and access, for example: the ability to vent one's feelings and demonstrate one's latent skills; to choose when to go to the toilet, go to bed, get up, say I love you, obey or disobey national laws, enter public buildings, travel by public transport from A to B at a chosen time; the ability to select a television channel and the chance to decide who to allow to enter their abode, are choices and chances most of us take for granted.

These kind of choices could, fairly simply, be extended to the disabled by empowering them through technology. By the same token, the limitations imposed on carers could be minimised by decreasing the burden created through the "knock on" effect of disability. Statistically, one in ten of the world's population have a disability of some kind during their lives. In pure numerical terms this amounts to 6.2 million in the UK and 33 million in Europe. Of course, not all of these will be severely disabled but even if you talk in terms of one percent and multiply by four, which is the average number of people affected by having a severely disabled person within the family, then we are talking about large numbers of people being denied full citizenship.

I have suggested that technology can afford citizenship to the above mentioned group, who represent a significant element in the cultural patchwork which forms the overall pattern of the canvas embroidered by the world's population. What then is the root cause preventing such technology being provided to all those who require it? In short, it is our sense of values. Market driven values and the imagery necessarily created for them to survive, has led to the concept of perfection equalling excellence. Thus we are bombarded with advertising called for to support such a philosophy.

The picture I have painted emphasises the challenge facing us and how we are able to affect the lives of people with disabilities. Surely we need to overlook the brainwashing of advertising which ignores all of us having afflictions. Such advertising concentrates in images of physical beauty, perfection and strength. In short, they are saying the superficial being, rather than the reality of Mr. Average, who probably cannot afford to own a top of the range car. Or the woman who cares more about paying her bills than the colour of her hair. Least of all, will you see the one in ten persons with a disability. When you do, it will be in a negative way, highlighting disability as opposed to ABILITY.

Riccado Patrella, Head of the European Union Fast Initiatives goes as far as to suggest that the vocabulary of the western world encourages stereo-typing and such senses of values. He maintains that key words of developed countries are along the lines of:–

PRODUCTIVITY
COMPETITIVENESS
EFFICIENCY
PROFITABILITY
OPTIMISATION
FLEXIBILITY
CONTROL
MEASURABILITY
MANAGEABILITY

Whereas, the language of lesser developed countries is inclined to be more altruistic, focusing on words like:–

HAPPINESS
BEAUTY
HOPE
STABILITY
CREATIVITY
WORKING TOGETHER
SELF IDENTIFICATION

Surely, the ideal society would achieve the aims implied by the capitalistic vocabulary through the philosophies suggested by the vocabulary of the more community based social structures. I will go so far as to suggest that it is within this kind of structure that people with disabilities, or indeed any minority group, would fit more comfortably.

You have probably gathered by now that I am not a capitalist, although I do believe in personal enterprise. Given the picture which I have painted thus far, I doubt, if born now, I could achieve the status and life-style which I have been able to build for myself. This concerns me because on the one hand I am promoting technology as being an empowering science, whilst on the other I am decrying the social and political systems which have created that technology. I have a dichotomy of ideas and therefore need to bring some logic to my thoughts.

Unfortunately, technology tends to lead to an introverted society in which individuals can happily lead their lives without much contact with their peer groups. Such societies tend to leave the physically and mentally disadvantaged to fend for themselves or via statutory agencies. This in turn leaves enormous gaps in the social knowledge of both abled and disabled persons in technology based societies, which is overcome by the more integrated nuclear societies of pre-technology.

I was born in 1943. Thankfully my parents had the courage to allow me to mix with my peer group, despite the fact that much scorn was directed on them from outside our immediate circle. My father also made me a chair in which I could manoeuvre myself by using my feet and therefore I could participate in games of football, cricket and so on. Not to mention the occasional kick that I dished out during the many childhood fights that occurred.

This whole process helped with my socialization process and I quickly learned that to enjoy life I had to learn to take the knocks of life. I seriously think that if you go through life without being hurt then you have not really been involved, therefore one message I would like to give to you is not to over-protect people with disabilities. What does need to be done however, is to provide the basic services, or the means to buy them. Technology is not that advanced to enable people with severe disabilities to survive without people power. As Henry James said,

> Live all you can; it's a mistake not to. It doesn't so much matter what you do in particular, so long as you have your life. If you haven't had that, what have you had?

and Grace Hansen,

> Don't be afraid your life will end; be afraid that it will never begin.

The social skills that I acquired during my early years became very useful as I grew older, went to University and then into a vocation. I knew that to make contact with a stranger I had to make more than 50 percent of the initial effort in order to put that person at ease. Once this is done, one's disabilities tend to become transparent and people see the inner you, allowing relationships to be formed. It was this socialization process which I believe would now be difficult to recreate in societies which are individualistic by nature. If a way can be found to overcome this by integrating and not marginalizing disability, then my mental dichotomy is solved and technology becomes an enormous bonus.

So what of technology? How can it facilitate citizenship?

Looking back again to my young days, one of my biggest problems was communication. I had a speech therapist who said to me *"however severe your physical disabilities are, it is your speech that will disable you the most."* She was realistic and right to be that hard on me, she probably did me the biggest favour of all in that I was naturally a lazy person. I did not take the time or make the effort to slow my thoughts down and deliver them at a pace and with the clarity to enable me to be understood. I had a waterfall of ideas cascading from my head but I had to build a few mental dykes to slow down the flow to bring it under control. Unlike power, communication does not require force, rather it can be likened to the gentle fall of dew from a tree. Each drop is an entity, clear and distinct.

If I were to truly practice what I preach, all my presentations would be given directly from a computerized text through a voice synthesizer with diagrams projected on to a screen. I could control this by the occasional tap of a switch whilst controlling a robotic arm with voice recognition to feed me a glass of whisky! This, of course, is quite feasible today. Excluding the robotic arm and glass of whisky, it is a procedure which I would be invoking for myself as soon as finances allow. Apart from the reasons already mentioned, such a method would equate to a dynamic demonstration of the liberating effect of technology.

It is this technology which affords people with disabilities a ray of hope by offering an opportunity to make the kind of choices which I believe equates to full citizenship. Of course, there is more but the over-riding feature of any technology is that it has to be user friendly and has to accommodate various means of human/computer interfaces. Such systems which gel the sciences of voice recognition/synthesis, cybernetics, optics, artificial intelligence, multi-media and virtual reality could surely form the embryo of systems which will crystallise to accomplish the empowerment discussed above.

FIGURE 1

ACTIVITIES

HUSBAND & PARENT

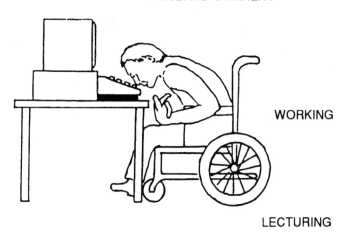

WORKING

LECTURING

LEISURE

We are now living in a global world requiring global solutions for mankind to survive. Disability is just one of the many problems facing man at this time but perhaps, providing solutions to disability and affording citizenship through technology, will in turn, solve some of our other social dilemmas. For example, much of the technology which could afford citizenship to the disabled evolves from research pioneered to meet the demands of the Arms race. I am pleased to say that this race has now diminished but in doing so, the research and creativity of mind required by the Arms industry is now to a large extent, being wasted. If nations were to think of providing citizenship to disability in a positive manner, recognizing the cost effectiveness of providing such solutions, then whole new industries could be created around these intellectual abilities of scientists previously engaged in producing tools of destruction. I cannot stop my mind wandering back to a visit I made to Iraq in 1986 when we were friends and united by the common enemy, Iran.

Primarily, my visit was to take part in a conference aimed at overcoming the vast difficulties created by the thousands of war wounded. By far the most stressful but intellectually valuable experience of this trip was the time I spent at a hospital. The majority of the patients had recently suffered lesions of the spinal cord at various levels and therefore it was not particularly "High Technology" that they were interested in. Rather they wished to bombard me with questions regarding how I coped with everyday life. I feel it was a pity that I could not have spent more time with these young people as they obviously gained from my experience.

> Any idiot can face a crisis–it's this day to day living that wears you out
>
> Anton Chekov

Being surrounded by thirty young men with bodies and minds mutilated, rejected and denied death by the weapons of destruction, created by man to destroy man, will be imprinted on my memory forever. For every one of these men there are thousands, if not millions, living or partly living memorials of the insanity of war and proof of man's inadequate intellect which cannot produce peaceful answers to national and international disputes. To discuss "High Technology" would have been nauseating and I could not do it. Instead I attempted to answer their questions which were all concerned with how I coped with life and how they could survive in the new world.

The fact that the Gulf war has completely reversed the situation with Iraq now being the common enemy of the west, and Iran an ally, emphasises to me the fickleness of fate. You must be aware that fate has no respect for colour, class or creed and nobody is immune from disability. In fact the very technology which affords or serves to increase citizenship will also prolong lives beyond that which fate or nature intended. It is therefore within your own interests to bring pressure upon your national Governments which lead to a "Coup de Tech."

> Imagination is more important than knowledge
>
> Albert Einstein

> Freedom is bold
>
> Robert Frost

A little rebellion now and then . . . is a medicine for the sound health of Government

Thomas Jefferson

This in turn will create societies in which abilities are recognised, not disabilities.

There is something that is much more scarce, something finer far, something rather than ability. It is the ability to recognise ability

Elbert Hubbard

The coup will provide the technology because manufacturers will recognise the financial expedience of doing so. If the propositions which I have made are true then the scenario which I put before you is–Can the world ethically reject the opportunity to facilitate the complete citizenship of disabled people and their carers? Historically liberation is something people have fought for and I trust that future generations will be more passive and pro-active in affording these fundamental rights to the whole of mankind. I call upon you to facilitate liberation in my life and the ever increasing number of people like me. At the moment I am like Steven Spielberg:

I dream for a living

I would rather my dreams were realities!!

The Computer Dilemma:
Harming the Helpers

Richard Reinoehl
Jack Coates
Diane Russell
Adam Engst
Tonya Engst
Gregory Stosuy

Richard Reinoehl is Affiliate Scholar with Oberlin College and Director of the
Human Development Consortium, Inc., a consulting group focused on informa-
tion technology and human development. He is a past faculty member of the
Social Work Program, University of Wisconsin, Superior, and is best known for
his work on computer literacy in human services.
 Jack Coates is Director of the Coates Chiropractic Clinic in Wellington, Ohio.
He has extensive experience in the diagnosis and treatment of occupational injuries. He is also a historian known for his multimedia presentations on General
Custer and the Battle of the Little Big Horn.
 Diane Russell is Director of Western Reserve Massotherapy and is on the
faculty of the Ohio College of Medical Arts. She has extensive experience in the
diagnosis and treatment of soft tissue dysfunction, such as Carpal Tunnel Syndrome and Myofascial Pain Syndrome.
 Adam C. Engst is Editor of TidBITS, a weekly electronic newsletter covering
the world of the Macintosh and electronic communications, and is the author of
Internet Starter Kit for Macintosh. He received a degree in Hypertextual Fiction
and Classics from Cornell University.
 Tonya Engst is Co-Editor of TidBITS and provides professional support for
Microsoft Word. She has a degree in Communications with a focus on publica-
tions, and a minor in the History and Philosophy of Science and Technology from
Cornell University.
 Gregory Stosuy is Administrator for the New Jersey Department of Human
Services, working with school based youth service programs. Also with NJDHS,
he has been an Assistant Administrator for the Ancora Psychiatric Hospital, and
Administrator for the Office of Institutional Services. He has been an adjunct
Professor at Rutgers University's Graduate School of Social Work since 1978.

[Haworth co-indexing entry note]: "The Computer Dilemma: Harming the Helpers." Reinoehl,
Richard et al. Co-published simultaneously in *Computers in Human Services* (The Haworth Press, Inc.)
Vol. 12, No. 1/2, 1995, pp. 21-36; and: *Human Services in the Information Age* (ed: Jackie Rafferty, Jan
Steyaert, and David Colombi) The Haworth Press, Inc., 1995, pp. 21-36 Single or multiple copies of this
article are available from The Haworth Document Delivery Service [1-800-342-9678, 9:00 a.m. - 5:00
p.m. (EST)].

© 1995 by The Haworth Press, Inc. All rights reserved. *21*

SUMMARY. As computer use in health and human service organizations increases, so does the number of workers susceptible to soft tissue and joint dysfunction. These problems can be manifested as low back, cervical, shoulder girdle, and wrist-hand related disorders. Some common, recognizable conditions are Tendinitis, Carpal Tunnel Syndrome, and Myofascial Pain Syndrome. An under-utilization of ergonomic principles for computer work stations is a primary cause but even strict adherence to ergonomic guidelines can result in disorders. Preventive actions, however, can be taken by introducing relatively simple systemic changes in organizational procedures. Such changes should be part of a broader, more holistic understanding of human relationships within organizations. *[Article copies available from The Haworth Document Delivery Service: 1-800-342-9678.]*

INTRODUCTION

It is ironic that most health, education, and human service organizations, dedicated to improving the quality of life for their consumers, are unwittingly damaging this quality for many of their workers. As we move toward a future of increased computer use, we also move toward a future of increased risk for computer related disabilities such as soft tissue and joint dysfunction. Often simply viewed as a physiological problem of individuals, this is a systemic problem with ramifications throughout an organization.

Studies show that the under-utilization of ergonomic principles for computer workstations will, over time, lead to physical disabilities such as Myofascial Pain Syndrome, Chronic Tendinitis, Carpal Tunnel Syndrome (CTS) and so forth. A review of computer use in health, education, and human service organizations in New Jersey also shows very little practice of ergonomic principles. A somewhat random checking of organizations in other states and countries suggests this is a problem of national, even international scope. Unfortunately, even the strictest adherence to ergonomic guidelines can lead (albeit more slowly) to the same end. To completely avoid these problems, one must also add frequent breaks and active exercises involving the affected muscle groups.

The medical interventions to treat these occupational diseases can be extensive, including surgery. Considerable expense can be involved in treatment of the diseases, in the form of worker disability payments, and in employee morale and turnover–as well as the physiological and emotional suffering of the affected workers. The fiscal drain and poor morale brought on by workers' disability and constant pain can also undermine the effectiveness of service delivery in an organization. When the latter is combined with anxiety, such as the stress from work deadlines, and inter-office conflicts, organizational dynamics can become similar to those found in dysfunctional families.

Fortunately, these debilitating physiological and organizational conditions can be prevented by introducing some specific systemic changes. It is clear that such changes also need to be part of a broader, more holistic understanding of the human and environmental relationships within organizations.

THE PROBLEM

When it would seem that information technology (IT) should be lessening our work load, we find that individuals working with IT are being plagued with physical and psychological stresses. In the average office most of the workers are unknowingly being set up for soft tissue (muscle tendon, ligament) dysfunction.

From an ergonomic view, this occurs through poor positioning of computers and other IT related equipment, and from poor posture from inadequate physical support. It is common to enter a health care or social service agency to find computers, keyboards, and related hard copy, at heights and angles which cause physiological stress in virtually all portions of the body. The disabilities caused by these stresses are being seen in numerous medical specialties with diagnosis from simple muscle strain to myofascial pain syndrome and degenerative joint disease.

As a model to better understand the complexity, we can see that external loads, or forces, on the musculoskeletal system will produce increased tendon, muscle, and joint tensional forces. Generally these forces will fall within the ability of the body to adapt, so long as the external loads are of a short duration, and adequate time is allowed for the tissues to recover. By prolonging the periods of stress, or increasing the frequency of exertion on the tissues, their ability to withstand the stress is greatly reduced. Initially the first result is muscle fatigue, and if the stress continues, acute pain will result. The latter is a clear warning, and pushing beyond this point can produce mechanical damage in the tendons and joints resulting in chronic pain and tissue degeneration (Cailiet, 1981).

The relatively recent research into these problems, and the fact that these disabilities can engage so many aspects of physical functioning and medical specialties, means that an integrated, holistic approach to diagnosis and treatment is still evolving. Thus, here, we integrate some of the literature of these diverse specialties.

MYOFASCIAL PAIN SYNDROME

Myofascial pain syndrome with associated trigger points and referral patterns is one of the most common disorders of the soft tissues, and most often mistaken for other disorders. "Myofascial trigger points are hyperirritable loci within a taut band of skeletal muscle, located in muscular tissue and/or its associated fascia, the sheath surrounding muscles and their tendons" (Travelll & Simons, 1983). The spot is painful on compression and will refer pain to remote areas of the body. These referral patterns are classic and palpation (applying pressure) reproduces the pain and symptoms of the patient. It is not uncommon for these patients to have a wide and varied diagnosis such as tennis elbow, cervical strain/sprain, tension headache, temporal headache, brachial neuralgia, bicipital tendinitis, lumbago, osteoarthritis of the spine, fibrositis, and so forth. The sufferers will in most cases have pain which is reported as constant, severe and sleep disturbing. These commonly go untreated long enough to become a vicious, self-sustaining cycle (ibid.).

The causal factors can be as simple as a desktop being positioned too high or low, copy being placed to the side, chair too high or low, poor support for back or arms, and poor lighting. Each of these conditions places a strain on specific muscle groups. For instance, if a computer screen is a little low, the user must tilt the head forward and hold it rigid, thus stressing cervical and thoracic muscle groups. Such strain causes the affected muscles to be in a shortened, contracted position for an extended period of time. As the muscles are held in contraction the vascular structures are constricted resulting in ischemic tissue. Ischemic tissue is tissue which lacks proper oxygen and blood supply, which results in pain, restricted range of motion, and a feeling of tightness and aching (Chaitow, 1988; Travelll & Simons, 1983).

Constriction of vascular and lymph channels also reduces the body's ability to remove metabolic wastes and toxic materials. These substances cause hyperirritability of nerve endings and hypertonicity (sustained muscle contraction) of skeletal muscles. This means that even after an individual stops working at a computer, the muscle contractions will continue, providing the effected individual with a chronic muscle spasm and tendon strain. Thus, simply taking a break from work will have no therapeutic effect (see Figures I and II). Repetitive movements in computer activities, as well as the muscular overuse just described, can also set the stage for microtrauma to the soft tissues repeating the effects of this painful and debilitating cycle (Chaitow, 1988; Travelll & Simons, 1983).

TENDINITIS, BURSITIS AND JOINT DEGENERATION

All muscles are connected to the skeleton by fibrous tissue called tendons. Tendons and related tissue, such as the synovia, and bursa membranes, are also subject to the same stresses as muscle. Continued exertion of already fatigued tissue causes separation of the tendon's collagen fibers, increased swelling, and pain in the region. This is commonly known as tendinitis. The tendon is now inflamed, and continued exertion will bring on degeneration involving the tendon, synovia, and bursa membranes (Bursitis) of the neighboring joints. Involvement of this area will produce limited joint mobility, and joint pain. Proceeding beyond this point with

FIGURE I. Disease Progression of Myofascial Pain Syndrome.

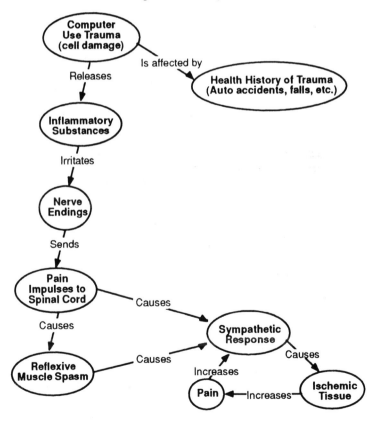

FIGURE II. Expanded Myofascial Pain Syndrome Cycle.

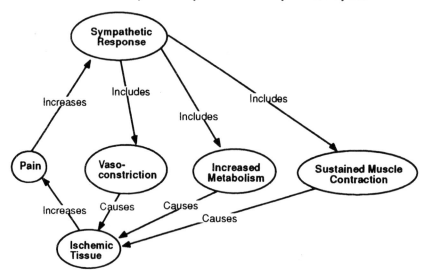

continued exertion results in permanent functional disability of the involved joints (Cyriax, 1982; Magee, 1992).

In the case of the spine, vertebra can be subluxated, e.g., moved from their seating, which can then create pressure on nerve tissue exiting the spinal cord. This can cause neck and back pain, which increase muscle contraction and tendon stress, adding again to the cycle of pain and dysfunction.

SPECIFIC DISORDERS AND THE CAUSAL RELATIONSHIPS

These physiological problems related to computer use can be grouped into four general categories of location and cause. They are: (1) low back related disorders; (2) cervical related disorders; (3) shoulder girdle disorders, and; (4) wrist-hand related disorders.

LOW BACK RELATED DISORDERS

When a person is seated, the weight of the body is borne by the ischial tuberosities (large rough bony eminence, on which the trunk rests) of the pelvis and surrounding soft tissue structures. The type of chair and individual posture determine how much stress is transferred to the seat and floor, and how much is borne by the body's supporting structures. Generally speaking, in an unsupported seated posture the pelvis tilts backwards and results in pressures that are greater than those encountered in a standing position. This increases risk of lower back pain and degenerative disease in predominately seated jobs, even though this type of work is of lighter variety (Chaffin & Anderson, 1991).

CERVICAL-DORSAL RELATED DISORDERS

Moving upward in the spine to the Cervical-Dorsal region (neck and upper back), we find that disorders in this area are interrelated with shoulder and upper arm problems for several reasons. Nerves supplying the upper arm initiate from the mid and lower cervical regions as well as the uppermost dorsal segments. These nerve components, along with accompanying vascular components, course from the Thoracic outlet region through the axillary region. Thus, many neck and upper back maladies will result in a pain referral into the arm. Also, excess loads on the neck and shoulder muscles will many times involve frequent, repetitive, contraction of the forearm muscles. A prime example of that is excessive keying on a keyboard that is set too high (Pheasant, 1991).

The head position and thus the neck posture is generally determined by the visual requirements of the job. Muscle fatigue and pain occur rather quickly when the head is tipped, especially when the inclination angle is significant. If the seat is too high or the work area too low the neck will flex awkwardly; this is also true if there is an intense visual demand (Chaffin & Anderson, 1991).

WRIST-HAND RELATED DISORDERS

The wrist-hand area contains the toughest of the work-related problems to treat. Disorders incurred in this region will frequently be categorized as: Repetitive Strain Injuries; Cumulative Trauma Disorders; or Overuse Syndrome. Whatever the name, the causative factors behind these maladies have shown to include: (1) fixed working posture; (2) Repetitive Motion, and; (3) psychological stresses (Pheasant, 1991).

Common problems in this region include:

1. Wrist tenosynovitis (Tendinitis)–The finger flexor/extensor tendons become inflamed and painful;

2. Ganglionic Cysts-Swollen–Painful, fluid-filled nodules develop in the wrist tendons or around the wrist or carpal bones, and;

3. Carpal Tunnel Syndrome–Eight carpal bones of the wrist covered by a fibrous sheath called the flexor retinaculum form the Carpal Tunnel, through which passes the finger flexor tendons and the Median Nerve. Irritation, inflammation, or poor compression in this area produce numbness and tingling along the thumb, through the middle fingers and can eventually spread to the rest of the hand. Sensation can be lost in these regions, making it difficult to pick up small objects, and the muscles may indeed atrophy, or, waste away (Chaffin and Anderson, 1991). Pain can be intense, so intense that simple everyday activities can produce great agony.

TREATMENT

The health care interventions most appropriate for treatment of the musculoskeletal system are usually effective, and can be as varied as the problems themselves. Ideally, early utilization of soft tissue therapies will economize on pain, time and cost of treatment plan. Several approaches to treatment, used in conjunction with each other, may give the best results. Medical doctors can prescribe anti-inflammatory and pain reducing drugs, as well as utilization of other therapies. Massotherapy, which is the manipulation of soft tissues by a trained medically licensed therapist, also can offer considerable relief. To be effective, the therapist must be trained in a wide range of techniques, such as: neuromuscular therapy, trigger point therapy, ischemic compression, massage, periosteal point therapy, postisometric relaxation exercises, acupressure, and various thermal modalities. The strengthening of precise muscles and joints must be carried out after the reduction of pain is accomplished. Flexibility and strengthening exercises will be a part of an efficient treatment plan. The strengthening and stretching of soft tissue functions as a preventive maintenance procedure as well as a rehabilitative procedure.

Chiropractic care also works well in unison with the deep muscular therapy to bring about and expedite a cure. Chiropractic doctors approach the problem at the level of the spine or the extremity where the injury has occurred, and through the use of manipulation, therapy, and preventative exercises and measures, most of these problems can be alleviated. However, no matter what the approach, Medical, Chiropractic, Osteopathic, or Allopathic, the earlier these problems are addressed, the better the outcome.

SELF TREATMENT

Self treatment can take a number of forms but should be discussed with one's primary health care provider. These treatments include the use of thermal modalities, splints, and massage.

Thermal Modalities

Current thought is that cold compresses are much better than heat for aid in healing of muscle and tendon tissue (Norman, 1991). The idea is that cold reduces inflammation, whereas heat may reinforce it. Also, since nerves are extremely sensitive to heat, heating aching hands may feel good, but it's deceptive because the nerves that are transmitting heat signals are simply overriding the pain impulses. Heat followed by cold may be the best approach, as heat brings oxygen and nutrient filled blood to the affected area, and cold then helps flush the metabolic waste and other toxic residues.

Splints

If CTS or wrist pain is the problem, wrist splints can help (ibid.). Wrist splints can be purchased in many drugstores and come in different sizes and shapes. They should be worn to bed and during times when working on a computer, or other activities (like driving a car without power steering or pushing a shopping cart) where there is stress on the wrist (Shellenbarger, 1991). The splints are generally called "cock-up splints" because the metal splint cocks the wrist at a 20 to 30 degree angle. This position is neutral, so one isn't compressing the carpal tunnel while wearing them.

Massage

Gentle massage of the hands, wrists, arms, shoulders, and back not only can feel good but also can aid in healing (Roel, 1991). Massage can help relax muscle tissue and stimulate blood flow. In the case of lesion (scar tissue) growth, around damaged tendons, for instance, massage can help establish the growth direction of the new fibers. This will strengthen the area as opposed to the formation of constricting interconnected tissue (Kellogg, 1975).

SERIOUS CASES

When soft tissue and joint damage is severe enough that less obtrusive treatment is not successful, cortisone injections may be tried. These injections are painful and a single injection may not solve the problem. Repeated injections of cortisone can help but the risk of detrimental side effects also increases. If the cortisone injections are successful, the pain will recede roughly three days after the injection. If not successful, surgery becomes the next option.[1]

In the case of CTS, for instance, the surgical principle is that slitting the carpal tunnel allows it to expand slightly thereby releasing pressure. Many people do well after this process and return to normal work after several months. However, there is no guarantee that surgery will be successful no matter where the joint dysfunction occurs. Additionally, whether the treatment has consisted of manipulation or an invasive surgery, what benefit exists for the employees if they are returned to the same situation which originated the disability? Hence, we must encourage communication between employer and the employee to bring attention to the causative factors, and possible preventions, of the problem.

PREVENTION

To recap, high levels of exertion or prolonged, frequent episodes of exertion will result in fatigue, pain, inflammation and degeneration proceeding through muscles-tendons-synovia-bursa-bone. Muscle fatigue is the first sensation, and if the stress continues, acute pain will result. The latter is a clear warning, and pushing beyond this point can produce mechanical damage in the tendons and joints resulting in chronic pain and tissue degeneration.

Avoidance of these problems can be summed up by three principles;

1. If frequent or sustained muscle exertion is required, external loads and unnatural positions must be minimized, e.g., an ergonomically designed work environment is essential;
2. Frequent breaks must be taken, and;
3. Active exercises which counter the effects of the stressed tissues should be used during breaks.

ERGONOMIC ISSUES

One of the best methods of reducing soft tissue damage is to work in an environment that minimizes physical stress. The height of the screen and keyboard, support for wrists, and so forth, are all important. However, most important is using chairs designed specifically for computer use, and using correct postural habits.

Chair Design

A major consideration in chair design is the backrest. The loss of the normal lumbar lordosis (low back curvature) in the seated posture (the curvature is decreased by an average of 38 degrees when going from standing to sitting) can be prevented with a well positioned backrest. There are three types of backrests in use. The low type supports the lumbar region alone. The medium type supports into the mid-dorsal region. The high type supports into the head-neck region. The style of backrest need will depend on tasks being performed (Chaffin & Anderson, 1991).

Most important is the design of the low back support. It has been shown that a lumbar curve resembling that of the standing posture can be produced in the seated posture by the use of a 4 centimeter lumbar support in front of the backrest. The exact position of the support is of little consequence as long as it is positioned in the lumbar region. Adjustable supports are best as they can adapt to changes in conditions or changes in employees (ibid.).

Another factor to consider with the backrest is the angle of inclination. Disc pressures decrease when the backrest angle is inclined from a vertical position to about 110 degrees. A free-tilting seat with a range of 15 degrees forward to 5 degrees backward is useful for the most seated activities. Too much forward tilt though may result in the individual continually sliding forward forcing them to support themselves with the calf and thigh muscles (ibid.).

Armrests, while awkward for some tasks, have also been shown to help in supporting the trunk and decreasing pressure. However, if they are positioned too high, the position raises the shoulder and abducts the arms, while if it is too low the individual must slump or slide forward (ibid.).

Another factor to consider is that support from the legs distributes and decreases the load on the buttocks and posterior thigh area. The feet need to rest on either the floor or a foot support so that the weight of the lower legs is not supported by the thigh resting on the seat. If a chair is too low the knee-flexion angle becomes uncomfortable, the pelvis rotates back and the spine flexes forward. If the chair is too high the feet do not rest on the floor, pressure on the back of the thighs becomes uncomfortable and the individual slides forward to the front of the chair. Here the feet find support on the floor but it is impossible to utilize the backrest properly, resulting in low back pain (ibid.).

The Screen, Keyboard and Posture

The work posture of an individual is determined by the height of the keyboard and screen relative to the seat. Generally the keyboard is too high and the screen too low. When the keyboard is too high it elevates the shoulder girdle and abducts the arms causing an increase in tension along the Trapezius and arm muscles. The sitting height of the individual then should determine how the work surface is organized and laid out. Care should be taken to ensure that the home row of keys is level with the user's elbow (Pheasant, 1991).

Wrist pads are important to use and can help in two ways. First, when an individual's wrists become tired, it is natural to rest the wrists on the work surface (Cobb, 1991). Unfortunately, that angle can compress the carpal tunnel, which increases the risk of damage. Secondly, when an individual stops typing to think or talk, he or she usually put their hands down, and it's better to rest them on a soft pad than on the hard corner of a desk. The latter can cut off circulation and compress the carpal tunnel.

An ergonomic approach to these aspects of a workstation would be something like this:

1. The trunk would have a backward angle of 100-110 degrees.
2. The arms would be held forward, relaxed, at the side, elbows at 80 degrees, forearms inclined slightly.
3. Padded wrist supports should be used to rest wrist upon and are available in various dimensions.
4. The keyboard should be about 30 centimeters thick, measuring to the home row of keys, and tilted to 10-15 degrees. Again, these dimensions are adjustable with various wrist pads.
5. The screen should adjust for about a 15 degree line of sight with an average distance from eye to screen of 60-95 centimeters.
6. A copy holder or reading stand should always be employed. Placement, again, should be adjustable, at about the height of the screen, near the side of the screen, and at the same distance from the eyes as the screen (ibid.).

Breaks, Exercise, Fluids, and Relaxation

Use of an adjustable, ergonomically designed chair and work station is a major factor in preventing physiological damage. However, this alone will not insure that a worker remains undamaged. It is also necessary that a IT user take frequent breaks and engage in active exercise.

Limiting times at the workstation is an important preventive measure. A worker should take a 5-15 minute break from the computer every 50 minutes or so. The length of break needed depends considerably on the quality of the workstation (one option to be considered is having computer users change jobs, to more physically active work, two or more times each day).

Useful software tools exist to help computer users take regular breaks. These programs monitor how long a user is typing, and then tells the user to take a break. The user sets the length of both the work and break time. Audible reminders or dialogue reminders suggest that the user do something else. One such program has a useful section on ergonomics and exercises.

When a worker takes a break he or she should not just rest but engage in physical activities which undo the stresses accumulated in the body. Also, since extended muscle contraction reduces blood flow, with a resulting build-up of toxins, it is important to maintain a high intake of fluids. Without a high level of fluids (four to six liters per day) a state of partial dehydration exists, and the body is hindered in its task of flushing out metabolic wastes and other toxins.

There are basically two approaches toward exercising. The first is to engage in deep breathing and slow, flowing movements which activate the various muscle groups and stretch the contracted muscles and tendons. Tai Chi and some forms of dance are quite good for this. The second approach is using specific exercises alternately activating specific body areas. Shoulder shrugs and hand flexes (Exercises #4 and #8, below), are exercises which should be done frequently, perhaps every 20-25 minutes. Either approach, or a combination of each, will aid in relaxing the irritated muscles, diminish stress, and lessen fatigue.

Specific exercises are:

1. Inhale deeply through the nose and exhale through the mouth, expanding and contracting the abdominal muscles at the same time.
2. Extend the arms above the head, reaching as high as possible, and wiggling the fingers, count to five, and bring the arms down to the side of the chair, and wiggle those fingers again.
3. Slowly, turn the head from side to side pausing on each turn for count of five, at the same time, try winking first one eye, then the other.
4. With the arms hanging at the side, shrug the shoulders as high as possible, and forward, and down, and back, outlining a circle with the top of the shoulders. Repeat this five times, and then try reversing the process for the same count of five.
5. Fold the arms, and bring the elbows to shoulder height, now stretch the elbows back, slowly, five times.
6. Place your hands on your lap, slowly bend forward, sliding the hands down your thighs, over your knees and down your legs. Bend

as far forward as you are comfortable with, don't fall out of your chair, hold for ten seconds, and slowly return to the upright posture.
7. Place both palms together, with the elbows pointing out and forward, gently press the palms together and feel a gentle stretch in the wrist area, as well as along the fingers.
8. With your hands in the front of you rapidly bend and extend the fingers into and out of the palm of the hand. Next, with the fingers extended, spread the fingers apart like a fan, very slowly.

The preceding demonstrates that there are many preventive actions which can be taken to reduce or eliminate the possibility of soft tissue dysfunction associated with computer use. Some of these actions can be taken by the individual without need for an organization to change from its business-as-usual format. However, if an organization wants to protect its workers from damage (and itself, from increased medical and worker disability costs), administration needs to lead in instituting and maintaining more healthful behaviors. The purchase cost of ergonomic chairs and work stations are minor when compared to costs of even the most minimal medical treatment. The break-time workers take to exercise, to consume fluids, and so forth, also provide considerable payback to an organization in a variety of forms. Actively embracing these preventive measures are part of an enlightened, holistic approach to human relationships and functioning within organizations.

CONCLUSION

A survey of human service organizations combined with other reports from health, education, and human service organizations show that basic ergonomic principles are not being integrated into IT workstation use. Studies show that the under-utilization of ergonomic principles will, over time, lead to painful soft tissue and joint dysfunction–which can become permanent disabilities. The lack of frequent breaks combined with active exercise are also important causal factors in the development of these conditions.

Early medical interventions can be effective treatment for these occupational diseases but the longer treatment is delayed the more extensive and costly the interventions become. Considerable expense also can be involved in the form of worker disability payments, and in low employee morale and turnover. Fortunately, these debilitating conditions can be prevented by introducing specific changes in workstation design, and in organizational policies and behavior.

NOTE

1. Confidential Interview with a Medical Doctor

REFERENCES

Anderson, Robert A. (1989). Vitamin B6 used in treating carpal tunnel syndrome, atherosclerosis, and other problems. *Health News & Review*, 7(6), 6-7.

Cailiet, R. (1981). *Shoulder Pain. 2nd Edition*. Philadelphia, PA: F.A. Davis.

Chaffin, D., Anderson, G. (1991). *Occupational Biomechanics, 2nd. Edition*. New York, NY: J. Wiley & Sons.

Chaitow, L. (1988). *Soft Tissue Manipulation*. Tochester Vermont: Healing Arts Press.

Cobb, Kevin (1991). RSI: the new computer-age health assault. *Prevention*, 43(4), 58-67.

Cyriax, J. (1982). *Textbook of Orthopaedic Medicine, Vols 1 & 2*. New York: Bailliere.

Kellogg, J. H. (1975). *The Art of Massage*. Mokelumne Hill, CA: Health Research.

Lacey, J. S. (1990). *How to survive your computer workstation*. Linden, TX: CRT Services Inc., 31-33.

Magee, D. (1992). *Orthopedic Physical Assessment*. Philadelphia, PA: W.B. Saunders Company.

Norman, Lee A. (1991). Mouse joint–another manifestation of an occupational epidemic? *The Western Journal of Medicine*, 155 (4), 413-16.

Pheasant, S. (1991). *Ergonomics, Work and Health*. Gaithersburg, MD: Aspen Publishers, 77-97.

Roel, R. E. (1991). Wrist watch. *American Health: Fitness of Body and Mind*, 10(6), 72-76.

Shellenbarger, Teresa (1991). When you're asked about carpal tunnel syndrome. *RN*, 54(7), 40-43.

Travelll, J. and Simons, D. (1983). *Myofascial Pain and Dysfunction*. Los Angeles, CA: Williams and Wilkins.

Viikari-J. E. (1983). Neck and upper limb disorders among slaughterhouse workers. *Scandinavian Journal of Work Environment and Health*, 9, 283-290.

_____ (1991). The perils of vitamin B6 megadosing. *Health News*, 9(1), 1-3.

Race Equality and Information Technology in Europe

Kish Bhatti-Sinclair

SUMMARY. This paper will focus on how Information Technology (IT) impacts on the quality of life of black people, with reference to the recent rise of racism in the European Union member states, and the potential of IT to improve their quality of life. *[Article copies available from The Haworth Document Delivery Service: 1-800-342-9678.]*

INTRODUCTION

This paper focuses on the quality of life of black people resident in the European Union (EU) and how it is affected by the Information Technology (IT) systems being developed to track cross border movements (the European Union was formerly the European Community or EC. For the sake of clarity the terms "European Union" and EU have been used throughout.). The issue of refugees will not be considered per se, although it will be acknowledged that refugees and black citizens and residents are being linked as groups which are directly affected by the tightening of immigration rules and the rise of racism and xenophobia within EU member states.

IT systems are not ideologically neutral, they raise fundamental issues

---

Kish Bhatti-Sinclair is a qualified youth and community worker and currently teachers in the Department of Social Work Studies at the University of Southampton, UK. Her main interests lie in the area of equal opportunities, anti-racist social work and computers in higher education.

[Haworth co-indexing entry note]: "Race Equality and Information Technology in Europe." Bhatti-Sinclair, Kish. Co-published simultaneously in *Computers in Human Services* (The Haworth Press, Inc.) Vol. 12, No. 1/2, 1995, pp. 37-52; and: *Human Services in the Information Age* (ed: Jackie Rafferty, Jan Steyaert, and David Colombi) The Haworth Press, Inc., 1995, pp. 37-52. Single or multiple copies of this article are available from The Haworth Document Delivery Service [1-800-342-9678, 9:00 a.m. - 5:00 p.m. (EST)].

about ourselves and our society, questions that inevitably lead to major concerns about their advantages and disadvantages. Rather than acting as a liberating force, IT can reinforce inequalities in society. There is growing evidence that groups which are discriminated against in society in general are further disadvantaged in two ways by IT. First, as potential users of IT they may not possess the resources which enable easy access to what is readily available to their better resourced neighbours (Glastonbury and LaMendola, 1993). Second, as citizens and consumers of services, IT developments do not take their needs into account. This paper considers how IT impacts on black people living in EU member states as the opening of the internal borders becomes a reality.

The EU is becoming increasingly concerned about the rise of racist activity within its member states (Council of Europe, 1992). This concern is a reflection of serious doubts amongst many members of black communities within Europe (Redmond, 1992) about the true benefits for black citizens of the single European market and for the estimated 12-15 million non-EU nationals rightfully living in the Union (Gordon, 1989, p. 4).

As signatories to the Treaty of Rome (1957), the International Convention on the Elimination of All Forms of Racial Discrimination (adopted by the General Assembly of the UN in 1965), the European Convention on Human Rights (1950), The European Social Charter (1961) and the Declaration on Racism and Xenophobia (1986), the majority of EU countries have made policy commitments aimed at combatting racism and xenophobia. This commitment, however, has been shown to be limited, difficult to enforce and implementation is left to individual countries, where progress (albeit limited) has been largely driven by domestic pressures (Forbes and Mead, 1992, p. 11).

This is set against a backdrop of tighter domestic immigration legislation in countries such as the UK, where the Commonwealth and Immigrants Act was enacted as long ago as 1962, and Germany, which passed the Foreigners Law in 1965 (Gordon, 1989, p. 16).

Although the many individual EU member states have made a paper commitment to combatting racism and xenophobia, the European Parliament has not legislated on this matter. On the contrary, it has moved swiftly towards cementing its identity as the White European Club. The aim of this paper is to introduce the range of ethical issues concerning IT and the part it will play in the quality of life of people who are unable to join the White European Club. It will also seek to consider how the EU and its member states can meet their responsibilities and avoid discriminatory practices.

DEFINITIONS AND TERMINOLOGY

It is clear that terminology needs to be defined in order to establish a common understanding as the same words can have different meanings within the EU as well as within its member states. The EU for example applies equal opportunities mainly to women and people with disabilities, whereas in the UK it has a far wider application.

Within the area of IT and human services, there is very little discussion of how words are used and understood. Teachers, researchers, program developers, reviewers, evaluators and workers within human services all have an imperative to extend personal and professional knowledge and change the status quo through tools such as language.

The terminology listed below is normally used with reference to black and ethnic minority people within this paper and, although by no means exhaustive, it exemplifies the terminology commonly understood and used within human services in the UK.

BLACK is a blanket term that embraces all members of minority ethnic groups within the UK who are non-white. It is a political term used to describe groups who because of their ethnic origin, language, cultural and religious differences share a common experience of discrimination and inequality.

DISCRIMINATION is a term that has legal status within the UK. It refers to unfair treatment based on differences in race, and/or gender, age, sexual orientation and so on. It is further divided into *direct* and *indirect* discrimination. The former is easier to challenge in law than the latter which is a more subtle and common form of discrimination.

RACISM occurs when prejudiced feelings, views and attitudes are translated into discriminatory behaviour, and describes a system of unequal power.

NON-NATIONALS is used to describe people without full citizenship who are unable to move freely within the EU and who are not offered the same social and welfare rights granted to EU-nationals. They have no rights to family reunion or access to housing and welfare benefits. It is generally acknowledged that the majority of non-nationals are black people, many of whom have been resident within the EU for many years (Birmingham City Council, 1991).

IMMIGRANTS is a generic term used by white Europeans to describe non-white people who are considered temporary, alien or foreign in any way. This term has been used systematically to discriminate against black people in some EU countries.

This paper will seek to focus on black people who live within EU member states. Black people in this context will be used to describe non-whites who fall into the categories of immigrant, migrant, guest, alien, foreign, temporary or non-national. Although each of these groups ought to be perceived separately from the others, black people are frequently placed into one or all of these groupings by white people whether they belong there or not. Black people are also frequently categorised as poor and disadvantaged, primarily because discrimination often leads to poverty and lack of citizenship. This label (along with all the others) stereotypes and is useful here insofar as it enables readers to conceive the additional barriers faced by black groups.

EUROPEAN POLICIES ON IMMIGRATION

In 1976 the EU Interior Ministers set up the Trevi Group to counter terrorism. The Group is supported by a temporary secretariat composed of senior officials from EU countries. It is not an institution of the EU, although membership is confined to EU countries. It meets in secret and little is known about its deliberations or decisions (Gordon, 1989, p. 10). The clandestine nature of the Trevi Group is echoed by The Ad Hoc Group on Immigration which was also set up by the EU Interior Ministers in 1986 (Bunyan, 1993, p. 144), which subsequently set up sub-groups on asylum policy, visa policy, border controls and data-processing. In addition to this, the Schengen Group set up in 1985 and is widely regarded as the initiator of immigration policies for the EU.

None of the above three groups are accountable to the EU and they all meet behind closed doors (Williams, 1992, p. 129). They are nevertheless instrumental in the development of policing and computerised information systems designed to stop terrorists, criminals, drugs and immigrants from moving freely across borders.

The EU has competence under Article 235 of The Treaty of Rome to legislate on the issue of race equality. In the absence of statute, however, two EU committees of inquiry have contributed to the debate on racism and xenophobia (Ford, 1992, p. 1). They are the Evrigenis Report, which made 40 recommendations and the Ford Report, which made 77 recommendations calling for social and human rights, increased resourcing and public scrutiny of the proceedings of committees and groups meeting in secret (Birmingham City Council, 1991, Sheet 6).

Some member states have introduced anti-racist legislation for the benefit of full citizens. Anti-racist legislation aimed at full citizens has been enacted in Belgium (Anti-racist Law 1981), France (Anti-racist Law

1972), Spain (Act No. 8 1980), and Denmark (The Racial Discrimination Act 1971). In addition race is mentioned in the constitutions of the following countries: France, Germany, Greece, Italy, The Netherlands, Portugal and Spain. However, inadequate and ineffective legalistic back-up and lack of institutional support make these provisions limited or meaningless.

Most EU countries do not have systems in place to record the citizenship status of their black residents. Many do not offer citizenship to non-indigenous residents even if they have been lawfully living there for 10 years or more. There is little or no protection for non-citizens in Denmark, France, Germany, Greece, Luxembourg, Ireland, The Netherlands, Portugal and Spain (Forbes and Mead, 1992).

Britain has stood alone within the EU in enacting effective and comparatively workable legislation. The 1948 British Nationality Act offered most British black residents access to some form of citizenship, and with it full rights as EU nationals. The 1976 Race Relations Act was significant because it outlawed both direct and indirect discrimination and created the Commission for Racial Equality which is responsible for dealing with discrimination and promoting equality of opportunity and good race relations. One of the Commission's duties is to keep under review the working of the Act, and when necessary to draw up and submit to the Secretary of State proposals for amending it. Britain is also exceptional within the EU because it offers voting rights to non-EU nationals in both local and national elections.

Lack of similar legislative support within other EU countries may prove a problem for black British people travelling, purchasing property or seeking personal social services, health and education on mainland Europe.

SOCIAL RIGHTS FOR EU RESIDENTS

It is argued that people have rights at a number of levels, as residents, as citizens and as users of health, education and welfare. Civil and political rights have traditionally been seen as valid societal concerns, whereas matters relating to health, housing, education and welfare are being pushed more into the domain of the individual by supporters of the market economy. One of the fundamental reasons for the formation and existence of the EU is to promote commerce and the market economy. It can be argued that unless residency and citizenship result in the right to welfare and social benefits, society cannot work in an equitable way. The entitlement to benefits should be available regardless of the person's citizenship, residence or contribution to the economy. This question is debated further by Plant (1992).

The idea that there is a right to welfare and to resources is a fundamental challenge to the idea that citizenship is only a civil and political status, and to the capitalist idea that a person's status in economic and social terms is to be determined by the market. The idea of rights to welfare has also become linked with the idea of social justice. According to this view, market outcomes should not be just accepted with all the resulting inequalities; rather, citizenship confers a right to a central set of resources which can provide economic security, health and education–and this right exists irrespective of a person's standing in the market (Plant, 1992, p. 16).

The justifiable societal debate on civil and welfare rights and how they impact on justice as discussed by Plant have been echoed by the EU in its attempts to produce a cohesive policy which begins to address the issue of social rights within the Social Chapter of the Maastricht Treaty. What is needed, however, are further instruments and a demonstrable commitment from the member states on the rights of black and non-EU nationals.

Current statistics indicate that there are approximately 12-15 million non-EU nationals resident in the EU who are unable to move freely to look for work or be reunited with family members (Gordon, 1989, p. 11).

The majority of EU residents with no legal rights have originated from developing countries such as India, the West Indies, Pakistan, Morocco, Turkey, Algeria, Tunisia, Vietnam and so on, as have many black EU citizens. Throughout recent EU history terms such as illegal immigrants, aliens, migrants and foreigners have been equated with people from these same developing countries. This labelling has been used to discriminate systemically against black people in some EU countries where black people who have been resident for 30 years are still regarded as visitors.

The 1989 Eurobarometer survey on racism and xenophobia carried out by the Commission of the European Communities and the European Parliament highlights white European attitudes and beliefs on immigration. The conclusions drawn were that within EU member states, the public makes a strong connection between foreigners and black people and that one third of all white Europeans maintain that there are too many people of *other* nationality or race in Europe (Commission of European Communities, 1989).

During the late 1980's a number of additional labels began to be applied to the *others*. Black people became linked to more undesirable and sinister elements in society by the UK Government when Mrs. Thatcher articulated her resistance to the raising of borders. The Prime Minister said, "We joined Europe to have free movement of goods . . . I did not join Europe to have free movement of terrorists, criminals, drugs, plant and animal diseases and rabies and illegal immigrants . . . " (Gordon, 1989, p. 8).

As 1992 and the opening of the internal borders approached, other European governments responded similarly and reacted inhumanely to black people and overtly breached all the anti-racist conventions previously signed by them:

> ... In France immigration and deportation laws have been tightened up to the extent that in 1987 several hundred Africans from former colonies were chained together and taken aboard an aircraft and deported with full media coverage ... In the first few weeks of unification thousands of guest workers in Germany were deported because of the increased availability of labour from the former East Germany (Birmingham City Council, 1991).

THE DEVELOPMENT OF IT WITHIN THE EU

Many European countries are moving swiftly towards computerisation within the human services sphere with the development of organisational, social security, employment and population registration systems. A number of ethical concerns emanate from the proliferation of IT such as the gathering and ownership of data on individuals and the widespread lack of awareness by the general public of data protection and privacy. There is evidence that possible infringement of democratic rights and misuse of information is innate within the systems being developed in some European countries which enable officials to cross-examine taxation and social security systems (Blennerhassett, 1988, p. 33). There is a further concern that the needs and rights of consumers of services are not being given due consideration either by developers of new technologies, service providers, politicians or civil servants.

The ideology behind the systems being developed in response to the abolition of internal border controls exposes the inconsistency of the EU which on one level is ready to impose social legislation on member states, and on another is encouraging member states to initiate and install tracking systems which may unlawfully impinge on the democratic rights of many EU residents. The Schengen Group (originally France, Germany, Belgium, Luxembourg and the Netherlands) first met in 1985 and agreed to abolish internal borders and strengthen external frontiers. The Schengen convention was based on increased surveillance at frontiers, more exchange of information, the development of a visa and refugee policy and the expansion of police co-operation. This agreement has been used as the basis for EU policy on border controls. Gregory (1991) discusses the significance of the Schengen convention and highlights Title IV which introduces the Schengen Information System (SIS).

This is envisaged as linking national law enforcement data bases to each other with a central technical support function (Article 92.3) located at Strasbourg. The aim, under many protective conditions, is to allow law enforcement agencies, "by means of an automated search procedure, to have access to reports on persons and objects for the purposes of border checks and controls and other police and customs checks carried out within the country" (Gregory, 1991, p. 150).

There is a clear EU policy that the border control systems being developed will serve a dual purpose. First, to track criminal activity and second, to curtail freedom of movement for targeted EU residents.

The British media are beginning to highlight the concern on the spread of cross border criminal activity with reports such as the following:

> **Busted Drugs Agency**-In a hut on the outskirts of Strasbourg, behind a triple ring of high wire mesh, senior police and customs officers of the European Community are planning the counter-attack against the spreading narcotics trade (The Guardian, 10 March 1993, p. 7).

Behind this lighthearted report is a serious message designed to introduce the person in the street to the EU-based policing body, Europol, in its embryo form. The Guardian report outlines Europol as 15 senior officers representing six member states coordinating the complicated constitutional and technical problems of police information exchange across national boundaries. The team is based within the secure complex where the SIS computer is located. SIS is the EU database used to store information on immigrants and criminals.

Europol is significant primarily because it is one of the products of agreements between EU member states stemming from groups such as Trevi and the Ad Hoc Immigration Groups which are not accountable to the EU Parliament. As stated previously, although controlled by member states, these groups are not subject to EU scrutiny, but are powerful enough to dictate how immigration policies are implemented.

The degree of anxiety about Europol and its activities has been highlighted by questions being asked in the UK House of Lords where Earl Ferrers, UK Conservative MEP, made a statement to allay the fears expressed by Lord Bethell. Earl Ferrers declared that Europol was launched on 1 September 1992 and the first assignment of the 15 senior officers was to establish a drugs unit and, under the direction of the Trevi ministers, to develop Europol's future role. The statement goes on to emphasise the part member states will play on data protection and stresses that private details will not be held within the system:

National data protection authorities will play an active role in the oversight of the Unit over the handling and protection of data which are received by it. The Unit will not, at any stage, hold a central database of personal information of any kind (House of Lords, 27 Jan 1993).

This statement confirms two fears, first, Europol's lack of accountability directly to the European Parliament; and second that data protection and with it the issue of confidentiality within such an arena may be outside the competence of the European Parliament. However, Europol has been constituted in Title VI of the Maastricht Treaty and is in the process of being set up with European-wide police powers (Bunyan, 1993, p. 27).

The importance of data protection was acknowledged by the EU in relation to cross border communications as long ago as the early 1980's when it invited member states to ratify the Council of Europe Convention 108 (1981) and the Organisation for Economic Co-operation and Development (OECD) privacy guidelines (1979).

In 1991 seven EU countries had domestic legislation on data protection in place. The laws vary considerably and may not only further jeopardise human rights, but may also hinder EU institutions from gaining free flowing information. As a result, the European Commission has issued a directive aimed at promoting data protection within the domestic arena. The directive has listed four interrelated goals: to ease the flow of information; to protect personal data; to stop the exploitation of data on nationals by third countries; and to enhance security for computerised information. The directive places particular emphasis on details such as race and other personal and political information: "particular attention is given to special categories of sensitive data revealing ethnic or racial origin, political opinions, religious or philosophical beliefs, trade union membership or concerning health or sexual life" (Baragiola, 1991, p. 26).

In response to the Council of Europe Convention 108, the UK enacted the 1984 Data Protection Act which applies to personal information held on computer. Data held in any other form is outside its remit, primarily because computer information was seen as the main threat to privacy. Evidence suggests that while most records are kept both on computers and on paper or only on computers, there is a significant amount of information kept on paper alone which is not regulated and may be open to abuse (Cornwall and Staunton, 1984, p. 96). There is a case to be made, therefore, for legislation on the protection of information held on paper.

The Data Protection Act does not cover the UK security services, and information passed to them by registered users is outside the remit of the Act. The police, customs and excise and any other law enforcement agency can exchange unregistered information, and citizens do not have access to the information held on them. The UK's Immigration Service is already using a linked computer system and although small, has significant input into immigration policy because it is headed by a Deputy Under Secretary of State who represents UK's interests at a European level.

The Deputy Under Secretary of State has been selected as the UK officials level coordinator for all border-control agencies' (police and customs) inputs into the EC states development of new order control systems related to the free movement of people and goods intra-EC frontiers (Gregory, 1991, p. 43).

There are indications within the UK that one of the answers to the control of movement across borders is through the adoption of personal identity cards or a numbering system similar to those which are already in use in Denmark, France, Germany and Italy (JCWI, 1988). In 1988 both Prime Minister Margaret Thatcher and Sir Peter Imbert, Metropolitan Police Commissioner, indicated that serious consideration was being given to the adoption of such a system after 1992. Further evidence of this thinking has been provided by the UK's Data Protection Registrar who warned in his 1993 annual report that there are covert moves by the Health Service to give additional personal identity numbers to every British resident.

In my Sixth Report I raised concerns about the possibility of the National Insurance Number becoming a de facto common identifier without Ministers and Parliament having the opportunity to consider whether a national identification system should be established. The same concerns now arise with the new NHS number. It will be issued at birth, will be well maintained, actively used and provide a unique identification number. Pressures are likely to arise for its use for non-NHS purposes. In effect it could become a de facto national identity number (Ninth Report of the Data Protection Registrar, June 1993, p. 17).

The NHS numbers can be transferred between Government departments and could promote a growth in the illegal use of private data. The Report further alerts the public to the lack of specific legislation to counter the proliferation of personal information (The Guardian, 16 July 1993.)

RACE AND INFORMATION TECHNOLOGY

There are a number of other ways in which black people will be affected by IT. First as residents and consumers within their own countries, and second, as EU residents. Black people are living within a Europe where personal computerised information is the norm. There is a danger, however, that they are being excluded from access to this information to a greater extent than white people, partly because of their relative lack of understanding and knowledge of the systems, and partly because of their powerlessness (Glastonbury and LaMendola, 1992, p. 134).

Within their countries of residence black people's access to employment, housing, education and personal social services will be recorded within computerised systems. They may or may not be conversant with these systems depending on whether the agency offers its clients information on its use and storage of what may be politically or culturally sensitive data. The empowerment of clients through access to information is not being demonstrably offered by many agencies to their clients. This may be because of the lack of strategic planning on the use of IT at a local as well as a global level within human service agencies. In Britain such agencies rank their services as first, to children, second to older people and third to people with disabilities (Glastonbury and LaMendola, 1992). Lack of strategy on IT creates problems for all consumer groups, but if a group is not a priority (such as black people), then its IT and human services needs are given an even lower ranking.

One of the main difficulties is that new technologies are mainly created and built by groups of white men, who are themselves comparatively small in number and who are a minority. They are champions of the information age and there is very little evidence to suggest that they have an understanding of user participation and empowerment. Nor do they take into account the needs of groups in society who are disenfranchised. The systems developed by them are monocultural and commercial in nature and therefore are not easily adaptable for use within agencies which strive to practice anti-discrimination.

Indeed, there are moves throughout Europe to curb civil and social rights and greater powers are being offered to agencies. In the UK, for example, housing officials are able to check the passports of black people, and in France the police are able to undertake arbitrary and unofficial identity checks (The Guardian, 26 May 1993).

The increased powers being given to agencies are heightening fears that black people will be susceptible to spot checks at every level, and that at each stage the information gathered on them will be fed into computers. This will increase in detail and will be available for use by people in authority. Black people as a visible minority are the only group in Europe who will be systematically and lawfully discriminated against in terms of information collection and storage in such a way.

Cross border travel will be the proving ground for many black citizens, who may have legitimate claims to travel in Europe, but may still be faced with discrimination because they belong to a visible minority. This is further evidenced by a report of the Expulsion Sub Group of the Ad Hoc Group on Immigration which agreed in 1991 to the External Frontiers Convention which advocated the need to develop a computerised common EU list of undesirable aliens (The Guardian, 27 May 1993).

The EU's visa policy is also being targeted as part of the External Frontiers Convention with the development of the Eurovisa system. The formation of the list has been a cause of concern to black people for a number of years because it will mainly include people who have originated from black developing countries as illustrated by Gordon in 1989.

At its meeting in Copenhagen in 1987, the EU ministers who make up the Trevi Group agreed on a list of over 50 countries whose nationals require a visa to enter any single EU state and it is likely that this will be extended. The visa list includes all the countries of the New (Black) Commonwealth. A study on the creation of a computerised system for handling data in connection with visa applications was also set in motion (Gordon, 1989, p. 12). Commonwealth nationals who are currently able to use their right to vote within the UK will be ineligible to vote for the EU Parliament.

CONCLUSION

The collection and dissemination of information is in the hands of white Europeans, as is the development of systems designed to manage this data. In a bid to maintain their power and status the EU member states are showing outward signs of pursuing their historical legacy of exploiting poor people from poor countries by capitalising on the use of guest and migrant labour.

There are, however, some possible avenues which can be followed which will allow equity to be seen to be delivered to all EU residents, not just to the powerful majority.

The EU has been attempting to work on the issues of immigration and asylum for a number of years and has recently published two communications. The immigration document stresses the importance of collaboration between European countries and countries of origin; that immigration will be strictly managed; that legal immigrants should be helped to integrate supported by positive policies; and that the EU must have an external migration policy (Commission of the European Communities-Background Report, 1992).

The effort to debate the issues and promote equality will bear fruit only if the political will exists. However, the EU and member states will have to avoid placing black citizens and residents who have lived and worked in their host countries for many years in the same category as the newly arrived guest workers, refugees and asylum seekers. Clearly the issues which are of immediate concern to the first group are not relevant to the second. The development of effective systems to empower both groups depend entirely on clarity of policies, and the ability to strategically target and implement such policies.

There are also concerns about the pervasive and indiscriminate connection between immigrants, terrorists and criminals. The experience in the UK shows that although such associations clearly breach anti-discriminatory policies and the 1976 Race Relations Act, they can nevertheless influence the workers who are delivering services. For example, social security officers and college administrators have asked only black applicants for personal identification when registering.

The Social Chapter Protocol of the Maastricht Treaty may play a central role in the development of equality policies. It has considerable potential to direct member states on working conditions and the integration of workers on the edges of the job market.

The Social Chapter has been rejected by the UK Government who are concerned with the expenses involved, and that it will make the UK less competitive. When the Treaty is fully ratified it will offer the EU a substantial increase in power to legislate for workers rights. This will have significant implications for women and non-EU nationals within the UK because it may not be able to escape such directives, more particularly because they will support the Treaty of Rome.

There is a danger that the EU and its member states may be immorally using IT in ways which will further discriminate against black people at the institutional and individual levels. Clearly IT serves the notion of the white European club admirably, it enshrines the status quo within newly developed IT systems.

The British National Council for Civil Liberties (NCCL) have produced guidance on data protection (Cornwell and Staunton, 1985, p. 95) which addresses the omissions within the 1984 Data Protection Act. It recommends that the Act is amended to include manual records, national security, crime and taxation and precautionary measures which safeguard personal information which are already within The European Convention. The NCCL further recommends the adoption of codes of practice which will augment the law.

The EU's existing equal opportunity programmes provide direct comparison in terms of resourcing for non-EU nationals. For example, the Helios II programme has been funded for four years until 1996 and has been awarded ECU 37 million to institute a third Community action programme to support creative, experiential annual projects for people with disabilities which will encourage user participation and involvement from close relatives, professionals and industry. A further task for Helios II is the development of a computerised information and documentation system, Handynet, for people with disabilities which will use national collection and information centres to collect and adapt information, and then disseminate it within Europe (Official Journal of the European Communities, 23 Feb. 1993).

Given the political will resourcing can also be made available to improve the quality of life of black residents within the EU with the development of IT systems. The possibilities are many and varied as demonstrated by an international computerised network operating from Geneva by the International Federation of Red Cross and Red Crescent Societies which has a membership 152 countries. It is currently using a grant from the Canadian International Development Agency to enhance communication between members. The Federation's sister body, the International Committee of the Red Cross (ICRC) works in areas of war such as Somalia and the former Yugoslavia. The ICRC is the core for the Central Training Agency which has in its possession 60 million refugee case histories some of which are from World War Two. The case histories are fed into computer networks and databases which locate refugees and prisoners of war and help to reunite families split by military or civil conflict (The Guardian, 3 Dec. 1992, p. 15)

As far as maintaining contact with families is concerned, many black residents and citizens are in situations which are similar to refugees. A significant number have been unable to have their families join them from their countries of origin because of the tightening of immigration regulations. Equity will dictate that in due course policies will change and the 12-15 million non-EU nationals will be able to settle and be joined by their families. When this happens an IT network can play a unique and important role in offering people their social rights.

There is a need to establish systems as a matter of urgency. The lack of established procedures and computerisation has led in many instances to the discretionary interpretation of rules and regulations by officials. For black people discretion usually equals discriminatory behaviour. Furthermore, computer information is more likely to be regulated and increasingly open to scrutiny and challenge.

REFERENCES

Baragiola, P. (July 1991). Standardization in information technology-piecing together the bits. XIII Magazine. Commission of the European Community, Directorate General XIII.

Birmingham City Council-Race Relations Unit. (Dec. 1991). 1992 and Race Equality-Fact Pack. Birmingham City Council.

Blennerhasset, E. (1988). Consumers, Computers and the Public Service: An overview of European Trends. In Glastonbury, B., LaMendola W. and Toole, S. Information Technology and the Human Services. John Wiley and Sons. Bury St. Edmunds, UK.

Bunyan, T. (Ed.) (1993). Statewatching the new Europe–a handbook on the European State. Russell Press. Nottingham, UK.

Commission of the European Communities. (Nov. 1989). Eurobarometer-Public Opinion in the European Communities. Directorate-General Information, Communication, Culture. Brussels.

Commission of the European Communities. (March 1992). Background Report–Immigration and Asylum. ISEC/B6/92.

Council of Europe-Standing Conference of Local and Regional Authorities in Europe. (Feb. 1992). Report on a new municipal policy for multicultural integration in Europe and the Frankfurt Declaration. ACPL8IP.17. 0502-3/2/92-3-E.

Cornwell, R. and Staunton, M. (1985). Data Protection: Putting the Record Straight. NCCL. The Yale Press. London.

Data Protection Registrar. (June 1993). Ninth Report of the Data Protection Registrar. HMSO. London.

Forbes, I. and Mead, G. (March 1992). Measure for Measure-A Comparative Analysis of Measures to Combat Racial Discrimination in the Member Countries of the European Community. Research Series No. 1, Employment Department/University of Southampton.

Ford, G. (1992). Fascist Europe–The Rise of Racism and Xenophobia. Pluto Press. London.

Glastonbury, B. and LaMendola, W. (1993). The Integrity of Intelligence–A Bill of Rights for the Information Age. MacMillan Press. London.

Gordon, P. ((Nov. 1989). Fortress Europe? The meaning of 1992. The Runnymede Trust. London.

Gregory, F.E.C. (1991). Police Cooperation and Integration in the European Community: Proposals, Problems, and Prospects. Terrorism, Vol. 14, (p. 145-155).

Gregory, F.E.C. (Spring 1991). Border Control Systems and Border Controllers: A Case Study of the British Police Response to Proposals for a Europe Sans Frontieres. Public Policy and Administration, Vol. 6 No. 1, (p. 9-50).

House of Lords. (27 Jan. 1993). Debate on Europol. Vol. 541 No. 85. UK.

Institute of Race Relations. (1991). Europe-variations on the theme of racism. Institute of Race Relations. London.

Joint Council for the Welfare of Immigrants (JCWI). (Nov 1988). Europe Without Frontiers? Bulletin Vol. 3. No. 8.

Official Journal of the European Communities. (Feb. 1993). Council Decision–establishing a third Community action programme to assist disabled people (Helios II 1993 to 1996). No L 56/30. European Community.

Plant, R. (1992). Citizenship, Rights and Welfare. In Coote, A. The Welfare of Citizens-Developing new social rights. Rivers Oram Press. London.

Redmond, R. (1992). Slamming Doors. Refugees V88, United Nations. Geneva.

The Guardian. (3 Dec. 1992). Battle Lines of Hope, (p. 15). London.

The Guardian. (10 March 1993). Busted Drugs Agency. London.

The Guardian. (26 May 1993). EC cracks down on migrants, (p. 1). London.

The Guardian. (27 May 1993). Fortress Europe prepares to wall in its racism, (p. 22). London.

Williams, S. (May 1992). EC Immigration Policy Post Maastricht. European Information Service, (p. 30-33). Issue 129.

The Legislation on Privacy Protection and Social Research

Erik Van Hove

SUMMARY. The heightened attention to privacy protection and the enactment of laws to control the flow of personal information is linked to developments in information technology. However, the awesome development in information technology is not the sole reason to give more attention to information control. Citizens have become alert and are more aware of their rights. A key role with regard to Automatic Processing of Personal Data is taken by the Convention for the Protection of Individuals adopted by the Council of Europe on January 28 1981. The twelve countries of the European Community have signed this treaty and implemented national privacy laws. These laws leave little room for the special requirements of social or epidemiological research. Removing scientific research completely from the scope of privacy laws is not a solution, nor is the full application of rules which were formulated with other problems in mind.

The introduction of powerful information technology in scientific research and progress in emancipation of citizens raises the problem of controlling that flow of information in the research context as well as in other spheres of action. The research community has a tradition of open communication which can easily come into conflict with the need to be careful with personal information. Clarification of rules of conduct and some external controls are advisable. *[Article copies available from The Haworth Document Delivery Service: 1-800-342-9678.]*

Erik Van Hove is Professor at the University of Antwerp, Department of Political and Social Sciences. He teaches social science research methods and his main research interests are in planning of social services. He is a member of the Commission for Protection of Privacy of Belgium.

[Haworth co-indexing entry note]: "The Legislation on Privacy Protection and Social Research." Hove, Erik Van. Co-published simultaneously in *Computers in Human Services* (The Haworth Press, Inc.) Vol. 12, No. 1/2, 1995, pp. 53-67; and: *Human Services in the Information Age* (ed: Jackie Rafferty, Jan Steyaert, and David Colombi) The Haworth Press, Inc., 1995, pp. 53-67. Single or multiple copies of this article are available from The Haworth Document Delivery Serivce [1-800-342-9678, 9:00 a.m. - 5:00 p.m. (EST)].

53

THE NOTION OF PRIVACY

The right to privacy can mean two things. First it indicates that a person has the right to a private sphere and, second, that a person has the right to control the flow of information about his private life. The second right only acquires meaning if there is a private sphere to talk about, but is seen as essential. The law is primarily concerned with information about a person's private life, with who is entitled to what information and for what purpose, and with how the flow of information should be organised and protected. The law presupposes the existence of a private sphere of life.

People are given the right to privacy on the assumption that such a right is an essential condition for self realisation and for happiness. Behind it lies a notion that society alienates people. Work, public life, politics and social services, are devouring threats preventing people from being themselves. Only in personal relations, within the family circle at home, one finds happiness and peace.

The first definition of the right to privacy was, following this logic, "the right to be left alone" (Warren and Brandeis, 1891). The right to escape from public life, to be oneself in private. This is a negative definition and reminds me of an old neighbour in my youth who had a sign on her front porch "Leave me alone." That sign had the attraction of a magnet to us, street boys. We threw little stones, we rang her bell, we did everything to get the woman to sally from the house in anger and to have the thrill of a chase we always won. That woman was extremely unhappy, disturbed and lonely. When the right to privacy is nothing more than the "right" to be lonely, to be ignored and excluded from care, it serves a very narrow purpose and there is little to protect.

A positive right to privacy presupposes a society which offers its citizens the possibilities to build a private life. Sufficient means to have a proper home, sufficient relational skills to have personal relationships, sufficient education and culture to develop the quality of life of the private sphere. It's only when such conditions are met that the purpose of the law, the protection of privacy, makes sense. A worthwhile private life is not realised by an individual against society, but as an integral part of our society and with a way of life, made possible by that society.

This situation leads to what at first sight looks like a contradiction: to make privacy possible society has to intervene in the private life of people, has to provide the material and spiritual means to foster it. This is impossible without knowledge of, and control over, the personal life circumstances of each and everyone. To make privacy possible, privacy has to be violated. This contradiction is, however, only superficial and implies a dichotomy of private life-public life which cannot be sustained. Private life cannot be a haven of humanity in a world which otherwise ignores humanity. Relationships are inherent in all spheres of life. Employees imply employers and the personal integrity of an employee as an employee should be respected at all times. A politician should recognise the human dignity of opponents. Even a car driver should be polite.

The purpose of the laws to protect privacy are not limited to shielding the private life of individuals from others. These laws can equally be seen as organising the legal infringements of privacy. These regulate how personal information should be handled, in all sectors of public life, so that at all times a humane perspective is maintained.

THE HEIGHTENED ATTENTION TO PRIVACY PROTECTION

The heightened attention to privacy protection and the enactment of laws to control the flow of personal information is linked to developments in information technology. Computers have evolved from mere high volume calculators into machines which can retain, process and make available enormous quantities of information. Not so long ago the mere cost of searching through large paper files limited the access to sensitive information. At present searches through databanks take only seconds and all kinds of information can be retrieved instantly.

Computers can now be linked into networks. Information is no longer tied to a single spot but can be available on-line everywhere in the world. I can know if space is available on any plane anywhere in the world by enquiring at any counter in any airport. Computers can also link information from several sources and process that information into in-depth profiles. Information on the type of purchases done by a person in one place can be combined with information on place of dwelling, family composition and so on, leading to rather penetrating marketing strategies.

The time that legislation on the privacy of the mail and against eavesdropping on telephone conversations was sufficient to secure the flow of communications has gone. The spectre of "big brother" looms and has stirred lawmakers into action.

However, the awesome developments in information technology is not the sole reason to give more attention to information control. The citizen has become alert and more aware of their rights. We have evolved from a rural society, where mutual control and pressure to conform were accepted, into urban societies where the individual prevails, where people are more educated and equipped to stand up for themselves. The possibilities for developing a private life have increased.

This more assertive citizen no longer accepts being treated as one of a crowd. People want to know why public authorities want to know such and such and to what end it will be used. The Dutch census of 1971 could only be carried through after extensive debate and will be the last one in the Netherlands. The German census of 1980 almost met the same fate. Fewer people are willing to cooperate in surveys, especially in urban areas. People have become much more selective in what they consider worthwhile becoming involved in and are wary of traditional forms of social engagement.

THE EMERGENCE OF PRIVACY LEGISLATION

On the 27th of June, 1980, after a preliminary hearing, a court in Antwerp ordered that the results of a survey done by our institute, should be destroyed. The survey of schoolchildren on learning difficulties had been conducted without prior consent of the parents. The court order developed the following arguments:

... Considering that we should at all times keep in mind the elementary principles of human dignity, given that more and more the individual is exposed to oppression by the media and all kinds of institutions for material or ideological gain, without adequate means of defense;

Considering that authoritative judicial doctrine has established that the right to personal integrity should be protected, including the right to physical integrity, the right to freedom, dignity and respect (De Page TI No. 235) and the rights implied in the exercise of parental authority, specifically the capacity of parents to decide what they consider proper for the education of their children (R.P.D.B. vb Puissance paternelle No. 61);

Considering that the Constitution takes the exercise of these personal rights so much for granted that no explicit mention was deemed necessary and that the Civil Code in art. 1166 B.W. only mentions them in passing when forbidding creditors to exercise the personal rights of their debtors;

Considering, however, that the Treaty on the Protection of Human Rights and Fundamental Freedoms, ratified by Belgian Law of the 13th of May 1955, explicitly in Art. 8 § 1 and 2 mentions what governs our system of law as an unwritten principle, i.e.,

1. Everyone has the right to respect for his private and family life, his home and his correspondence.
2. There shall be no interference by a public authority with the exercise of this right except such as is in accordance with the law and is necessary in a democratic society in the interest of national securi-

ty, public safety or the economic well-being of the country, for the prevention of disorder or crime, for the protection of health or morals, or for the protection of the rights and freedoms of others.

Considering that a Family Council or a University or any other body, no matter how praiseworthy their intentions are, has no authority whatsoever to infringe on those personal rights without being mandated by law; . . .

This court order is noteworthy in that an international principle of law is invoked to take a very drastic and concrete measure, the destruction of social research data. This notwithstanding the fact that the judge has to agree that no Belgian law provides specific rules which implement the international norm. The unmediated application of the international norm works as a very blunt axe. If the reasoning of this judge were followed through, all social research involving the collection of personal sensitive data would have to be prohibited.

Since the European Treaty to Protect Human Rights, 4th November 1950, further developments in legislation both international and national, have been inspired by two concerns, the protection of privacy, but equally important, the protection of an open flow of information and the safeguarding of further technological developments in the field of information processing. The Convention for the Protection of Individuals with regard to Automatic Processing of Personal Data adopted by the same Council of Europe on January 28 1981 opens with the following declaration of intent: "the necessity to reconcile the fundamental values of respect of privacy with the free flow of information between peoples."

Previously, in 1971, the European Commission expressed its concern about the possible hurdles to the further expansion of the European informatics industry that an unchecked growth of national privacy legislation could be (Nugter, 1990).

Such an unchecked growth has not happened. The deliberations and discussions within the Council of Europe, the European Parliament, the European Commission and the OECD, have led to a consistent body of rules and concepts which have been codified into broadly similar national legislation.

The key role is taken up by the Convention for the Protection of Individuals with regard to Automatic Processing of Personal Data adopted by the Council of Europe on January 28 1981. The twelve countries of the European Community have signed this treaty. Ratification by each country presupposes the implementation of a national privacy law. All EC-countries, with the exception of Italy, have adopted such legislation.

THE NATIONAL LAWS FOR THE PROTECTION OF PRIVACY

The system of protection with a central commission supervising the treatment and flow of personal data and clearly defined sets of rights and duties of registered persons and keepers of personal data files is called by Westin the Continental European model. He compares this to the United States approach in the establishment of codes of good practice under guidance of the courts. Most European countries have adopted laws fitting this mould. We will start out with a discussion of the recent Belgian law, as we are most familiar with it, emphasising those features which are commonly found in most national legislations. Later on, we compare this law to the laws on privacy in neighbouring countries. Finally, we will take a look at the concept directive of the European Commission which should be the keystone of the whole edifice.

The Belgian Law for the Protection of Privacy

It took twenty years for a privacy law to get adopted in Parliament. This long period of gestation does not indicate the peculiar controversial nature of the matter, there were no major political differences between parties. To the contrary, the problem is so far removed from the daily hustle of politics, fundamental and very technical at the same time, that it never got on top of the agenda. Only at the moment that Belgium risked becoming isolated in the group of countries which co-signed the treaty of the Council of Europe, was the effort finally made to adopt a law which conformed to the stipulations of that treaty.

This long period of preparation provided ample opportunity to learn from the experience and insights of neighbouring countries, especially France and Germany.

The Object of the Law

The law applies to *treatments of personal data*. By "treatment" is meant the whole cycle from data collection to the end usage of data, be it manually or by computers. The law regulates, actions on and handling of, personal data, not the data by itself. Both the public and the private sector are envisaged. A unity of treatment is defined by one or more consistent objectives. The entire set of actions carried out in relation to these objectives becomes the object of regulation under the law.

The definition of the concept "personal data" is left rather vague: "the data concerning a natural person who is or can be identified." Three categories of personal data are given special attention:

- "Medical personal data," those data from which information can be derived on the past, present or future state of physical or mental health of the person;
- The so called "sensitive personal data," defined by enumeration: personal data on race, ethnicity, sexual behaviour, opinions or activities concerning politics or religion, membership in unions or mutual aid societies.
- "Judicial personal data," criminal records and records on all kinds of judicial measures applied to the person.

Not all treatment of personal data comes within the scope of the law. Strictly private records on natural persons for personal use are exempted. The actions of the national statistical bureau are also exempted and the files kept by security services come under a special category. Automatic data treatments abroad, but directly accessible in Belgium, are brought within the scope of the law.

The Actors

The law establishes a national Commission for the Protection of Privacy. This commission is given a central role in the operation of the law, acting as an advisory board to policy makers and acting as a mediator between registered persons and keepers of personal data files. In addition to this commission, the law defines the following actors:

- The *keeper of a file:* the physical or legal person who keeps and exploits a manual or automated file with personal data;
- The *registered persons:* those natural persons on whom information is kept;
- *Third parties,* that is, all other persons or institutions.

Each party is given a set of duties and rights concerning the treatment of personal data.

The Duties of the Keeper of a File

- The keeper of a file has the obligation to register, with the Commission for the Protection of Privacy, each automated data treatment s/he intends to undertake.
- At the moment of data collection the registered person must be informed on the identity of the keeper of the file, the legal base for the

data collection, the objectives pursued and the inclusion in the national register.

* The keeper of a file is bound to take all measures needed to secure the privacy of the persons included in his files: physical security measures, internal monitoring, control measures to deny access to unauthorised persons, etc. Moreover, the data treatment should be proportional to the objectives and not excessive.
* Communication to third parties is forbidden in principle. This does not mean that all transmission of data is excluded. Such transmission should follow the rules established for data treatments.
* More strict rules apply for sensitive data. Such data can only be collected and treated by a specific legal disposition advised by the Commission. Medical data can only be treated under supervision of a medical doctor and cannot be communicated to third parties except by legal disposition. The treatment of judicial data also requires a legal measure. The law provides such legal grounds for a national and municipal penal register.

The Rights of a Registered Person

The duties imposed on the keeper of a file and the supervision of the Commission provide for a certain degree of protection of privacy. Under this law, however, it is mainly the individual concerned exercising their legal rights who must defend their own privacy. These rights are as follows:

* *The right to know.* Both at the moment of data collection as at the moment of inclusion in a new treatment, the person concerned has to be informed of the fact that a record on them is kept, by whom, and to what end. A person has the right to refuse to give information but cannot prevent the use of exact information on him which has been legally obtained.
* *The right of access.* A person can at all times check what is known about them in a given treatment. In some cases this right is exercised indirectly through the Commission.
* *The right of correction, deletion or to block use.* Everyone can have incorrect information on them corrected. If certain data are excessive in relation to the stated objectives of the treatment, their deletion can be ordered.

These rights are in the first place exercised by the registered person towards the keeper of the file. If they meet difficulties, they can ask the Commission to intervene and, as a last resort, obtain a court order.

COMPARISON OF BELGIAN LEGISLATION
WITH THAT OF SOME OTHER EUROPEAN COUNTRIES

The German Legislation

The German law *Bundesdatenschutzgesetz* came into force on January 1 1978 and underwent a major revision in the law *Gesetz zur Fortentwicklung der Datenverarbeitung und des Datenschutzes* of December 20 1990. Compared to the Belgian law, this law is much more detailed. More parties are defined and all steps which can be distinguished in a data treatment are elaborated. A disadvantage of this approach is the need to adapt the law regularly to the changes in technology of information processing, as was done in 1990.

Supervision, is distributed over three agents. The federal commissioner supervises the federal treatments of personal data, the state commissioners exercise control over other public and private data treatments and within firms an agent is made responsible for privacy protection by the firm. The federal commissioner for privacy protection has the same advisory powers towards the federal authorities as are entrusted to the Belgian Commission.

The duty to register treatments of personal data is less extensive than under the Belgian law. Only public data treatments and commercially exploited personal data need to be registered. The provision of within-firm responsible agents indicates the emphasis on self-regulation.

The Dutch Legislation

The Dutch law on the registration of persons was also long in the making and was finally adopted on January 6 1989. Following the commotion around the census of 1971 a state commission on the protection of privacy was established which published its findings in 1976. After five years, a draft law was submitted to parliament which followed the recommendations of that commission. In the meantime, however, times had changed, de-regulation was on the public agenda and the draft law was seen as an example of excessive state meddling. The draft law was withdrawn. Only in 1985 a new draft was reintroduced, and it took until 1989 before it was adopted (See Nutger, 1990).

In the Dutch law the object of regulation is the personal data file itself and not the data treatment as in most European countries. This leads to a more static approach which to many is considered less appropriate in a rapidly changing technological environment.

In relation to those data files, approximately the same actors, with similar rights and duties, are defined. The main initiative to secure privacy also belongs to the registered person who must exercise rights of access, correction, deletion and control over transmission to third parties. Supervision is the task of the "Registration Chamber." This body receives the notifications of the keepers of personal data files and makes them accessible to the general public in a register.

The law allows for a large number of exemptions to the duty to register: data files in the context of internal management of firms, membership and subscription files and files limited to identification data. In principle this should not lead to the conclusion that these data files fall completely outside of the scope of the law. A number of special data files which in other countries give rise to special measures of protection, legal registers and police and state security files, are not covered at all. The Dutch law was not too well received (see Kuitenbrouwer, 1991).

The French Legislation

The French law, *Loi No 78-17 relative a l'Informatique, aux fichiers et aux libertés,* became operational on January 6 1978. France was the second European country, after Sweden, to have a legal framework for privacy protection. This law has served as a model for many European countries and even for the European Convention (Fauvet, 1988). Certainly the Belgian law was greatly influenced by the French example and the ten years of experience with it. The principles, the rights and duties of the different actors, and the procedures established by the law are identical to what was said earlier about the Belgian law.

The most striking feature of the French experience is the central role of the "Commission Nationale de l'Informatique et des Libertés" the CNIL. That supervisory body has over the years transposed the vague principles of the law into workable procedures and regulations, supported by a large staff of more than fifty specialists in law and informatics. Contrary to the Netherlands or Germany, where a large number of common data files are exempted from registration, France works with simplified notifications for those treatments which come within the scope of "simplified norms" worked out and published by the CNIL. If the person responsible for an intended treatment can fit their treatment in one of the thirty models provided, a summary registration is sufficient. To date more than 150.000 such simplified notifications were received by the CNIL.

A EUROPEAN DIRECTIVE IN THE MAKING

On October 15 1992 the Commission of the EC published a revised proposition for a directive of the Council concerning the protection of natural persons in relation to the treatment of personal data and concerning the free flow of these data. This revision comes after a first draft of 1990 which was rather critically received and severely amended by the European Parliament.

The objectives of this directive are twofold. First, to harmonize the rules concerning privacy protection in the twelve countries of the EC. Second, through this harmonization, secure the free international flow of information throughout the Community. A third important aspect is not mentioned in the commentary to the directive. When this directive comes into force, the realization of a system of adequate privacy protection at the European level itself will put an end to an increasingly embarrassing situation. Countries with operational legislation were compelled to transmit personal data to EC-bodies, while such legislation normally forbids transmission of data to unprotected environments.

The harmonization achieved by the draft directive should be taken with a grain of salt. In fact the directive takes over the schemes adopted by those European countries with the most experience, leaving open as alternatives points of divergence. For example, both the system of exemptions from registration used in Germany and the system of simplified notification used in France, are considered acceptable.

THE CONSEQUENCES OF THESE LEGAL DEVELOPMENTS FOR SOCIAL RESEARCH

The Position of Social Research Under the Present Belgian Law

Most social research clearly involves setting up automated data files with personal data. Prior registration with the Commission on privacy protection is required. Moreover, most surveys will include one or more data items of the so called sensitive type. If so, the study requires a legal authorization.

At the time of data collection, interviewing or otherwise, the researcher is also obliged to inform fully the prospective respondent. The objectives of the study, by whom the study is commissioned, the registration number with the Commission, the legal grounds for the study or lack thereof, all have to be stated, together with the voluntary nature of the respondent's participation. One can imagine an increase in the non-response rate with all the consequences this has for representativeness.

At the time this law was debated in Parliament, the problem of scientific research, more specifically medical research, was brought up (July 1992). The Minister for Justice declared at that time that indeed the law created a problem for scientific research, but that a solution will have to be found in the European Directive under discussion. However, even if the European Directive were to address the problem, which is not the case at the moment, a Belgian legal measure will still be required. As things stand at the moment, most social research would have to cease when the present law becomes fully operational, in about a year.

How the Problem Has Been Met in Other Countries

In 1988, the CNIL in France published a report on its ten years of existence (Vitalis, 1988). A full chapter is devoted to the scientific research problems the CNIL has had to resolve.

In its recommendations the CNIL has been guided by the following principles:

- The unmistakable value of scientific research for the acquisition of knowledge, policy-making and planning;
- The need to safeguard the rights of registered persons under the law: the right to be informed, the right to refuse cooperation and the need for explicit approval by the respondent when sensitive data are recorded.

The CNIL has accepted the fact that the rights of the individual cannot be fully maintained in all research designs. Sometimes the nature of the research requires a degree of secrecy on its objectives, even towards the respondents. The CNIL has weighed case by case, and in some cases the rights of the individual have been waived in the name of a higher good.

From the stream of recommendations some general rules can be derived which constitute a code of good practice which can be applied in most research projects.

- Identification data and scientific data should be kept in separate files. The identification data files should only be preserved for the limited time needed to collect the scientific data. In some cases, longitudinal research and epidemiological registers, this "limited period" could become very long indeed.
- Prospective respondents should be informed on the objectives of the study and on the voluntary nature of their cooperation. However, in some cases, the individual information can be replaced by general information to the public.

- A certain flexibility is introduced for the transmission of medical data or administrative data to research institutions. This is considered more an "extension of the objectives" for which the data originally were gathered rather than "new objectives." This legal construction allows foregoing the duty to inform the registered persons of their inclusion in a research project.

It is clear that the CNIL had to interpret the law rather extensively in order to make valuable scientific research still possible.

Art. 33 of the Dutch law stipulates that for personal data files that are established for the sole purpose of scientific research the usual rights of registered persons do not apply. Notification of the transfer of data for scientific research need not be made. Given that the concept of scientific research in itself is rather vague, this is a sweeping exemption from external control for the many data files that go beyond the direct operational processing of persons. The implied assumption is that the ethics and self-regulation of the research community are sufficient to safeguard privacy.

The State of Affairs at the European Level and for Transnational Research

The treaty of the Council of Europe which provides the framework within which the European countries have developed their privacy legislation, allows in art.9 that the rights of registered persons can be restricted in the case of automated data files established for research purposes. As stated earlier, the Dutch law has made a very extensive use of this possibility.

The draft directive of the EC (art.14) does not go that far. The rights of registered persons can only be restricted in the case of temporary files that are only statistically treated. The draft directive also allows for special guarantees which can be stipulated for the historical preservation of data files for scientific purposes (art.3, § 1, (e)). This summary treatment of the problems of scientific research is in sharp contrast to the care taken in the draft directive to preserve journalistic freedom or to preserve the possibility for ideological organisations to process sensitive data. The research community apparently has not the same lobbying capacity at the European level.

Concerning the transnational transmission of personal data, the draft directive established the general principle that such transmission should be completely free between countries that have realised an adequate legal system of privacy protection. The directive provides mechanisms for the recognition of countries as such.

CONCLUSION

Is There a Problem?

I know of no cases where harm was done to people by the infringement of their privacy through scientific research. That does not mean that such cases do not exist, it only means that the problem is not at the foreground of public debate. Problems like aggressive direct marketing or unobtrusive monitoring by security firms are much more alive and are matters of complaints brought to the attention of supervisory bodies.

Neither is the fact that scientific research often involves in-depth observation of the private lives of people in itself a problem. Quite often it is a prerequisite to making such privacy possible. Only supported by this type of research can society fulfil its mandate to provide people with the space and means to build their private lives. Scientific research provides the knowledge and techniques for better health care, better methods of psychosocial support and more equality in the distribution of wealth and well-being. Researchers provide the building blocks of privacy, rather than destroying it. For exactly this reason, they should also be more aware of the need for privacy protection.

A Good Practice

The introduction of powerful information technology in scientific research and progress in emancipation of citizens poses the problem of controlling that flow of information in the research context as well as in other spheres of action. Furthermore, the research community has a tradition of open communication which can easily come into conflict with the need to be careful with personal information. Clarification of the rules of conduct and some external control are advisable. Removing scientific research completely from the scope of privacy laws is not a good solution, nor is the full application of rules which were formulated with other problems in mind.

Based on the practical experience, mostly acquired in France, the following rules could be formulated.

1. The person who gives information to scientific research has a right to know about it, has the right to be informed about the research objectives and has the right to refuse cooperation. Any deviation from this rule should be motivated and sanctioned by an agency that is independent from the researchers: an ethics committee or a privacy commission.

2. Identifying information should be kept separate from scientific information with special measures of security and restricted access. Identifying information should be deleted as soon as possible.
3. Research projects which involve the collection of personal information should be registered with the national register, to allow for control on practice. This register should not lead to any restrictions on the freedom of research.

The research community should take up the responsibility of enacting a code of conduct and not wait for legal measures. This should not be done in a spirit to escape from the law by invoking self-regulation. A legal order is always to be preferred to free-floating voluntary systems. In that sense it is a pity that the voice of the research community has been heard so little when the different national legislation and the European directive were formulated.

REFERENCES

Belgische Kamer van Volksvertegenwoordigers, Buitengewone zitting 1991-1992, 2 Juli 1992, Verslag namens de Commissie voor \judyiyir, p. 39.

Fauvet, J. (1988) Statement by the President of the French Supervisory Commission, the preface to: Vitalis, A. et al., *Dix ans d'informatique et libertés*, Economica, Paris.

Kuitenbrouwer, F., *Het Recht om met rust gelaten te worden*, Uitgeverij Balans, Amsterdam. pp. 161-176.

Westin, A.F., New Issues of Computer Privacy in the Eighties, in *Information Processing* 83, R.E.A. Mason (Ed.), IFIP 1983, pp. 735-736. Expanded on in:

Nutger, A. C. M., (1990) Transborder Flow of Personal Data within the EC, *Computer/Law Series* No. 6, Kluwer Deventer-Boston, pp.29. pp. 145-167.

Warren, S. D. and Brandeis, L. D., The Right to Privacy, in *Harvard Law Review*, *1890-1891*, Vol 5, pp. 193-220.

LEARNING
AND EDUCATIONAL TECHNOLOGY
IN SOCIAL WORK

Introduction

Jackie Rafferty

Teaching and learning take place in a complex, interacting system. The outcomes of learning depend on the combined effects of the whole learning environment . . . and what is required are supportive learning environments which capitalise on both educational technology and other innovations in teaching and learning (The Committee of Scottish University Principals, 1992).

The history of the use of technology in learning is, in technology terms, a long one but it is only in the last ten years that social work training and education has begun to address how it may support the social work learning process. Even then developments have tended to be piecemeal and isolated and remain so in most countries to date. Social work training and education has had to overcome its reluctance to use educational technology and has

Jackie Rafferty is Senior Research Fellow at the Centre for Human Service Technology, University of Southampton, UK.

[Haworth co-indexing entry note]: "Introduction." Rafferty, Jackie. Co-published simultaneously in *Computers in Human Services* (The Haworth Press, Inc.) Vol. 12, No. 1/2, 1995, pp. 69-73; and: *Human Services in the Information Age* (ed: Jackie Rafferty, Jan Steyaert, and David Colombi) The Haworth Press, Inc., 1995, pp. 69-73. Single or multiple copies of this article are available from The Haworth Document Delivery Service [1-800-342-9678, 9:00 a.m. - 5:00 p.m. (EST)].

only now reached a position where there is a critical mass of interest in creating new and relevant ways of harnessing the power of the microchip. The 1990's have seen the world of technology open up to social work teachers as more "friendly" tools have become available which allow teachers to bend the technology to the needs of the students rather than the students bending to the demands of the technology. As we approach the end of the century current thinking is pragmatic whilst remaining creative about the place of technology in teaching and learning. A survey of use of new technology in UK higher education institutions outlined that educational technology was being used in a number of different ways:

> . . . developing courseware for computer based learning; buying in commercial software for teaching; promoting computer literacy/IT skills; enhancing presentation of teaching; and for electronic communication/library automation (ibid.).

The role of Information Technology in human service education has been a recurring theme since the first HUSITA conference in the UK in 1987, with a watershed in 1990 with Dick Schoech's publication of *Human Service Computing Concepts & Applications* (Schoech, 1990). Schoech set out and addressed the use of information technology in the Human Services and in Part 3 explored the application of computing in social work education and training. Schoech described the concept of "professional computing competency" which he defines as "knowing how to use the software of one's profession effectively" which would focus on students accessing software in use in the human services as part of their core curricula. It is only when Schoech turns to the future that he envisages new forms of education and training where

> . . . the task turns from students trying to find information to information trying to find students . . . the tasks of finding information will be replaced by the tasks of synthesizing and applying information . . . and interactive video simulations of human service delivery systems will be used by professional education . . . (Schoech, 1990).

The focus of the papers in this chapter is on using educational technology to teach social work rather than teaching social workers about information technology. They represent a geographical spread and the current state of development of the use of educational technology in social work. The three papers from western societies (North America and The Netherlands) have had every opportunity to take advantage of the developments in educational technology, yet it is also clear that the relative newcomer from

Romania in Eastern Europe is going to develop the use of technology for education in a much shorter time span. The papers also represent different conceptual approaches to the use of educational technology and provide a spectrum of views which mirror the debate in the subject generally.

The first paper written by Poliana Stefanescu is particularly welcomed as one of the few contributions to the field we have had from Eastern Europe. It is a pertinent lesson to those of us in countries where change appears fast but is often marginal to our everyday lives to read the matter of fact way Stefanescu writes about the abolition of social work schools in 1969, followed by the abolition of psychology and sociology departments in 1978 and the eventual reopening of the social work department in 1990. It is clear from her paper that she supports the definition outlined by Grebel and Steyaert in their report "Social Informatics–Education on the vocational use of Information Technology in Schools of Social Work" (Grebel & Steyaert, 1993). They describe the vocational use of information technology in the Human Services as: "our concept of what to teach about IT is based on the use of information and only in the second place on the use of technology to handle information." Stefanescu's paper deals with the introduction of a new course in Social Informatics in the Department of Social Work at Bucharest with the support of the Dutch Ministry of Welfare, Health and Culture. The curriculum whilst concentrating on handling social work information, does include students needing to learn BASIC programming and therefore places an emphasis on what Schoech would call "computer literacy" rather than "computer competency." Stefanescu describes the course "as a beginning" and admits to a secondary agenda of motivating students to argue for the need for computerisation when they move from training to practice.

In contrast the next paper sits firmly as a support to the traditional core curriculum of social work training. Less than three years after Schoech's prediction on interactive video systems Satterwhite and Schoech's paper "Multimedia Training for Child Protective Service Workers: Initial Test Results" describes the initial use of "Keisha," probably the first interactive, Windows based, multi-media simulation program within human service education. The paper first gives a useful context to the specific application by describing computer based learning (CBT) and summarising the studies showing that CBT "can offer a cost-effective, non-judgmental, confidential, and safe learning experience." The paper's main content however, outlines the rationale for producing "Keisha," its contents and approach and its development and initial testing including the trainees responses to it. Though the paper describes the "discovery instructional" approach of "Keisha," the very nature of multi-media with its mix of sound, graphics and text means that words alone cannot do it justice and although the program was developed specifically for the local context anyone contemplating developing CBT should acquire at least the demonstration version. Whilst much is written on CBT very little has been developed specifically for social work education and training. Earlier developments, other than for the Apple Macintosh community, have had to rely heavily on text based DOS supported programs, or specialist hardware such as interactive video players. This Windows based program sets a new standard for those of us following similar paths.

Albert Visser's paper is set in the context of a proactive approach to the use of educational technology by the Ministry of Education and Science in The Netherlands which has been funding various projects since 1984. Visser concentrates on the contribution that computer assisted learning (CAL) can make to learning and the situations in which it is relevant to use CAL. He describes the characteristics of CAL and then illustrates these by giving us a case study of a CAL Law Tutorial, "ZAO." The paper is not though a description of the program but concentrates on dealing with the important issues surrounding the implementation of CAL such as strategies to enhance the acceptance of CAL amongst teachers and students and the role of the change agent. Visser argues that what is needed is "a structural embedding of IT in curricula."

So far the emphasis in the papers has been on using technology to teach information skills and to teach elements of the core curriculum. The next paper adds another dimension as Paula Nurius synthesises these two approaches and adds others in her paper on "Critical Thinking: A Meta-Skill for Integrating Practice and Information Technology Training" where the computer is used as "a medium of thought and expression." Her focus, similarly to Stefanescu's is an educator's perspective on what students need to know about information processing. However, she takes a much more in-depth look at the integrative framework required and encompasses and differentiates amongst others: *substantive* and *procedural knowledge, modularised* and *embedded approaches, information processing* and *information management.* The theme which binds together the framework is the clarification and the place of *critical thinking* and Nurius leads us through this complex domain. This is a thought provoking paper which hopefully will continue to stimulate discussion and adds a vital element of theoretical analysis to this growing field.

Nurius concludes that "In coming years as entering students are increasingly computer facile, we will see a shift in learning curves less toward hardware and computer commands and more devoted to concepts and ideas." The papers in this chapter show that a good start has been made in this direction.

REFERENCES

Committee of Scottish University Principals, *Teaching and Learning in an Expanding Higher Education System*, Report of a Working Party of the Committee of Scottish University Principals. ISBN. 0 9519377 2 3, CSUP, 1992 (pg.ix & 67).

Grebel, H., and Steyaert J., *Social Informatics*, Hogeschool Eindhoven, The Netherlands, June 1993. Research report presented at HUSITA 3, Maastricht, 1993.

Schoech, D., *Human Service Computing Concepts & Applications*, The Haworth Press, Inc., NY, 1990.

Using a Computer Network for Social Work Training

Poliana Stefanescu

SUMMARY. The social worker needs basic knowledge about human behaviour, the economic and social structure of society, law and regulations, etc. In recent years, knowledge about new methods and techniques for registering, reporting and analysing data and information has become necessary for the social worker. This paper deals with the introduction of a new course in Social Informatics in the Department of Social Work at the University of Bucharest. This department was established at the University after December 1989. The paper describes the starting point and motivation for a course in Informatics and contains a short presentation of the curriculum and gives information about the computer network and software used by the students. The results during and after the first year of teaching are mentioned and there is also a discussion about the opportunities the graduate students will have to use IT in social work practice. Finally, the conclusions lead to an optimistic approach regarding the utility of "Social Informatics" courses. *[Article copies available from The Haworth Document Delivery Service: 1-800-342-9678.]*

INTRODUCTION

In Romania the profession of social worker ("asistent social") is almost unknown to the people. During the communist regime, social work had a

---

Poliana Stefanescu is Lecturer at the Faculty of Sociology, Psychology & Education, University of Bucharest, BD Mihail Kogalniceanu 64, Bucharest, Romania.

[Haworth co-indexing entry note]: "Using a Computer Network for Social Work Training." Stefanescu, Poliana. Co-published simultaneously in *Computers in Human Services* (The Haworth Press, Inc.) Vol. 12, No. 1/2, 1995, pp. 75-80; and: *Human Services in the Information Age* (ed: Jackie Rafferty, Jan Steyaert, and David Colombi) The Haworth Press, Inc., 1995, pp. 75-80. Single or multiple copies of this article are available from The Haworth Document Delivery Serivce [1-800-342-9678, 9:00 a.m. - 5:00 p.m. (EST)].

75

passive and bureaucratic character because the political leadership gave the impression that they could provide solutions to every problem. In this situation most of the population was provided with minimum but secure living conditions, wages, sick benefits, family allowances, medical care free of charge, old age pensions and other social benefits. This had a double effect:

a. The social work services have been reduced to a minimum;
b. Social work has been deprived of professionalism; professionals were replaced by employees.

In these circumstances, the communist regime abolished the Social Work Schools in 1969 and also abolished the Psychology and Sociology departments of the University in 1978.

Since the events of 1989, we have had the chance to rebuild social work as a profession and a service. It is the duty of the Social Work Department of the University of Bucharest to prepare future social work professionals. This process commenced in 1990 with the opening of a 3 year course that was turned into a 4 year course in 1992. Social Work was included as a separate department in the Faculty of Sociology, Psychology and Pedagogy. The reorganisation of the social work system in Romania includes not only a legislative basis and the (re)definition of the social worker profile, it also means new methods and modern technical resources. In this context, a computer is a common instrument for a social work office. The graduating social workers will have the opportunity to move from training to practice and we hope they will have the ambition and motivation to improve their knowledge. If their office has no computer they will hopefully be persuasive enough to get one.

In starting this new department, we received a great deal of help from the Dutch Government that financed the PSO 1 and POS 2 projects, "Professional education for social work in Romania" (We have to mention the policy of the Dutch Ministry of Welfare, Health and Culture on Eastern-Europe and one of the priorities in this policy is the support for professional education for social work).

Briefly the objects of these projects are:

• curriculum development and research
• retraining in social welfare systems and social work systems
• retraining in specific professional and didactical methods
• producing manuals and translating textbooks
• organising an international seminar
• supply of equipment.

We also have to mention here the TEMPUS programme financed by the European Community that helped us to develop an exchange programme for students and teachers and the acquisition of a new computer network.

In Romania, the economic and social crisis have transformed social needs. The redefinition of social needs involves collaboration with people from very different areas. The social worker must be prepared to be confronted with different kinds of groups, from for example, neighbourhoods, schools and minorities and also has to manage a lot of information about clients. The use of computers will lead to the improvement of social worker's activity. A very specific tool and an aid would then be, the computer.

The ability to record, send and retrieve information quickly is very useful for the social worker. That is why a special course in Informatics has been started at the Department of Social Work. Including this course in the curriculum was agreed by the Ministry of Education and supported by the leadership of the Department of Social Work.

TECHNICAL RESOURCES

The students in Social Work study Informatics in the second school year. They use a Novell computer network with 10 work stations that belongs to the faculty. Every work station has only 1MB RAM and a 3.5″ floppy drive. The file-saver has 4MB RAM, 120MB hard-disk and 2 floppy drives (3.5″ and 5.25″). All the monitors are monochrome. We use the Novell V2.2 and DOS 3.3 operating systems. At the beginning of the next school year the Department of Social Work will use its own computer network.

THE CURRICULUM

The curriculum for social informatics is divided into two parts spread over two terms (one term is about 14 weeks). Every week the students have a course (2 hours) and a seminar (2 hours) in the computer room. The students may also practice on the computer during their spare time.

In the *first term* the curriculum includes:

- introduction to the development of informatics and the computers
- some areas of applications, related to social work
- the main steps in problem solving

- the statement
- the analysis
- algorithm "step by step"
- the computer programme
- BASIC programming language and very simple programmes
- recording data from questionnaires and interviews in files.

At this stage the students had to solve the following problem: A company is looking for a person to be hired in certain conditions. How can the computer be used in this situation?

The students programmed the interview questions for hiring and also the analysis of the answers. They had the opportunity to create several alternatives of questions and answers and at the end, to take the decision (as a manager).

After finishing their computer programmes I let the students invite each other to answer their questionnaires. It was a good opportunity for me and for them to collect their ideas and impressions and to see that the students introduced questions applicable not only for getting a job but also for assessing social help or care for unemployed or elderly people.

With these examples in mind, the students will be able to solve practical problems involving computer processing. Another kind of exercise was the use of data files; for instance:

1. Create a date file for registering people including information like: name, age, occupation, income, etc., and display the individual's information.
2. Read the file with the students of the department and find those who are married and have children, in order to get financial support.

In the *second term* the students learn how to use software packages for writing reports, processing data or creating a database. For didactical reasons I used an integrated package: *Microsoft Works* that includes a text processor, a spreadsheet and database.

The students learned very fast how to use the text processor and now they are able to type their work. The spreadsheet module was more difficult to learn, but I used many practical examples:

- the calculation of the new salaries in the economy;
- the calculation of the expected income of a middle class family;
- the analysis of the number of school children versus the number of students for every district of the country.

These are only some examples that the students analyzed and made graphical representations.

The database module was easier to access, having in mind the experience that the students got with the BASIC files and the Works Spreadsheet. Then I asked them to create a database with the students from their department. This database must include all the information necessary for the administration and the secretary of the faculty.

While carrying on their job, the social worker will often see or collect data about the private conditions of various persons or about the relations between groups of institutions. The social worker has the obligation to deal with all data confidentially. The professional secret is a very strict duty of a social worker. Even when social workers use the computer for registering clients they have to ensure the confidentiality of the data. That is why the curriculum includes a special lesson about how to protect data in order to preserve the secrecy of information. The ethics of this profession includes keeping the professional secret unless the social worker has discovered serious abuses that will "force" them to talk.

CONCLUSIONS

Some of my students are working in nongovernmental organisations or foundations and they come to the seminars with their own problems. In their organisations they had computers and they had a large amount of data to process but they have not started yet. The computers were almost always used for text processing.

After the first steps in informatics, my students realised how to use the computer in a more efficient way like organising a data base and recording all the data they have. Those who were not able to do this by themselves, have enough knowledge to ask a professional in computer programming what to do, so they were able to describe:

- the problem
- the kind of data they have
- the kind of reports or answers they need
- other kinds of data processing.

I think it is good to offer to the social workers such a useful tool like computer but it is equally important to train them in how to use it efficiently and effectively. This is possible only by giving them an appropriate knowledge during professional training.

My students have neither computers at home, nor specific documentation. It is the task of the teacher to cover this lack and to provide them with the most useful and up-to-date information.

The curriculum and the examples that I used are only the beginning of an important activity in the Department for Social Work. We intend to explore the first steps made in social work practice and to find the situations that require the use of computers in administrating data or in testing human abilities and demands. Thus we can offer to our students new examples and exercises in order to stimulate them to link the theoretical methods with the practical techniques. The *feedback* will be of as great importance for the teacher as for the students. If the attitude of the students towards the computer is based on interest, knowledge, and recognising its necessity, the department will have done a good job.

REFERENCES

Lieshout, H. van (ed.) (1991). *Leerplan sociale informatie-kundesao VIT-leerplan*, s-Gravenhage, HBO-Raad.

Vim van Rees et al. (1991). *A survey of Contemporary Community Development in Europe*, The Hague.

Zamfir Elena (1992). *Romanian Social Work Education Today*, pre-print, Univ. of Bucharest.

Professional Profile of the Social Worker, Committee on Professional Questions Regarding Social Work, The Netherlands.

Microsoft Corporation (1989). *Microsoft Works, Reference Manual*, Microsoft Corporation.

Multimedia Training
for Child Protective Service Workers:
Initial Test Results

Rosemary Satterwhite
Dick Schoech

SUMMARY. Child protective service agencies are showing increasing interest in computer based training due to factors such as deskilling of worker tasks, high turnover, and court orders to improve worker performance. Recent developments in computer-based multimedia offer new potential for computer based training. This article describes a child protective services case simulation and the results of preliminary testing. Fourteen users with a variety of experience responded very favorably to the design and learning that occurred by

Rosemary Satterwhite MSSW, is Supervisor in the Texas Department of Protective and Regulatory Services and was the subject matter expert for the case simulation.

Dick Schoech, PhD, is Professor and Project Director. Others involved in developing the simulation were Monica Williams, MSSW, simulation programmer and Ann Wilder, resource base developer.

Contact the developers at the University of Texas at Arlington, School of Social Work, Box 19129, Arlington, TX 76019-0129. The project was funded by the Texas Department of Protective and Regulatory Services, Child Protective Services Program through the Children's Protective Services Training Institute, Center for Social Work Research at The University of Texas at Austin. A demo version of the simulation is available free from the developers. The demo will run on any computer that runs Windows 3.1.

[Haworth co-indexing entry note]: "Multimedia Training for Child Protective Service Workers: Initial Test Results." Satterwhite, Rosemary, and Dick Schoech. Co-published simultaneously in *Computers in Human Services* (The Haworth Press, Inc.) Vol. 12, No. 1/2, 1995, pp. 81-97; and: *Human Services in the Information Age* (ed: Jackie Rafferty, Jan Steyaert, and David Colombi) The Haworth Press, Inc., 1995, pp. 81-97. Single or multiple copies of this article are available from The Haworth Document Delivery Service [1-800-342-9678, 9:00 a.m. - 5:00 p.m. (EST)].

working the simulated case. Issues concern the lack of informal guidance while working the simulated case and the need to tailor the complexity of the simulation to the intended audience. *[Article copies available from The Haworth Document Delivery Service: 1-800-342-9678.]*

INTRODUCTION

In the US the deskilling of human service jobs has increased the importance of training to insure quality services. This was especially true in Child Protective Services where studies estimate 24 months are required to become a proficient worker, yet the average length of stay of new hires varies from 9 months in major cities to 18 months in rural areas. To address the training issues, the Texas Department of Protective and Regulatory Services (TDPRS), Child Protective Services (CPS) Program joined with the Schools of Social Work in Texas to establish the Children's Protective Services Training Institute. The Institute's goal was to develop, implement and monitor a CPS curriculum and certification program. One part of this goal was to explore how technology could support CPS training.

A statewide committee developed a five year plan in the Spring of 1992 to explore the use of technology for CPS training. One major planned effort was to illustrate the potentials of multimedia for computer based training (CBT) and to guide the Institute's future use of technology. Two development projects were funded. One was an interviewing strategies module developed by Patrick Leung, Ph.D., Associate Professor, at the University of Houston School of Social Work. The second was a case simulation on "failure to thrive" developed by the authors at the University of Texas at Arlington School of Social Work.

This article describes the case simulation, its supporting research and rationale, and the results of preliminary testing after 6 months of development. The case simulation was called "Keisha" after the child in the case. The case simulation will be integrated into worker training in several TDPRS offices in 1994.

COMPUTER BASED TRAINING (CBT)

The Emergence of Multimedia CBT. CBT is where a computer plays an integral role in delivering curriculum. Computer assisted instruction (CAI) is a more general term. For example, in CAI a computer may be used to test trainees but not deliver curriculum. While the computer and educational technology behind CBT are not new, new tools provide the capacity to develop CBT far superior to previous developments. Especially important are tools that incorporate multimedia, such as sound, graphics, pictures, video, and animation. Multimedia allows dual coding, a process by which memory traces are etched simultaneously by several stimuli, such as visuals, text, and sound (Rieber, 1989). Dual coding can enhance retention (Rieber, 1989; 1991; Rieber, Boyce and Assad, 1990). Banyan and Stein (1990) found that students recalled more details from CBT when they received speech plus video. However, in spite of their increased performance, students reported that they preferred the use of only video, text, or speech. Other researchers also cautioned not to overwhelm learners with too much stimuli at once. Patterson and Yaffe (1993) contrasted a linear presentation of screens containing numbers and text to teach diagnostic criteria in the Diagnostic and Statistical Manual (Ver. IIIR) to a multimedia presentation that provided multiple methods of encoding material and sustaining user interest. They found that computer assisted instruction was equally effective as the traditional paper based instruction in increasing students' diagnostic speed and accuracy. Students reported that they found the computer training harder, but they "liked it better."

Simulation as a type of CBT. Other forms of CBT exist besides the traditional "drill and practice" where information is followed by practice sessions and quizzes. One of the most complex forms of CBT is a simulation. Schoech (1990) defined a simulation as "an experimental method which attempts to replicate a system or activity without building or operating the actual system or performing the activity." In a policy simulation developed by Flynn (1985), students influenced a particular community goal by taking various roles in the simulation. Flynn found that "learning by doing" was an effective way to master knowledge and skills.

Petry (1990) described a computer simulation designed to teach strategic decision making in a group. The program was tested by political science students assigned either to conventional teaching methods or to the computer simulation evaluation group. Petry inferred from preliminary data that the computer simulation was more effective than conventional classroom methods.

Sussman and Lowman (1989) found that students felt greater satisfaction in actively engaging in the learning process through a simulation versus the printed materials. The key variable did not appear to be a matter of control but the degree of realism in the simulation programs.

In a simulation by Chan, Berven, and Lam (1990), students were able to develop improved problem solving skills by modeling their approaches and strategies after the practices of successful rehabilitation counselors. Evaluative statements provided feedback for actions taken by students. Ill-advised actions resulted in the client losing confidence in the counselor. The client could even terminate service if too many ill-advised actions were taken. This simulation illustrates that inappropriate case management actions taken by students can be corrected without detrimental effects to actual clients. Despite these positive findings, authors typically caution that case simulations are in their infancy and norms for evaluation have yet to be established.

   CBT in Child Protective Services. In June 1992, TDPRS conducted a national survey on the use of CBT in child protective service. Thirty-four of the 50 states and the District of Columbia responded. Fifty-one percent of those responding indicated they will use technology in CPS training in the next 5 years. Another 43% was interested in the possibility of using technology in their CPS training. Topics to be covered by CBT included computer literacy, system overview, workload management, indicators of physical abuse, indicators of sexual abuse, communication skills, interviewing skills, and others. Respondents considered multimedia the best long-term, cost-effective, technology-based instructional strategy at present. States that had developed CBT indicated that resistance to CBT comes primarily from administrators and trainers not familiar with CBT, not from workers.

   In 1992, MacFadden developed a CBT program for sexual abuse assessment and tested whether the CBT improved the knowledge of new CPS workers in child sexual abuse. The training group's mean knowledge score was significantly higher (9%) than the control group. Short, medium, and long term retention rates indicated that the advantages of CBT may weaken over time. MacFadden describes an unexplained finding that older workers appeared to benefit more from CBT than younger workers.

   Leung, Cheung, and Stevenson (in press) note that computers were mostly used by the trainer, not the trainee. Trainers used computers to prepare training materials, to conduct research, and to manage staff development activities. Leung et al. (in press) described a collaborative project between the Colorado Department of Social Services and the Graduate School of Social Work at the University of Denver to develop and implement a 7 module CBT curriculum for new workers. The CBT was to train all new workers in their offices, before classroom training, on the basics of law, policy, and procedures. The project found that CBT was effective in helping workers master both knowledge and skill. Limitations included the high cost of translating existing training into CBT and the lack of mandated use (Colorado Department of Social Services, 1991).

Pittman (1992) designed and pre-tested a multimedia application to help workers attain entry level competence in the performance of child abuse and neglect investigations. Pittman's CBT consisted of five modules. Each module contained training objectives; learning activities including readings, interactive exercises and video; and performance appraisals for use by the evaluator. Pittman pretested the CBT on experienced CPS workers who also were familiar with computers and a convenient sample of five CPS students who were somewhat familiar with child abuse and neglect. Preliminary results indicated that sustained interest was low and that users took exception to some of the CBT material and suggested changes. Pittman discussed the importance of a pretest during the development process to increase the likelihood that the final project will achieve its stated goals.

In summary, studies suggest that CBT can offer a cost-effective, nonjudgmental, confidential, and safe learning experience where workers can experiment at their own learning pace without harm to the client. In addition, the CBT can capture and store an immense amount of information to compare prior and current performance of individuals or groups. The key factors spurring CBT in Child Protective Services agencies is that CBT technology is rapidly improving while forces resulting in inconsistently and insufficiently trained workers are increasing. Currently, most CBT uses a text based drill and practice format. While CBT holds much promise, it must be put in perspective. Leung et al. (in press) cautions that CBT is only part of an integrated program of training and cannot stand on its own.

RATIONALE AND DESCRIPTION OF THE CURRENT SIMULATION

Rationale for the case simulation. The Training Technology Advisory Committee of the Children's Protective Services Training Institute indicated that the CBT developed was to:

• Illustrate the costs and potentials of multimedia CBT to address a significant TDPRS training need so the Institute can make intelligent decisions about the role of technology in future CPS training.
• Not discover new knowledge, but contain existing knowledge that would be consistent over time.
• Research the CBT design and development process for an organization as large, diverse, and decentralized as the TDPRS.
• Run on current technology while having the capacity to use technology that will be common 3-5 years in the future.

- Be based on workers' needs and conceptually display information in ways that are typical of how workers view their work world.
- Be designed for new workers under instructor guidance at TDPRS learning centers.

Given these criteria and the fact that the University of Houston was designing drill and practice multimedia on basic job skills training, the UTA development team chose to create a case simulation. A case simulation would allow the developers to make maximum use of multimedia technology with the exception of video which required more sophisticated hardware than was available.

Failure to thrive (FTT) was chosen as the subject of the simulation because FTT has a fairly circumscribed and consistent set of medical and clinical (behavioral and physical) characteristics (Goldstein & Field, 1985; Lozoff, 1989). FTT intervention was also commonly agreed upon. A literature search revealed only one treatment model for neglect families whose children were either in foster care or in their own homes (Harris & Alexander, 1982). It was advantageous that the model was used in Dallas, Texas for treating neglect families with children in their own homes. FTT was also an area of expertise of the author of this paper who was the subject matter expert for the CBT. A real FTT case was chosen as the basis of the simulation to add as much realism as possible. The case was of a newborn infant where neighbors reported the mother using crack cocaine and seeming incompetent to parent.

Description of the case simulation. The entire simulation consisted of 4 modules that took 30 to 45 minutes each to complete. The modules were: (1) the referral, (2) the home visit, (3) casework activity, and (4) forms and feedback.

The CBT simulation was based on a "discovery" instructional approach that allows the user to "discover" the best way to "work" a case. All actions in the case were connected, for example, trainees could not go out on the home visit until they analyzed the intake and called the complainant. The simulation opens with the user providing their name, selecting a gender and ethnic specific graphic of a worker to represent themselves, and selecting whether an owl or shark should be used during the simulation to represent their supervisor. After initial instructions, the trainee was placed in an office where icons represent the actions that could be taken (Figure 1). Trainees moved the mouse over an icon to see the options associated with the icon. Trainees mouse clicked an icon to see and do the actions associated with the icon. To begin the simulation, trainees would first click the pencil icon and receive a list of available reports. Trainees would then click on the block called night intake report and analyze the

FIGURE 1

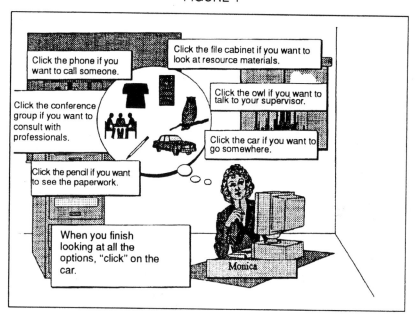

intake for risks to the child, work safety issues, and case priority level. Trainee analysis of the intake was then compared with the analysis of three experts. The experts did not always agree on every observation. Similar analysis and feedback occurred as trainees worked the case and viewed pictures of the house and child (Figure 2). Sound was used to add realism, for example, dogs barked while viewing the outside of the home and the telephone rang with unwelcomed calls when returning to the office.

Through the "discovering" of information, the user completed an investigation. The simulation ended when the paperwork was completed. By making choices throughout the simulation, the user accumulated knowledge that was used to complete forms such as a risk assessment form. On all forms, the user received feedback on the correctness of the answers and where the information for the answers was or could have been obtained when working the case.

It was anticipated that the simulation will need to be modified to fit the needs of each training site. For example, some sites may want to print trainee analysis of the pictures of the child for evaluation and discussion (Figure 2).

Hardware and Software Platform. The simulation ran on any computer

FIGURE 2

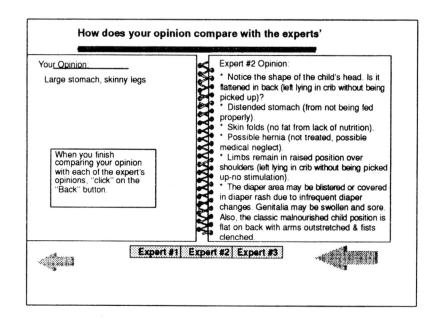

capable of running Windows 3.1, although the faster the computer, the better. A super VGA monitor with monitor card and drivers to achieve 800×600 resolution with 64,000 colors was required for good quality pictures. A Soundblaster Pro compatible audio card was also required. Currently, TDPRS does not have computers on workers' desk or at the training sites. Thus, the simulation was developed to run on future PC hardware. Multimedia ToolBook was chosen as the authoring system due to its low cost, free run time version, and because it was easy enough for a non-programmer but technology literate social worker to use.

Simulation Objectives. The simulation had the following objectives.

- To allow users to experience the complexities of working a real FTT case.
- To allow users to make mistakes while working an FTT case without harming a client or themselves.
- To reinforce good judgment in the order of events when working an FTT case.

- To allow users to discover and apply the knowledge required to work an FTT case.
- To allow users to apply what is learned in CPS training to an FTT case.
- To allow users to complete required forms from the knowledge base discovered while working an FTT case.
- To provide constant monitoring and feedback while working an FTT case.
- To improve judgment in working an FTT case by comparing user judgment to expert judgment in:
  1. Analyzing an intake for priority, risk to the child, and worker safety
  2. Viewing the outside and inside of a house for worker safety and health and safety hazards to the child
  3. Viewing an FTT child for risk indicators

INITIAL TESTING SAMPLE AND PROCEDURES

The purposive sample consisted of eight trainees and six non-trainees. The trainees were in their third or last month of training at the CPS Training Academy in the Dallas-Fort Worth area. Trainees were assigned by trainers on a voluntary basis as their training schedules permitted. The six non-trainees consisted of three trainers, one program director, and two experienced workers who were slotted into night appointments so as not to interfere with casework.

Due to scheduling difficulties, the four modules were completed in one session of approximately two hours. The CBT evaluation instrument consisting of 43 statements was administered by computer. In order to capture spontaneous comments and provide closure to the user, the subject matter expert debriefed users immediately following their completion of the modules.

RESULTS OF TESTING

The average age of the sample was 34.2. The sample contained 10 females and 10 individuals who had human service related degrees. The sample was very similar to what was expected, except in the area of computer experience. A few trainees had spent substantial time working on a computer, however, the mode score for days of computer experience for trainees and non-trainees was 1 day.

Table 1 presents the results on the 43 evaluation questions where a response of 1 = strongly agree, 2 = agree, 3 = neutral, 4 = disagree, and 5 = strongly disagree. Table 2 presents open ended comments that have been edited for brevity. The overwhelming response to the case simulation was more positive than anticipated. Eleven of the 43 responses to the questions were in the strongly agree range, 27 were in the agree range, and the 5 remaining were in the neutral range. Most of the neutral responses concerned the preliminary nature of the simulation or were expected due to the nature of the question. Each group of evaluation questions of Table 1 will be briefly discussed following an analysis of trainee versus non-trainee responses.

Trainees Versus Non-Trainee Responses. The debriefing revealed that both trainees and non-trainees found the two hour simulation a long and difficult experience. The common response was that the simulation was as hard as working an actual case. For the trainee, working a simulated case was hard but an experience they sought. For non-trainees, working a case was simply more work. As was expected, non-trainees perceived the simulation to be less realistic than trainees and made suggestions to make the case more accurate.

The mean scores of trainees and non-trainees were compared for significance differences. However, given the very small sample size, few significant differences were expected. Trainees and non-trainee responses were significantly different on three questions (in Table 1). The three questions indicated that the sophistication of some of the material may be an issue. For example, trainees felt the time constraints were significantly more realistic and their judgment increased significantly more than non-trainees on use of time and viewing a client's room for child health and safety risks. Anecdotally, two experienced workers laughed at the picture of a client's room indicating that they had seen much worse and had to "reach for it" to find much that really "endangered" a child. These findings indicate that sophistication of the user should be an important factor in developing a realistic simulation. Since few significant differences existed between trainees and non-trainees, the term respondents will be used to discuss the remaining findings.

Relevance of The Computer Based Training to Your Work. With the exception of the time constraints mentioned above, all the questions measuring CBT relevance were in the agree direction. Since future implementation requires the simulation have face validity, it was important that both trainees and non-trainees found it relevant. While trainees may have found the simulation relevant due to their learning, non-trainees may have found the simulation relevant because it validated their opinions about the case. Caseworkers often share "war stories" to obtain other's reactions to cases that involve difficult decisions and painful emotions. Future research is needed to investigate what makes a simulation relevant as relevance is important for designing CBT for the intended audience.

Impact of Computer Based Training on Your Future Judgment. Responses indicated the most powerful portion of the simulation was examining the pictures of the FTT child and comparing one's responses to those of several experts (Figure 2). Even non-trainees who were nonchalant about the simulation became quiet and interested as they compared their observations with those of experts. Other pictures were not as dramatic, but all pictures positively impacted future judgment. The previous findings of dual coding (Rieber, 1991) and the lack of a long term effects of CBT (MacFadden, 1992) suggest future investigation to determine whether the improved judgment scores on the dual coded parts of the simulation had any long term effects.

Learning as a Result of Completing the Computer Based Training. Overall, respondents strongly agreed that they gained knowledge about an FTT case and were satisfied with the learning that occurred. However, these opinions about learning should be interpreted with caution. Combining non-trainee with trainee responses may have lowered the estimation of the overall learning that occurred because the "experienced" sample should not have learned as much as novice trainees. Another complicating factor was that newly hired trainees may be reluctant to indicate that they are not learning in their initial training.

Evaluation of the Computer Programming. The computer programming of the simulation received high marks, with the exception of the weaknesses the developers knew existed. The use of pictures, graphics, and sound was especially appealing as indicated by many positive comments.

Evaluation of the Design of the Training. Respondents strongly agreed that the simulation held their interest and they liked the discovery approach. Respondents would have preferred working the simulation in small sessions rather than the approximately two hour time frame used in this initial test. The finding that user control was less important than realism was consistent with the Sussman and Lowman finding mentioned earlier. Not surprisingly, respondents disagreed with the need for their performance to be graded. Monitoring is a difficult issue, because trainers and managers usually see grading as one way to weed out unsuited workers. The issue of grading and feedback will be addressed more thoroughly as the simulation is implemented in several sites in 1994.

Suggestions for Improving the Design of the Case Study. Respondents

TABLE 1. Number of respondents, standard deviation, and mean scores for the evaluation questions.

	N	SD	Mean
Relevance of the computer based training to your work			
The material covered in this case study seems relevant to my job	13	.48	1.31
The comments I received while working the case study were appropriate	14	.77	1.86
Working this case study seemed "true to life"	14	.77	2.14
The resource information presented when using the file cabinet icon seems accurate	13	.80	2.15
*The time constraints provided in this case study seem realistic	13	.85	2.69
Impact of computer based training on your future judgment			
Due to comparing my judgment with the judgment of experts, I can better do the following:			
Assess a suspected FTT child	14	.52	1.50
View the outside of a client's house for child health and safety risks	14	.55	2.00
View the outside of a client's house for worker safety concerns	13	.69	2.15
*View a client's room for child health and safety risks	14	.43	2.21
View a client's room for worker safety concerns	14	.73	2.29
Learning as a result of completing the computer based training			
I gained knowledge about an FTT case by completing this case study	14	.50	1.64
Overall, I am satisfied with my learning from completing this case study	14	.53	1.86
Due to the feedback on the completeness of the knowledge base I accumulated in this case study, I can construct better knowledge bases when working CPS cases	13	.49	2.08
I better understand the appropriate sequence of activities when working a case	14	.94	2.50
*Due to feedback on my use of time when using this case study, I will better use my time in working CPS cases	13	.73	2.77
I better understand how to complete sections of the risk assessment form	14	.70	3.21
Evaluation of the computer programming			
The presentation of the case study was visually appealing	14	.61	1.29
Information in this case study was presented in a clear manner	14	.78	2.00
This case study was easy to use	14	.73	2.07
Using this case study was a pleasant experience	14	.95	2.14
The instructions for using this case study were clear	14	.91	2.29
This case study was polished and relatively free of defects	14	.86	2.86

Evaluation of the design of the training

	Mean	SD	n
This case study held my interest	1.79	.43	14
I liked the free form "discovery" approach taken by this case study	1.93	.73	14
I received an adequate number of comments while working the case study	2.00	.55	14
The case study allowed me to make mistakes in a non-judgmental environment	2.00	.39	14
Information was presented in a manner that is consistent with my learning style	2.21	.97	14
I was in control and able to guide my learning experience	2.57	.94	14
The time it took to complete the case study was appropriate	3.00	.96	14
Trainers should be allowed more opportunity to grade my performance during the case study	3.00	.95	12

Suggestions for improving the design of the case study

	Mean	SD	n
I prefer more snapshots (still pictures) in the case study	2.29	.91	14
I prefer more video (moving pictures) in the case study	2.46	1.05	13
I prefer more sound in the case study	2.54	1.05	13
I prefer more graphics (drawings) in the case study	2.86	1.10	14
I prefer more text in the case study	3.21	.70	14

Your Perception of Technology Delivered Instruction

	Mean	SD	n
Due to completing this case study, I have more positive perception about the potentials of technology for training	1.50	.65	14
Due to completing this case study, I have a more positive perception about the potentials of technology to support me in my job	1.71	.73	14
I would like more training that uses computer based training techniques	1.78	.44	9
Computer based case studies such as this can be most effective if completed as an integral part of training at the Training Academy	2.00	.71	13
I would like more of my training at the Training Academy delivered by computer	2.25	.62	12
The computer based training techniques used are better at imparting knowledge than traditional training techniques	2.50	.94	14
I prefer computer based training materials, such as this case study, to traditional training materials	2.62	.87	13
Computer based case studies such as this can be most effective if completed before receiving training at the Training Academy	3.58	.90	12

- - - - - - - - - - - - - -
* = -Significant at .05 or greater

93

TABLE 2. Selected open ended comments.

What users liked about the case simulation:

- The ability to seek and gather information from all sources while at the computer.
- The help in organizing information appropriately for the case. The feeling you were working on a real case, thus got more involved.
- Held my interest. Sort of like a CPS role playing game. Was fun.
- The information was thorough and it was helpful to have several expert opinions and the backup resource information. I think it helps people to understand that the answers are not absolute, but that there are a lot of factors in making each case decision.
- The graphics are wonderful and truly contribute to the attention-keeping quality of the entire program. This program allows a new worker to learn dynamics in the context of more realistically based casework practice than in traditional lecture-type training. Also, the training is provided in a very non-threatening manner which is conducive to learning by doing without fear. As a whole, the program gives a potential caseworker a better understanding of what it can be like to respond to an actual case in the field, and this can help to alleviate some of the fears that new workers feel about "being out there." The pictures, especially those of Baby Keisha, are extremely vital to the learning process by giving an example of what FTT really looks like.
- The addition of photos made the entire exercise much easier to "connect" with on a human level.
- I enjoyed having the opportunity to get an actual feel of what I would have to do in case of a real emergency removal.
- I really enjoyed the different graphics used in the case study. The combination of still pictures and computer graphics were neat and helped bring the case to life.
- Many physical identifiers were mentioned which I had not read of or learned in class. The opportunity to practice the sequencing of events in a removal case without the actual pressures of time and child safety is an excellent training device. This sequence should be (mentally) in place prior to an emergency arising. The addition of photos of the child made the exercise much easier to "connect" with on a human level. The photos turned a computer game into the biography of a real human infant. The graphics were great! The icons were accessible and altogether, this program is extremely user friendly. Even computer novices should not be intimidated by this piece of software.

Suggestions for Improvement

- A few more prompts when wandering off course would have been helpful. A few extraneous phone calls would have made it more realistic and frustrating.
- At times, it was very unclear what I should do next. As a new worker, I need more guidance and was sometimes unable to figure out what I needed to do. I became "stalled" several times.
- The only thing I can think of is a "help" or "hint" menu when students get stuck
- The sequence of events is not completely accurate. We need additional opportunities to interview the mother after leaving the house. We wanted to call some people more than one time. Perhaps the supervisor could have her own menu which could include topics of discussion, such as requesting permission to remove, who the ongoing worker will be, further case actions and plans, placement and permanency issues, and court. We want noise! CPS is a noisy place.

preferred (slightly) more graphics, sound and photographs. Respondents were neutral in their response to the preference for more text. As the multimedia hardware and software improve, simulations will be able to offer trainees more exciting and innovative ways to learn, for example, full motion video.

Your Perception of Technology Delivered Instruction. Respondents strongly agreed that they were not only more positive about CBT for CPS, but wanted more training by CBT. They were slightly less enthusiastic, but still agreed, that they wanted more training at the Academy delivered by computer. This finding was very positive considering that a number of the respondents were trainers at the Training Academy. However, trainees might have worried that a "disagree" answer would be interpreted as a negative response toward the Training Academy. Respondents were neutral on whether CBT was better than traditional training techniques. We expected disagreement with this statement because we believe that CBT techniques are better for some types of training, but worse at others, for example, getting at the emotional content of being a CPS worker. We feel that respondents may have been overly enthusiastic about multimedia and not appreciative of the value of a good trainer.

Open Ended Comments and Observations. Comments and observations from the preliminary testing of this CBT indicated the important role of supervision for trainees (Table 2). While the trainees averaged 74 days at the Training Academy and 2.6 months CPS experience, they did not have the experience to work a case without close supervision and direction. At work, this direction and supervision may come in casual conversations while socializing. However, in the simulation, the only way to obtain detailed guidance was from the supervisor. Due to this reaction, the supervisor's role in the simulation was greatly enhanced. This finding may also indicate that helping supervisors learn to supervise is an area that needs further examination.

The comments and data indicated trainees were "hungry" for a casework sequence that is orderly and structured. However, non-trainees asked for a change in the process to interview and telephone people more than once and to confer with superiors about many things. Non-trainees generally seemed more comfortable with less structure and a less routine sequence of activities. This finding suggested that developing a case simulation for training experienced workers may be an unrealistic task.

CONCLUSIONS

Overall, this study found responses to the multimedia case simulation overwhelmingly positive in its ability to teach trainees. Non-trainees learned as well, but may have found the module lacking sophistication in certain areas involving casework process. However, a dilemma exists. As the sophistication of CBT content increases, the consensus on the content often decreases. We avoided areas where casework as it is taught may conflict with casework as it is practiced in an agency. As multimedia CBT becomes more common in detailing practice, these dilemmas will have to be addressed. Whether we like it or not, the power of multimedia CBT is here and so are the challenges.

REFERENCES

Banyan, C. & Stein, D. (1990). Voice synthesis supplement to a computerized interviewing training program: retention effects. *Teaching of Psychology, 17*(4).

Chan, F., Berven, N., & Lam, C. (1990). Computer based, case management simulations in the training of rehabilitation counselors. *Rehabilitation Counseling Bulletin, 33*(3).

Flynn, J. (1985). MERGE: Computer simulations of social policy process. *Computers in Human Services, 1*(2).

Goldstein, S. & Field, T. (1985). Affective behavior and weight changes among hospitalized failure to thrive infants. *Infant Mental Health Journal, 6*(4).

Harris, J. & Alexander, K. (1982). *Group therapy for neglecting mothers.* Texas Department of Human Services, Austin, Texas.

Leung, P., Cheung, K. M., & Stevenson, K. M. (in press). Advancing competent social work practice: A computer-based approach to child protective service training. *Computers in Human Services.*

Colorado Department of Social Services. (1991) Competency-based child protection training: Final report. Denver, CO: Author.

Lozoff, B. (1989). Nutrition and behavior. *American Psychologist, 44*(2).

MacFadden, R. (1992). Computer-assisted instruction in sexual abuse assessment: Does it work. *Computer Use in Social Services Network Newsletter, 11*(4), Available from the U. of Texas at Arlington.

Pittman, S. (July, 1992). Development of a Multimedia training prototype: Automated training for child welfare workers. Paper delivered at the NASW World Assembly, Washington, DC.

Patterson, D. A. & Yaffe, J. (1993). An evaluation of computer-assisted instruction in teaching axis II of DSM-III-R to social work students, *Research on Social Work Practice, 3*(3), 343-357.

Petry, F. (1990). Learning outcomes of game-theoretic computer simulation: An evaluation. *Social Science Computer Review, 8*(3).

Rieber, L. (1991). Animation, incidental learning, and continuing motivation. *Journal of Educational Psychology, 83*(3).

Rieber, L. (1989). The effects of computer animated elaboration strategies and practice of factual and application learning in an elementary science lesson. *Journal of Educational Computing Research, 5*(4).

Rieber, L., Boyce, M., & Assad, C. (1990). The effects of computer animation on adult learning and retrieval tasks. *Journal of Computer-based Instruction, 17*(2).

Schoech, D. (1990). Human services computing: Concepts and applications. NY: Haworth.

Sussman, D. & Lowman, J. (1989). Hard copy versus computer presentation of the supershrink interview simulation. *Teaching of Psychology, 16*(4).

Computers in Education:
Added Value
Leading Towards Better Quality

Albert Visser

SUMMARY. The reasons why students work with computers in social work education are threefold: computers and software are increasingly general tools, as well as tools in professional practice and educational technology is supplying schools with more computer-based learning materials. The use of computers in the learning process is leading to better quality professional preparation of students, in that they have to learn to cope with innovations in professional practice. Computers are increasingly used for word processing in practice, but also in managerial and financial information systems and not least in being an aid in directly helping clients (for instance in assessing processes, in interviewing and calculation of benefits). Computers are also improving the quality of the learning process itself. This article will not only highlight the didactics of

Albert Visser, PhD, has a background in sociology and social psychology, he started social work teaching in 1972 and since then has had experience in community development and adult education, as well as studying educational technology and applied informatics and teaching the application of IT. Since 1989 he has had responsibility for coordinating all computer based training for the Faculty of Social Professions of the Midden Nederlands Polytechnic. Visser is also engaged in several projects about development and implementation of educational software in higher education, conducted by the Council for Higher Professional Education and the Open University and has published extensively in both Dutch and English.

The author would like to thank Henri Roosdorp for his contribution.

[Haworth co-indexing entry note]: "Computers in Education: Added Value Leading Towards Better Quality." Visser, Albert. Co-published simultaneously in *Computers in Human Services* (The Haworth Press, Inc.) Vol. 12, No. 1/2, 1995, pp. 99-108; and: *Human Services in the Information Age* (ed: Jackie Rafferty, Jan Steyaert, and David Colombi) The Haworth Press, Inc., 1995, pp. 99-108. Single or multiple copies of this article are available from The Haworth Document Delivery Service [1-800-342-9678, 9:00 a.m. - 5:00 p.m. (EST)].

99

courseware but also give some strategical hints about effective implementation of computers for better social work education. *[Article copies available from The Haworth Document Delivery Service: 1-800-342-9678.]*

INNOVATIONS IN LEARNING

Learning is not a static phenomenon; over the ages it has taken place in different forms. Learning can take place by experiencing what is going on (learning by doing) or by talking and reflecting. The invention of printing was a great leap: it became possible to write down thoughts and experiences and spread them out to a large number of people. Recent visions in learning philosophies led to developments like programmed instruction and language laboratories, some with more, others with less success.

One of the trends is problem oriented learning: present a practice problem to students and teach them how to solve the problem. Students learn to solve problems and are learning by doing. For social work students field practice is also very important in the educational process and this raises a serious problem because when you are dealing with clients there cannot be much experimenting as work has to be highly reliable and professional. This is of course not easy when you are in a learning situation and therefore fieldwork is often simulated in the classroom. Recent technology such as audio and video recorders are good tools for practice simulations.

Developments in computer technology and programming made it possible for parts of learning and teaching to be presented with new technological media. Courses were developed for transferral into software and presented to students on computers. This development is sometimes technology-driven and unfortunately not content-driven. Still there are reasons to accept computer assisted learning as a useful tool in learning, especially when driven by content.

What contribution can software have to learning, what are the situations in which it is relevant to use these programs, from now on called CAL (Computer Assisted Learning)?

CHARACTERISTICS AND TYPES
OF COMPUTER ASSISTED LEARNING

There is something strange about CAL; the value and acceptance of CAL is often discussed as a myth, leading to the inevitable consequence that one is in favour or one is against it. But it cannot be emphasised enough that this is complete nonsense in the same way that one cannot be in favour or against books in general. There is however the question of WHEN to use books or other learning tools in the learning process.

If a trainer or teacher is responsible for the development of a new course on any subject, he or she will compare several alternative learning strategies and tools and choose the ones that fit best in the course. Computer assisted learning should be treated in the same way. In a concrete case it either has advantages or it doesn't, if it does, select it. On the other hand, of course, it is important to mention the specific features of CAL, although you should be aware that a specific CAL product seldom possesses all the features of the ideal learning tool in one.

TYPES OF CAL (COURSEWARE)

Computers can be used as a learning tool, together with books, readers, video and lectures. The type of tool (the medium) that is to be chosen should depend on the goals that have to be reached. Elementary knowledge can be learnt from a book, difficult situations can best be explained by a teacher in a lecture. Also, practising mathematics requires another concept of a course than practising vocabulary. If computers are used as a learning tool, the program consists of certain knowledge (the course) and of a computerised representation (the software). This is often called the courseware and is produced in different types:

- Drill and Practice: programs developed in order to supply a large number of *exercises* can be mentioned as one type of CAL. Computer assisted learning is highly effective as a tool for practising and exercising. A good example here is practising the grammar of a language.
- Tutorial: Another type of a computer assisted learning program is the *tutorial*. The most important difference between the first type and a tutorial is the fundamental emphasis on explaining procedures, structures, relations and processes. In making a tutorial, a developer will have to create a subtle balance between interactive working and reading texts presented on the screen. Many programmes have failed in their educational objectives by presenting an overkill of information on the screen. These educational software programmes do not add value compared to a book. So one should always avoid the so-called electronic page turning tutorials. Examples are: tutorials about social legislation (like the "ZAO" program that will be discussed later) and about client interviews.

- Simulations: The third type of CAL to mention is the *simulation*. This type is used for very different subjects. Some good examples are the simulations of information systems which are developed to instruct employees in working with new applications introduced in the organisation.

Not only are there different types of courseware, there is also a major distinction between traditional learning materials and computer assisted learning materials. As the computer can contain so much information, one can make all kinds of resources, like dictionaries, references, overviews available to the user. This will be explained in the next section.

What are the specific *characteristics* of computer assisted learning? In short:

- flexible education–CAL makes it easier to present a course when and wherever you like and the course is continuously available which is why CAL fits well in modular educational systems. It preserves flexible course programming. Like all examples of standardised teaching, CAL makes it possible to guarantee the same contents, level and quality for a large number of students.
- individualized education–using a CAL-based course, the student has a lot of freedom. She or he studies at her or his own speed and is able to repeat the learning tasks as much as (s)he wants.
- reducing costs–depending on the circumstances CAL can be more efficient and cheaper than the usual methods of education, especially in commercial companies. For example, instead of hiring several trainers from a commercial training centre over two days for twenty groups of twenty people one can use in-house professionals to run the course with the support of a computer-based program.
- interactive learning–using CAL the student has to deal with several learning tasks in a dialogue with the computer. The student is constantly encouraged to be active in thinking and responding. Of course the character of the dialogue itself depends strongly on the subject(s).

LEARNING ABOUT LAW: A CASE STUDY

The HMN polytechnic has recently had experience with newly developed tutorial courseware called "ZAO." Its content is the introduction in matters of law about social legislation within the areas of health and disability of employees. Until recently students had to learn the rather boring contents of legislation from books. The teacher tried to improve students' understanding by giving several lectures for large groups of students (150 at a time). The teacher did not really like this method and the students were bored by the contents and the way they had to learn it. Because of the good chance of success of courseware in this situation we decided to develop a dedicated courseware program. We decided on the contents ourselves, CMN (a courseware company linked to the polytechnic) did the specification and programming of the software.

The *reasons* for developing this program with these contents are as follows:

- the contents are highly cognitive.
- the contents are very dull.
- it is normally represented theoretically (lectures) and even the cases from practice are mostly taught in a theoretical way.
- the number of students that have to learn these contents is increasing rapidly, because of socio-economic circumstances (economic recession and unemployment rates) and because of a shift in the professional education towards more knowledge of legal matters.

We hesitated for one reason, laws are subject to regular changes every year, this means that every year there needs to be at least one update. We agreed on this with CMN.

DIDACTICAL ASPECTS

Particularly compared with the traditional lecture (where knowledge transfer takes place in a one-directional verbal session) the courseware is a totally different medium. The learning process has changed from one direction to interactive, from single-source to multi-source, from static to dynamic learning. An example can clarify this:

The courseware we design is offering a complex and flexible, multi-directional resource learning environment. The student can start the course at any desired point (chapter or paragraph), move forward or backward and stop at any time. In this respect it is not any different from books. The difference is in the following features:

- the student can start with a test and end with a test. Sometimes the student even gets advice as to what chapters should be studied;

- a large number of cases are presented in the courseware, the professional practice is coming more directly into the classroom;
- students have different learning styles: those who want to learn theory first and then apply it to cases, and those who want to try to solve practical problems from cases first and then compare it to the theory. The courseware offers both possibilities;
- the student can activate several resources by pressing function keys (in later versions those will most likely be by clicking icons with the mouse). These resources are in the case of this courseware ("ZAO," as mentioned above):
  - a dictionary, with explanations of all the jargon words that are used in the course;
  - the texts of the laws that are under consideration in the relevant paragraph (contextual information);
  - all the texts of all the laws of the course, not restricted to the actual context;
  - information about additional literature, relevant organisations, actual political issues concerning the content matter, overviews of the whole system of social security laws and expectations of future developments.

The student can moderate the course to his or her own needs in a flexible multi-resource learning environment. For students this is a great advantage.

Teachers have more problems with it. At the start they have to be convinced that courseware has nothing to do with informatics, but everything to do with their subject: social legislation. Then it is not easy for them to let the students go through the contents by themselves, they feel they are losing control. They can also miss the reduction in face-to-face contact with students, although this can easily be repaired by giving "response lectures." In these lectures, the teacher answers questions that arose when students went through the courseware. This can be favourable for both teachers and students, because they can explore the content in greater depth. With extra attention to the role of the teacher these "problems" can be overcome.

IMPLEMENTATION

Implementation is not an autonomous process. It needs careful attention, planning and sufficient resources. In this case there were some very favourable conditions for implementation:

- senior and middle management were highly positive about innovation of curricula with new technology;

- there was a change agent (the CAL-coordinator) who had the full support of senior and middle management;
- there was a reasonable amount of computer equipment available;
- there was technical support by a technical assistant and a systems operator;

and, not least:

- the courseware was designed by "our own" teachers.

When the courseware was ready the implementation had to start. This was done in four steps:

1. The teacher had to become very familiar with the courseware and anticipate the questions and problems that might arise for students with the material.
2. Then the students were informed by the CAL-coordinator about different learning tools and styles. Actually this was more a lecture with demonstrations about learning methods and theories.
3. Students had to work with the courseware. They had full assistance from the people mentioned before and the teacher was available for content matters.
4. Then it was evaluated with the students and the teacher.

The results were the students were enthusiastic, they loved the new medium, they thought it was a good addition to the learning tools they already knew and most of all they appreciated the large amount of case materials. They felt more involved in field practice by working with these materials.

The teacher was also very positive: she thought it was very good for students who were more independent in their learning and it is a good gain in the mix of learning materials. What was very supportive was that the results of students in exams were certainly not worse.[1] Although we could not reliably establish whether they improved results, the gain was particularly in the motivation of the students. And in this field (law) that is a major achievement.

The gain for the teacher was that she won time to update her other learning materials and found time to give specific support for those students who needed it.

CHANGES IN THE LEARNING PROCESS

What are the differences when you use CAL in social work education?

1. CAL adds a new and different learning process. The process of knowledge transferral is split into two different actions:

- the individual part, in which the student sits in front of the computer and is experiencing the learning software (courseware), with apparently no teacher available (although some technical assistance is useful). This has some resemblance to an individual reading a book, but with the difference, that courseware is interactive and has several resources available during the course. Until now the interactivity came from the teacher or from other students. This is new and students and teacher have to get accustomed to new things.
- the group part, in which the teacher has a "response lecture" to discuss questions which were raised by the courseware. This usually is more in depth than the teacher was used to. Highly motivated teachers tend to get more professional satisfaction from this, while the less motivated think it is too great a challenge and they prefer the previous situation.

2. There is a higher rate of use of technological tools in the professional training of social workers. This is more or less a culture shock that has to be overcome. Students came to learn to work with people and now they have to work with computers.

The changes look more massive than they actually are. A main reason for this is that with the introduction of computers in professional practice also came the introduction of computers in educational practice and to make it even more confusing and threatening, computers also came into the offices of administration, management and teachers. It was a new tool that suddenly appeared everywhere. With the coming of the computer as a tool, the work procedures did not change much, only the printed paper got a companion, it had the computer alongside. Even with computers on every desk the paperwork was not replaced by the computer, the paperless office is even farther away than ever. However, working through electronic networks could change this.

In fact we can state that the computer is just a tool to do the same things in a slightly different way, the real possibilities and capacities of the computer still have to be elaborated, although in the example mentioned above we already have had some promising experiences.

STRATEGICAL NOTES TO GET CAL ACCEPTED

Schools as organisations are peculiar, Mintzberg called them "professional" bureaucracies, which means in respect to change processes they have to be treated in a special way. Changes cannot just be imposed upon by the management, although they can be very much in favour of the use of information technology in education for various reasons: it can be cost effective; can enable better competition with other schools; or can even be to keep up with universities. A more top-down treatment may possibly only work in the schools administration or as Mintzberg calls them "the support staff and technostructure."

The teaching process however is conducted by professionals, the teachers. They are absolute authorities in their field. They are trained in their discipline and no manager can tell them they have to change their contents or their ways of teaching.

Changes and innovations have to be reached in a different way. Literature about change processes (like Lippitt, Watson and Westly, 1958) can be applied to changes in respect to adaptation of new technologies in education. The change process mainly consists of two phases:

- unfreezing the pattern where teachers do not really think about the learning tools that are best to reach certain learning goals.
- establishing a new pattern of working to ensure the quality of the learning process: choosing the best learning tools in specific learning situations, regarding the tools you want to reach.

This major change process is initiated and maintained by a "change agent" (a highly esteemed teacher) and by a "champion" at management level, who favours the efforts of the change agent.

Teachers have to become convinced of the new tools by themselves, at their own speed. This means that a strategy of unfreezing mainly consists of supporting those professionals who in one way or another are in favour of the new technology. They should get all the support they need. In terms of a strategic approach we call this "let 100 flowers grow." Those teachers who are willing to experiment with the new technology should get all the facilities they need, software, hardware and support and training; really on a basis of "no questions asked." They are the prospectors, the innovators, the pioneers; the reward they get is the freedom to experiment. But this is only a stage: after a year or so, there are some teachers using IT and there is some infrastructure. Now it is time to move to the next stage. What is needed is a structural embedding of IT in curricula on the basis of perceived advantages and of their quality aspects. Now the implementation of IT is no longer haphazard, but it is part of the institutional policy, budgets are located for implementation of IT in the curricula of the different departments.

To reach the stage of structural use of information technology in education, the following ingredients are needed:

- *Students* who are curious and want to learn;
- *Teachers* who are open to various media to transfer knowledge and skills to students, and
- *Management* who are willing to support all this with sufficient money and infrastructure;
- *Support and assistance* of skilled personnel;
- *Good learning software.*

When the above conditions are met computer use can contribute to a better learning environment for students and also for continuing education for practitioners achieving higher quality of the learning process and improved practice.

NOTE

1. Although not significant we have a promising experience: Last year, when the course was in lecture form, only 45% succeeded in the test of the course the first time, this year, when the course was in courseware 70% passed the test the first round.

REFERENCES

Mintzberg, H. (1983). *Structure in fives: designing effective organisations*, Prentice Hall.
Lippitt, Watson and Westly. (1958). *The dynamics of planned change*, Harcourt.
More than computers (1993) in *Human Welfare and Technology*, papers from the HUSITA-3 conference, Bryan Glastonbury, pp 230-240, Van Gorcum, Assen, 1993.

Critical Thinking:
A Meta-Skill for Integrating Practice
and Information Technology Training

Paula S. Nurius

SUMMARY. Human services are at a developmental stage that requires less orientation to the computer as a machine and more to the computer as a medium of thought and expression. We now have advances in cognitive research on information processing and technological experience with agency information management to inform and guide training that supports such an orientation. This paper first presents a framework for identifying needed elements, using critical thinking as a meta-skill to integrate training related to practice and technology. A series of examples are presented to illustrate integrative, critical thinking training at three different skill levels. *[Article copies available from The Haworth Document Delivery Service: 1-800-342-9678.]*

Paula S. Nurius, PhD, is Professor at the University of Washington School of Social Work. Dr. Nurius directs the doctoral program as well as teaches research and practice courses. She is active in consultation to social agencies and to editorial boards, and has published extensively in the professional literature. In addition to critical thinking in practice reasoning and the use of computers to support practice, her current areas of research include self-concept and the role of social cognition in coping, particularly related to violence against women. Address: Paula S. Nurius, PhD, Professor, University of Washington, School of Social Work JH-30, Seattle, WA 98195.

The author gratefully acknowledges the helpful input of Walter Hudson, Cindy Riche, and Virginia Senechal on earlier versions of this manuscript.

[Haworth co-indexing entry note]: "Critical Thinking: A Meta-Skill for Integrating Practice and Information Technology Training." Nurius, Paula S. Co-published simultaneously in *Computers in Human Services* (The Haworth Press, Inc.) Vol. 12, No. 1/2, 1995, pp. 109-126; and: *Human Services in the Information Age* (ed: Jackie Rafferty, Jan Steyaert, and David Colombi) The Haworth Press, Inc., 1995, pp. 109-126. Single or multiple copies of this article are available from The Haworth Document Delivery Service [1-800-342-9678, 9:00 a.m. - 5:00 p.m. (EST)].

As we shift from a stage of revolution to evolution of computers in the human services, we naturally begin to look at different issues, and to look at issues differently. One aspect of this evolution is an increasing orientation away from the computer as a *machine* per se–and thus an operation skills emphasis–to the computer as a *medium* of thought and expression.

As a medium of thought and expression, we begin to consider more fully the relationship of this technology to how we conceptualize the mission and tasks it is expected to support; how we communicate and accomplish that mission and those tasks; and how we go beyond extant tasks and technology to envision and create new possibilities. Bedrock functions such as information processing and information management then begin to take on changed meaning as we build upon machine contributions, that have greatly augmented our capacity to store and manipulate information, to focus on the potential of the medium to optimize meaningful use of information.

In this paper, I will be talking primarily as an educator concerned with these issues. Clearly, however, there is considerable overlap between student/curriculum issues and practitioner/agency issues. Many of us have been dismayed by the sluggishness with which social work education overall has moved forward in preparing social work students for the technological realities of their future professional roles. I will argue that we are presently in a position wherein preparing students to engage information technology as a dynamic medium is both essential and achievable. Goals such as these, however, require an integrative approach where factors such as mission, task, context, and machine must simultaneously be considered (see Colombi, Rafferty, & Steyaert, 1993; Glastonbury & LaMendola, 1992; Schoech, 1990, for related discussions).

I will first present a framework for distinguishing current emphases and deficits in teaching human service practice and information technology. Within this framework, critical thinking is identified as a useful meta-skill to help integrate training related to practice and technology, for both substantive and procedural forms of professional knowledge. After identifying three levels of critical thinking skills relative to the integration of information technology and practice, a series of examples will be presented to illustrate these skill levels and educational possibilities.

MENTAL MAPS

Consider the following. You are trying to lay out–for a student or supervisee–your mental map of how it is "you can get from here to there" (in how you undertake some complex task such as reasoning through a risk assessment or reasoning from assessment to service plan or from agency outcome objectives backward to program and personnel planning), and it quickly becomes clear that a lot is getting lost in the translation. How is it that we know what we "know"? How is it that we pull a lot of complex information together into a coherent picture? These are among the biggest challenges in training.

We have talked for a long time in social work about the importance of this essential but elusive reasoning capacity. We have talked in terms of instinct, intuition, practice wisdom and the art of practice. These have remained compellingly important notions. But we have not yet achieved the kind of understanding of this more procedural (reasoning) component of practice relative to the more substantive (content) component, and this gap is evident in the training, supervision, and decision supports typically available to direct service providers.

We are, however, now at an exciting convergence point. Part of this convergence involves advances in the study of knowledge structures, cognitive processes, memory functioning, and so forth that govern our mental maps and methods of information processing. Another part of this convergence involves the increasing potential of computer technology toward better understanding how we build and apply these information processing guides as a crucial part of effective service. And finally, ready or not, we all recognize that social agencies are in the midst of a rush to automate; which presents an unprecedented window of opportunity to better support this relatively hidden element of quality services–that is, critical thinking and effective use of information.

AN INTEGRATIVE FRAMEWORK FOR TRAINING

In Figure 1, I lay out a framework for training that is intended to capture the prevailing emphases and deficits in information technology and practice training, as well as the potential for information processing and information management to inform instruction of critical thinking as a coalescing meta-skill. This is followed by a brief description of each of the framework components:

- *Substantive Knowledge*: concepts, beliefs, facts, descriptors (e.g., about social problems, societal groups, service or intervention methods); the "what's" of professional knowledge.
- *Procedural Knowledge*: the "how's" of professional knowledge; guidelines or rules about what activities are associated with what conditions (e.g., "if . . . then . . . ") and how activities are done (this

includes mental activities such as observing, interpreting, reasoning, and decision-making as well as behavioral action).

- *End User Competencies*: knowledge and hands-on skills directly related to machine and software operations; this can include a range of skills such as using basic operating systems, accessing and storing material on networked systems, and gaining facility with any number of specific software applications.
- *Analytic Competencies*: abilities related to analytical, problem-solving, and conceptual capacities (e.g., ability to identify and to evaluate computer applications in light of appropriateness for a given client group or service goal).
- *Modularized Approaches*: generally involves a limited presence of information technology training in the curriculum (e.g., in introductory research courses, finance-related courses, stand-alone course on computers in social welfare); generally involves lack of sequenced or coordinated training across courses.
- *Embedded Approaches*: information technology is integrated into courses across the curriculum; information technology training tends to be treated as a professional skill or content area meaningful across service roles and contexts.
- *Critical Thinking*: a growing zeitgeist in education around this concept has spawned a variety of definitions–some of the common elements include: disciplined, responsible thinking; the skill and propensity to engage in an activity with reflective skepticism; an orientation to search for evidence, be sensitive to context, and strive for corrective feedback (see Gambrill, 1990; Gibbs, 1991; Halpern, 1989; Kitchener & Fischer, 1990; the contributors in Norris, 1992, for overviews).
- *Information Processing*: the cognitive schemas, scripts, and associative networks that we develop to represent our understanding of reality as well as the ways in which these direct our observational, inferential, judgmental and action processes; the information processing paradigm in the study of cognition has drawn heavily upon computer-related metaphors (long- and short-term memory storage, memory buffers, nodal networks, activation, subroutines, etc.)
- *Information Management*: an encompassing concept of ways through which information technology can support and strengthen our individual and institutional capacity to handle volumes and complexities of information that would otherwise be overwhelming; here it refers to the mechanisms through which information technology gathers, organizes, stores, retrieves, and manipulates information through software applications.

FIGURE 1. A Framework for Planning Practice and Information Technology Training in Social Work Education.

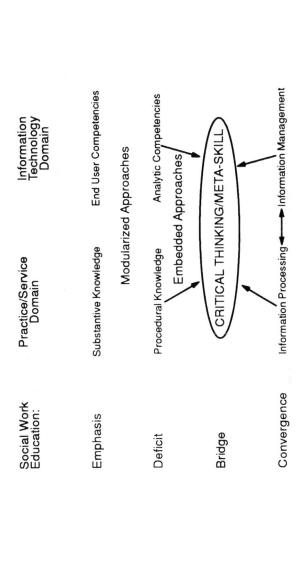

The above necessarily reflects an abbreviated overview of these key components. It is not my purpose to argue for a bifurcated perspective: that analytic competencies are more important than end user competencies, for example, or that embedded approaches are better than modularized approaches per se. Social agencies and schools of social work (and allied human services) have widely differing needs and resources. Rather than looking for a silver bullet solution, I am arguing that we need to support a critical thinking capacity in human service professionals to assist them in determining on an ongoing basis what types of information technology supports are available, appropriate, viable and sustainable relative to the needs, resources, and context at hand.

Ultimately, information technology in varied forms and to varying degrees will be a mainstream element in the life of social agencies. Thus, ultimately, information technology will be a fundamental component of training for work in these social agencies. At present, however, we as educators need conceptual vehicles for binding together the different "pieces" of computer use that we may individually include in our courses so that we collectively support a coherent and meaningful experience for students. Moreover, this instruction needs pragmatic grounding if it is to be useful in agency life. For example, creative thinking about what computer tools, theoretically, *can do* needs to be combined with understanding the resources required to implement that vision to enable a realistic evaluation of whether the benefit (e.g., improved service) justifies the investment and is sustainable. To this end, I will organize my remaining points around three aspects of critical thinking:

1. the ability to mentally move back and forth between concepts, language, functions, and so forth of multiple frameworks (UNDER-STANDING DIMENSION)
2. the ability to be use constructively critical observations in recognizing weaknesses and engaging in problem solving (APPLICATION DIMENSION)
3. the ability to create; to move beyond what is to see and contribute to what could be (GENERATIVE DIMENSION)

CRITICAL THINKING: UNDERSTANDING DIMENSION

An initial aspect of critical thinking that ties together the domains of practice and information technology training in social work is the ability to "translate" back and forth in concepts, lingo, functions, etc.: of being able to think integratively between practice tasks/needs and what available technology can and cannot do.

Part of what has reinforced my emphasis on critical thinking skills has been input from the field. For example, in a survey of Seattle agencies, my colleagues and I found that the aspect of computer skills that agency heads most valued in social workers was their conceptual understanding of the computer functions (Nurius, Hooyman, & Nicoll, 1988). They reported that they could teach specific software packages and hands-on tasks fairly quickly (although practical skills were an advantage). By contrast, the ability to "get on board" in terms of understanding as well as attitudinal comfort took considerable time to develop and was sorely needed as a starting point.

Many schools explicitly examine some of the conceptual linkage steps involved in translating between service tasks and computer supports as part of research training: how to operationalize your question in terms of a data base, how to retrieve and manipulate relevant data appropriately, how to interpret and appropriately qualify findings, how to translate findings back into practice and policy terms, and so forth. However, we now need to extend this training *across* the routine functions that make up human service providers' daily work lives.

Consider the array of tasks and activities typical for the direct service provider (e.g., social history and related intake interviewing, determining eligibility status(es), risk screening, psychosocial assessment and diagnosis, goal setting and contracting, baseline and ongoing case record recording, service provision and management, routine reports and activity recording, client tracking, agency networking, case termination and referral, case and unit evaluation). By and large, these tasks and activities are all part of our foundation curriculum. The ability to discern the ways through which the information technology of one's agency can or cannot realistically support each of these functions reflects critical thinking at the understanding level.

In pursuit of this goal of "thinking in the interface" between the social work practice world and the computer world, Ram Cnaan (University of Pennsylvania) and I developed a classification system to help social workers orient their thinking regarding how information technology can support practice goals and tasks (Nurius & Cnaan, 1991; see also Reinoehl & Hanna, 1990 for related points). This involved a grid wherein one identifies (1) the different classes of software or computer functions and where any given computer tool would be categorized as well as (2) what any given tool can and cannot realistically do relative to the different types of practice activities such as those noted above. Thus, rather than stopping at classifications such as database management tools, spreadsheets, or statistics packages, one adds the question of intervention relevance: what practice tasks does this tool help accomplish, and how well suited does it appear to be?

Something of interest emerged from working with this classification system. It helped students see some of the vagueness in how we use many important terms. For example, "assessment" encompasses an enormous diversity of activities (e.g., detailed psychosocial history, mental status exam and diagnosis, inventory of risk factors and environmental supports, etc.). This diversity in turn reflects the need for clear definition about what each practice task or function involves and requires if it is to be useful in informing software selection and use.

In a related vein, we encountered a lack of consensus regarding what constitutes "good practice." Differences in how good practice is defined and conducted hold direct implications for decisions about how *computer use in practice* is conceived as relevant or appropriate–if at all–and the extent to which implementation of that tool will result in *improved practice*–if at all. This kind of exercise highlights our need to further clarify our thinking about the appropriate roles of information technology in varied service and practice tasks and the circumstances under which investment in any given tool appears warranted. If a certain software cannot be classified according to a relevant social work practice task, or if its use does not appear to meaningfully improve or strengthen that task or a related aspect of practice, this software may be regarded as interventionally irrelevant. We focused on direct practice tasks in this classification due to their relative neglect in the literature, and, of course, there are parallels to many other messo and macro tasks.

CRITICAL THINKING: APPLICATION DIMENSION

A second aspect of critical thinking at this interface of practice and information technology involves the ability to be constructively critical; to recognize limitations and potential problems and, optimally, to be able to engage in creative problem-solving.

Whether they are on-line or paper-and-pencil form, we generally rely on a plethora of forms, reports, and accompanying procedures to capture and utilize information in human service agencies. Thus, one set of training exercises that I have found very useful does not involve direct use of the computer at all. It involves students bringing in stacks of the forms they and others routinely deal with in their practicum agencies, and engaging in a constructively critical analysis.

Information processing research tells us that we all rely upon a number of cognitive heuristic and biasing strategies to make sense out of and efficiently deal with the otherwise overwhelming amount of stimulus we encounter (see Brower & Nurius, 1994; Fiske & Taylor, 1991, for overviews). We look for and generally find what we are expecting and we are prone to quickly sort people, places, and events into categories. While this may be normative and even very useful, it also poses a number of serious risks (Berlin & Marsh, 1993; Nurius & Gibson, 1990). Grasso and Epstein (1987) also noted this double-edge with respect to management by measurement. That is, we look for and use what our attention is directed to, and the forms, procedures, and norms (e.g., what questions and issues are typically raised in supervision and case consultation) that make up daily life for the direct practitioner play crucial roles in where attention gets directed. Thus, analyses of agency forms, norms, and procedures with these issues in mind can be important steps in increasing a constructively critical consciousness.

Insights might involve something as simple as noticing that placement of financial eligibility questions early in intake or assessment forms biases workers to think of service plans only within the range of what that agency provides given the client's financial status. Another example involves critique of what our attention is and *is not* directed to (an example of the latter being environmental contributors that would help offset normative person-focused searches for information about problems) via forms and protocols.

A similar question is whether we are using our information technology tools to collect information in forms that are truly useful and that support critical reflectiveness. For example, categorical data is far easier to handle from a software perspective relative to multifaceted, contingent, qualitative forms of information. Given our inherent cognitive bias to search and sort on the basis of categories, consider the risks posed by an increasing orientation toward a narrow measurement approach (e.g., heavy reliance on yes/no and checklist systems that are easily codified and sensor scanned but that may amplify natural tendencies toward syndromatic thinking about people and problems).

Finally, consider what may be the single most complex practice task: synthesizing disparate pieces of information into a meaningful analysis. Again, information processing research tells us that we all tend to be notoriously unreliable in our even handling of information: what we notice, in what form we store it in memory, and what we do and do not recall (Ashcraft, 1989; Kahneman, Slovic, & Tversky, 1982), and the pressured, "messy" contexts of social service agencies too often serve to exacerbate these vulnerabilities (Fasano & Shapiro, 1991). Thus, another question we can pose of our computer-assisted information management tools is how well they support users' information needs and thus, quality of both data and decisions.

Synthesizing information can, of course, take many different forms. Figure 2, for example, illustrates the capacity to retrieve selected information from multiple sources and integrate it into a single source, such as a summary report (Nurius & Hudson, 1993). If the data are incomplete, inaccurate, or in a reductionistic form ill-suited to the practice task, technological tools that search, sort, and synthesize will be of little real value. Thus, critical thinking at this juncture requires substantive knowledge about the practice domain in question, procedural knowledge about how relevant practice decisions and actions are undertaken, sufficient technological knowledge to evaluate how the computer operation relates to the practice elements, and, optimally, the capacity to troubleshoot and identify alternatives if problems are detected.

Other forms of synthesis are based on information across rather than within cases. We are all naturally prone to developing generalizations about "types" of people or situations and drawing upon these generalizations to make inferences, judgments, and decisions. Thus, information technology tools that can assist us in drawing upon our broader information base can serve as an important critical thinking support in this regard. Again, I have found from my own teaching and consultation with direct practitioners that this aspect of critical thinking need not involve high level technological expertise. In some instances, practitioners have requested aggregate information about background and outcome variables presumed characteristic of certain problems in living and found the data did not support the underlying theory, triggering an examination of both the measurement tools and the clinical assumptions. Another illustration involves a practitioner's response to the question of how available client data and technology tools could better support reasoning and decision-making in risk screening. A list of risk indicators was identified, weighted according to their importance, and aggregated across clients to provide a profile of variables associated with high, medium, and low risk, which then guided both individual service planning as well as program planning about how best to triage and anticipate differing needs (Nurius, 1992; see the contributors in Grasso & Epstein, 1992, for further examples).

CRITICAL THINKING: GENERATIVE DIMENSION

A third aspect of critical thinking at the interface of practice and technology has to do with a CREATIVE ability to not just see the connec-

FIGURE 2. An Illustration of Computer-Assisted Information Integration. Reprinted by permission from *Human Services Practice, Evaluation and Computers: A Practical Guide for Today and Beyond* by Paula S. Nurius and Walter W. Hudson. Copyright by Wadsworth, 1993.

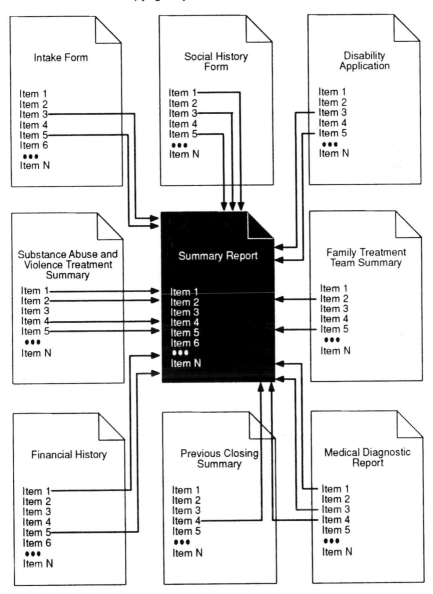

tion and not just see the problems, but to also see beyond what is to what could be.

One of my longtime concerns about critical thinking in practice is the fuzziness about what our interventions and services actually "are" and how we tend to think about the relationship of interventions to outcomes. It is generally very difficult to determine from case records exactly what a given practitioner actually did. Consequently, it is a leap of faith to generalize about and decide what is and is not effective. Single-system design methods have been explored for a number of years toward better operationalizing interventions and their relationship to change, or the lack thereof, over time (Bloom, Fischer, & Orme, 1993). In some settings, these designs can be very useful toward identifying what constituted the services received, when changes in services were made, what a client's status is relative to some referent (e.g., their preintervention level, their goals, clinical cutting norms).

In some settings, however, this kind of client monitoring is not realistic. So, we need to use a little ingenuity to develop computer-assisted aids from routinely collected databases that actually aid practitioners in critical thinking about their clients' needs, their service planning, and their ongoing adjustments and decisions based on changing information. An innovative example of this kind of creative thinking comes from a hospital discharge planner. The practitioner's goal was to more clearly operationalize what exactly constitutes effective service as a discharge planner, and what type and form of information would support this service, approached realistically given the multiple time and role restrictions (Nurius, 1992). The result was a standardized form that involved rating the degree of satisfactory completion of (1) a series of tasks that were common to most if not all cases as well as (2) case specific tasks that helped to communicate important individual client needs to other members of the service team as well as to build a clinical database of intervening factors that otherwise tended to "get lost in the shuffle."

As a profession, we tend to be very verbally-oriented. We are inclined to ask clients questions and, not surprisingly, our computer aids reflect this semantic, inquiry bias. However, information technology today offers rich and dynamic alternatives for how to go about getting needed information. Various forms of multimedia tools that are far more intuitive and appealing for many people offer extraordinary possibilities. I have repeatedly been impressed by students' ability to generate creative alternatives; for example, use of cartoon style assessment tests regarding knowledge of child safety and good parenting for use with at-risk parents with limited reading skills. Critical thinking training needs to pair support of such creativity with consideration of the costs, training, and situation factors needed to realistically and appropriately implement any given creative idea. But, like any other skill, the ability to conceive practice relevant technological alternatives needs to be practiced with feedback in order to be strengthened.

Finally, let us touch on reasoning and training possibilities that are more centrally focused on *processes* of reasoning. We all develop theories that undergird our mental maps about how the world works: what goes with what, what causes and/or results from what, and so forth. However, we are often not consciously aware of either developing or drawing upon these implicit theories (Fiske & Taylor, 1991). Because one aspect of critical thinking involves mindful reflection, we need to acquire greater awareness as social workers about what theories and assumptions we hold and use in our work with clients. Several of the prior examples will assist with this goal. Increasingly, a variety of computer tools can assist us in understanding and managing how we think (e.g., Carlson, 1993; Semke & Nurius, 1991).

Although we are still a long way from what could properly be called expert systems in the direct practice arena, there are some inviting possibilities for increasing users' awareness of their reasoning models and habits. In our own experience (Nurius & Nicoll, 1992), we found many of the knowledge inquiry and knowledge representation strategies very useful in this regard. One project involved assessment and early service planning related to domestic violence. Figures 3 and 4 illustrate the mental maps that a collaborative practitioner[1] held about what domains are important for assessment, how observable facts are related to inferred states and conditions, and how these are related to reasoning about service planning. Simplified versions could be incorporated into routine information management systems, such as queries to the practitioner as to what variables they are basing a conclusion on, what factors would possibly disconfirm their conclusion, were these factors investigated, and so forth.

Practitioners, like all people, approach situations with a practical need to filter out relevant from irrelevant information and to read and assign meaning to behavior and events. Concern with "process" variables in social work has been long-standing, but there has been limited success in delineating what these factors are or how best to manage them. Although allied professions such as medicine, nursing, psychology, education, and psychiatry have been more vigorous than social work in building upon new findings and technology in training regarding procedural knowledge, critical thinking, and integrative approaches, social work is increasingly taking an active role (as reflected in several contributions to the recent HUSITA 3 Conference; see *New Technology in the Human Services*, Spring

FIGURE 3. An Example of Modeling A Practitioner's Mental Schema of Domestic Violence. Reprinted by permission from Paula S. Nurius and Anne E. Nicoll, 1992, "Capturing Clinical Expertise: An Analysis of Knowledge 'Mining' Through Expert System Development", *Clinical Psychology Review, 12*, 705-717. Copyright by Pergamon Press, 1992.

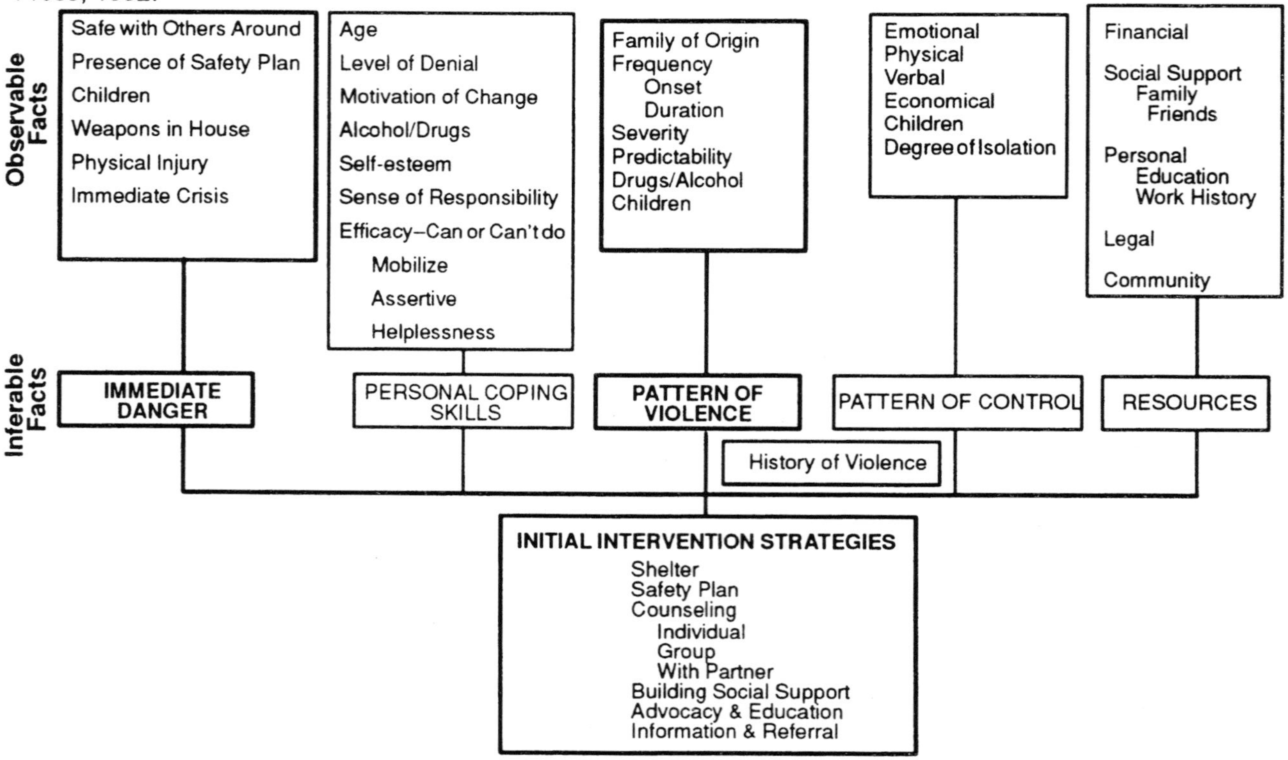

Observable Facts

IMMEDIATE DANGER
- Safe with Others Around
- Presence of Safety Plan
- Children
- Weapons in House
- Physical Injury
- Immediate Crisis

PERSONAL COPING SKILLS
- Age
- Level of Denial
- Motivation of Change
- Alcohol/Drugs
- Self-esteem
- Sense of Responsibility
- Efficacy—Can or Can't do
  - Mobilize
  - Assertive
  - Helplessness

PATTERN OF VIOLENCE
- Family of Origin
- Frequency
- Onset
- Duration
- Severity
- Predictability
- Drugs/Alcohol
- Children

PATTERN OF CONTROL
- Emotional
- Physical
- Verbal
- Economical
- Children
- Degree of Isolation

RESOURCES
- Financial
- Social Support
  - Family
  - Friends
- Personal
  - Education
  - Work History
- Legal
- Community

Inferable Facts

History of Violence

INITIAL INTERVENTION STRATEGIES
- Shelter
- Safety Plan
- Counseling
  - Individual
  - Group
  - With Partner
- Building Social Support
- Advocacy & Education
- Information & Referral

122

FIGURE 4. An Example of Modeling A Practitioner's Mental Schema for Risk Assessment. Reprinted by permission from Paula S. Nurius and Anne E. Nicoll, 1992, "Capturing Clinical Expertise: An Analysis of Knowledge 'Mining' Through Expert System Development", *Clinical Psychology Review, 12,* 705-717. Copyright by Pergamon Press, 1992.

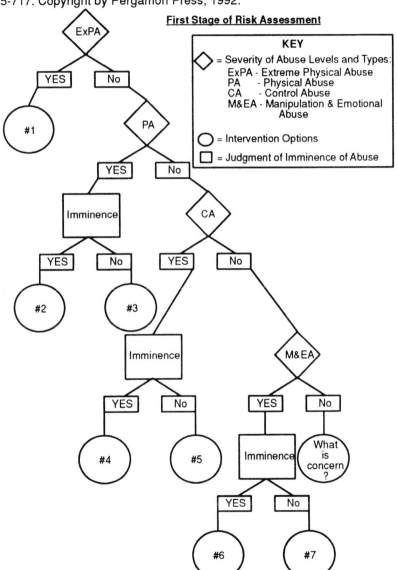

1993; Gambrill, 1990; Nurius & Gibson, 1994; Oyserman & Benbenishty, 1993; Seelig, 1991, for overviews).

CONCLUSION

In coming years as entering students are increasingly computer knowledgeable, we will see a shift in learning curves less toward hardware and computer commands (the computer as a machine) and more devoted to concepts and ideas (the computer as a medium); more toward the computer as a reasoning resource than a giant calculator. How can we best prepare for this?

There are neither simple nor universal answers to this question. Recently revised requirements in the U.S. Council on Social Work Education regarding the incorporation of information technology into foundation courses and the requirement that students demonstrate an ability to evaluate their own practice as a requisite for graduation are examples of useful catalysts. The increasing presence of information technology in social agencies will likely increase administrators' and educators' sense of need to generate effective training responses. We are at a juncture point where significant changes in the face of information technology in the human services will, ready or not, evolve. My premise is that we balance the powerful potential of the computer as a machine with its potentially even more powerful possibilities as a medium of thought and expression.

NOTE

As system developers, Anne Nicoll and I gratefully acknowledge the generous contributions of time and practice expertise by Ms. Ginny NiCarthy in this work.

REFERENCES

Ashcraft, M. H. (1989). *Human memory and cognition.* Glenview, IL: Scott, Foresman, & Co.
Berlin, S. B., & Marsh, J.C. (1993). *Informing practice decisions.* New York: MacMillan.
Bloom, M., Fischer, J., & Orme, J. G. (1993). *Evaluating practice: Guidelines for the accountable professional* (2nd ed.). Englewood Cliffs, NJ: Prentice-Hall.
Brower, A. M. & Nurius, P. S. (1994). *Social cognition and individual change: Current theory and counseling guidelines.* Newbury Park, CA: Sage Pub.

Carlson, R. W. (1993). From rules to prototypes: Adapting expert systems to the nature of expertise in clinical information processing. *Computers in Human Services, 9*, 339-350.

Colombi, D., Rafferty, J., & Steyaert, J. (1993). Human services and information technology. In D. Colombi, J. Rafferty, & J. Steyaert (Eds.), *Human Services and information technology: A European perspective*. ENITH.

Fasano, R., & Shapiro, J. J. (1991). Computerizing the small non-profit: Computer consultants' perspective. *Computers in Human Services, 8*, 129-145.

Fiske, S. T. & Taylor, S. E. (1991). *Social cognition* (2nd ed.). New York: McGraw-Hill.

Gambrill, E. (1990). *Critical thinking in clinical practice*. San Francisco, CA: Jossey-Bass.

Gibbs, L. E. (1991). *Scientific reasoning for social workers: Bridging the gap between research and practice*. New York: Merrill.

Glastonbury, B., & LaMendola, W. (1992). *The integrity of intelligence: A bill of rights for the information age*. New York: St. Martin's Press.

Grasso, A. & Epstein, I. (1987). Management by measurement: Organizational dilemmas and opportunities. *Administration in Social Work, 2*, 89-100.

Grasso, A. & Epstein, I. (Eds.). (1992). *Research utilization in the social services: Innovations for practice and administration*. New York: Haworth Press.

Halpern, D. E. (1989). *Thought and knowledge: An introduction to critical thinking* (2nd ed.). Hillsdale, NJ: Lawrence Erlbaum.

Kahneman, D., Slovic, P., & Tversky, A. (Eds.) (1982). *Judgment under uncertainty: Heuristics and biases*. Cambridge, MA: Cambridge University Press.

Kitchener, K. S. & Fischer, K. W. (1990). A skill approach to the development of reflective thinking. In D. Kuhn (Ed.), Developmental perspectives on teaching and learning thinking skills. *Contributions to Human Development, 21*, 48-62.

New Technology in the Human Services, 6(Spring); ENITH presents HUSITA3 Conference Abstracts.

Norris, S. P. (Ed.). (1992). *The generalizability of critical thinking: Multiple perspectives on an educational ideal*. New York: Teachers College Press.

Nurius, P. S. & Cnaan, R. (1991). Classifying software to better support social work practice. *Social Work, 36*, 536-541.

Nurius, P. S. & Gibson, J. W. (1991). Clinical inference, reasoning, and judgment in social work: An update. *Social Work Research & Abstracts, 26*, 18-25.

Nurius, P. S., & Gibson, J. W. (1994). *Practitioners' perspectives on sound reasoning*. (Manuscript under review).

Nurius, P. S., Hooyman, N. R., & Nicoll, A. E. (1988). The changing face of computer utilization in social work settings. *Journal of Social Work Education, 24*, 186-197.

Nurius, P. S. & Nicoll, A. E. (1992). Capturing expertise: An analysis of knowledge "mining" through expert system development. *Clinical Psychology Review, 12*, 705-711.

Oyserman, D., & Benbenishty, R. (1993). The impact of clinical information systems on human service organizations. *Computers in Human Services, 9*, 425-438.

Reinoehl, R., & Hanna, T. (1990). Defining computer literacy in human services. *Computers in Human Services, 6*, 3-20.

Schoech, D. (1990). *Human services computing: Concepts and applications.* New York: Haworth Press.

Seelig, J.M. (1991). Social work and the critical thinking movement. *Journal of Teaching in Social Work, 5*, 21-34.

Semke, J., & Nurius, P. S. (1991). Information structure, information technology, and the human service organizational environment. *Social Work, 36*, 353-361.

Introduction

David Colombi

The five papers included in this section cover a broad spectrum of communication themes with the common thread of assisting and enabling people to communicate via technology to achieve their personal goals or social aims. It includes development of general skills through communication camps for young people in Finland, or specialist needs such as people in isolated rural communities in Scotland, and research undertaken at Kauserslautern University in Germany on assisting disabled people to communicate. At a wider level, an authoritative paper on computer networking takes a global perspective on new ways of communication and opening up networking to ever wider groups of participants. Finally this section finishes in Finland, where it began, with an account of a particular application to assist planning services for the elderly. This focus on technology as a means of communication is still relatively new for many who use computers either alone or on small local networks. The analogy of it being the difference between owning a car and taking it out onto the roads is perhaps a useful one, even if to overstate the case. Even a "stand alone" computer can become a powerful means of communication.

David Colombi is Information Manager of West Sussex Probation Service, UK.

[Haworth co-indexing entry note]: "Introduction." Colombi, David. Co-published simultaneously in *Computers in Human Services* (The Haworth Press, Inc.) Vol. 12, No. 1/2, 1995, pp. 127-131; and: *Human Services in the Information Age* (ed: Jackie Rafferty, Jan Steyaert, and David Colombi) The Haworth Press, Inc., 1995, pp. 127-131. Single or multiple copies of this article are available from The Haworth Document Delivery Service [1-800-342-9678, 9:00 a.m. - 5:00 p.m. (EST)].

127

Ritva-Sini Härkönen's account of "Communication Camps–The Real Utopia" takes a refreshingly and unashamedly optimistic perspective that perhaps challenges those brought up on the dictum that *social workers don't like good news*. The paper is a relatively short one that succinctly summarises the aims, activities and achievements of the communication camps. These camps seek to encourage and enable children to develop personal skills and use technology as a means of communication and self expression. The concept of mixing camps in the woods with use of information technology is in itself an interesting and different notion. However the value of the paper is not just in the account of the diverse activities involved but also in the theoretical perspectives which frame those activities. Not least of these is the idea of information technology as shaping cultural change with the camps in a microcosm in which a group of young people can build their own culture. This experience is contrasted with the external world where the author questions the dichotomy and tensions between apparent opportunities for citizens to participate and a more restricted reality. What we find is concentration of ownership and control of all forms of media in the hands of fewer and fewer unaccountable multinational companies.

At an individual level, the paper effectively challenges an assumption we all too easily make. We assume that growing up with computers somehow gives children intuitive understanding of their use and potential, rather than that as something that needs to be nurtured. Children may display a natural aptitude in using computers that can leave their parents feeling clumsy and stupid. However, all too often these skills are narrowly focused and fail to develop, with many children excluded from the start. The camps seem to be a way of taking the natural skills, curiosity, creativity, and enthusiasms of children to harness these in a way that is about living together and developing personal and social skills as well as understanding. Härkönen provides an intriguing and valuable insight into this unique and exciting project and, for those who wish to know more, the paper provides reference to a fuller account of the work.

The second paper in this section is also about communications in a rural setting, but moves on from education to an experiment in provision of services. Jenny Brogden and Cara Williams write about "Using Advanced Communications and Multimedia Applications to Provide Real Life Benefits to Remote Rural Areas: BARBARA." This paper is an account of the application in the Scottish Highlands of the BARBARA (Broad Range of Community Based Telecommunications Applications in Rural Areas) Project. BARBARA is a pan-European project which operates in Ireland, Greece, and Germany as well as in Scotland. The two principle strands of the paper encompass a description of the aims and concepts involved in the project and of the detailed participative research involved. The research was integral to the aim of ensuring that it was user-led rather than technology-led. The first strand draws on modern tele-communications possibilities, on application of multi-media systems and concepts from teleworking as the practical and theoretical basis to the project. Thus, the project is at the technological forefront of IT developments in the human services. These elements are adapted in an innovative way to form "tele-units" or information access locations. The tele-units have some parallels with established public access systems such as the street information points in Antwerp or the Minitel data services in France. However the approach goes much further with video-link access to people providing services as well as to information about these services and possibilities for developing links between communities.

The criteria for success of the project is not provision of a service but use of that service. This led the project into the research methodology used to ensure that the project would be responsive both to users needs and to service providers. Brogden and Williams describe the theoretical basis of the research, the processes involved and the outcomes achieved. This strong focus on user's needs places the paper firmly in the tradition of the best of work on community work and on developing information systems. Such an approach should be a *sine qua non* of all such projects, but is all too often neglected or treated cursorily. Overall the paper presents a valuable perspective on an important area of development. It has not just to do with the economic case for delivering particular services but to do with the whole quality of life in rural communities.

Addressing a different set of special communication needs, the paper by Harald Weber, Gerhard Zimmermann and Klaus Zink at the University of Kaiserslautern in Germany focuses on "Computer Access for People with Special Needs." The emphasis here is not on a particular computer application or a particular piece of hardware to meet a specific need. The approach used is a careful analysis across a whole range of disabilities to identify ways in which access to all computers can be increased. The way in which this is planned is through systems that mediate at an operating system level between the machine and the program to increase the flexibility in how the computer can be controlled. It moves us away from the notion of a "standard user" with a standard way of operating a computer into diverse approaches to meet diverse needs. The people analysis involves attention to the dimensions of physical, sensitive, and cognitive functioning associated with special needs. The system analysis encompasses a wide range of inputting devices, such as scanners and speech recognition, and output devices such as speech synthesis, braille, and enlarged text for the visually impaired.

The work presented is detailed, thorough and particularly notable for bringing together expertise from different disciplines within Kaiserslautern University such as vocational rehabilitation, computer architecture, system design, ergonomics and work organisation. Work so far reported is at a conceptual rather than a practical level and such a fundamental analysis and approach does not bring short term results. As though with a number of other contributions in this book, the step from localised thinking about particular solutions towards wider perspectives marks a new stage of development and of sophistication.

Taking this theme of wider perspectives to its ultimate conclusion of a global perspective on a particular subject is Thomas Hanna's paper on "Towards Consensus in Human Services Computer Networking." This paper tackles the theme of networking both as access to local networks and between networks, chiefly via the Internet and emerging use of the World Wide Web (WWW). To address such a theme presents considerable problems in writing to a mixed audience. Many of that audience use networks as a daily tool of their work for communication and accessing data, whilst for others the world of networking is alien, anxiety inducing, and intensely confusing. To some extent the division is between insiders working in academic environments, and outsiders working in agencies. However Hanna extrapolates from survey work in New York State to indicate the extent of access to computers and to modems in agencies in that part of the world. He shows how the barriers have moved, for the richer world at least, from accessibility and cost, to those of knowledge about what is available and understanding about how it can be used.

Hanna writes as someone who has been involved at a practical level with the development of networks for human services and enabling "gateways" between them as part of *HumanServe* and other initiatives. As such he brings an insider's knowledge and awareness of the bewildering diversity of developments and of the technical complexities. However he conveys the issues in a non-technical way that is both accessible and geared to the needs of current and potential users alike. As such this paper is a remarkable and comprehensive contribution that deserves to be and should be widely read by anyone who wants to understand how the human services fit into one of the "megatrends" of the future. One network in England was memorably described as a "Ferrari being driven in first gear" and this paper can perhaps help people in human service agencies, as well as academics, to find and join the fast lane.

Finally in this section we return to another Finnish contribution with

Marja Vaarama's account of the Evergreen project for strategic planning of welfare and health services for elderly people. Here the emphasis has moved on from young people into projections of demographic changes and the consequences for provision of services. As with many other countries, Finland is facing a sharply rising proportion of elderly people in its population. The Evergreen computer software works with those demographic changes to evaluate the demands placed on society through four different forms of modelling future services. These models–the laissez-faire, normative, humanist and economic–are described along with descriptions of how the software handles them. There is also technical information about the program and about experience of its successful use in practice.

Of particular interest is that the software can be used at different levels for national, regional, and local planning of services. Vaarama identifies that further development of the program can be seen in the context of pan-European planning on "Ageing and Technology" with Evergreen as a potential base for this work. This aspect of wider use of applications, whether from local to national contexts or from national to international levels is a continuing theme both within this section and in the next.

Building The Future:
Communication Camps–
The Real Utopia!

Ritva-Sini Härkönen

SUMMARY. The most important skills of the future would be communication skills–that is why communication camps for children
and youngsters are implemented. The camp is more than mere media
technology, it is a way of living and learning together. At the camp,
children take part in five activities: press, video, radio, telecommunications and catering. The theory behind the activities stresses such
constructs as interaction, non-hierarchy, cultural change, equal
rights, internal luxury and media literacy. The main goal of the camp
is to educate children (and adults) to be active builders of the future who
work for a better interactively-communicative world. *[Article copies available from The Haworth Document Delivery Service: 1-800-342-9678.]*

According to the laws of evolution a healthy generation will renew
the views of the previous generation and introduce essential reform.
As long as a nation is reborn in this manner it will have a great life.

Santeri Alkio 1893

Ritva-Sini Härkönen completed her doctoral dissertation on media education
at Helsinki University and is Senior Adviser to the National Board of Education
in Helsinki. She is also Chairperson of the Finnish Communications Education
Society. With many years teaching experience, Ritva-Sini's main field is media
education as a whole and she has published many research reports and articles as
well as her doctoral dissertation.

Address correspondence to: Ritva-Sini Härkönen, National Board of Education, P.O.Box 380, 00531 Helsinki, Finland.

[Haworth co-indexing entry note]: "Building the Future: Communication Camps–The Real Utopia!" Härkönen, Ritva-Sini. Co-published simultaneously in *Computers in Human Services* (The Haworth Press, Inc.) Vol. 12, No. 1/2, 1995, pp. 133-140; and: *Human Services in the Information Age* (ed:
Jackie Rafferty, Jan Steyaert, and David Colombi) The Haworth Press, Inc., 1995, pp. 133-140. Single
or multiple copies of this article are available from The Haworth Document Delivery Service
[1-800-342-9678, 9:00 a.m. - 5:00 p.m. (EST)].

133

The need to do something serious to improve the basis of future tele-communications and media as a whole was realized on cold winter day (−30°C) at a colloquium, where the theory of media education was dis-cussed. We realized that the most important skills of the future would be communication skills–and the Communications Education Society was founded. We decided to act empirically: a communications camp was a dream that came true in the middle of a hot (+30°C) summer in 1987.

The main idea behind a media camp is that communication skills are present everywhere in the society and belong to everybody. Activities in the camps provide participating children and youngsters experiences of a new way of life, involving self-expression, participation and taking re-sponsibility. The camp is more than mere media technology: it is a way of living and learning together, combining mutual responsibility with indi-vidual initiative. The basic value taught and learnt is justice, which in-cludes both the right to self-expression and the duty of sharing responsibil-ity with others. Summer media camps aim at being models for future growth towards individual action, initiative, and the ability to master one's own life. This all proceeds from open communication. From a researcher's point of view the camp is based on testing of different action models and experiments with the functioning of social insight and ideas. The camp measures the functionality of social innovations. This is why we may use well the term "laboratory of the future."

ACTIVITIES IN THE CAMP

The children stay at the camp for a week. They start by constructing the networks and setting-up the equipment. These are used as means of self-expression: newspapers are edited, videos and radio programmes are pro-duced and data and messages are recorded in databanks and electronic mail systems. Telecommunication technology is utilized in daily chores by ordering food from the grocer using E-mail and by seeking data about the nutritional values of foodstuffs from a databank. Equipment is at hand all the time and everyone is free to use it. Use of the equipment is learnt by watching and copying pals, but above all by experimenting and trying independently. During the camp children do what good journalists do, according to a dynamic approach to knowledge: they use information, examine facts, analyse ideas, practice source critique, exchange ideas in small groups, analyse, summarise, edit and report. For more information see "The Story of the Communications Camp" (Luokola, 1991).

The Press Group

The aim in the press group is to learn the process of newspaper making. The task of the press group is to produce a morning paper for the camp. The stories are written into the micro-computers and lay-out is carried out with the lay-out programme (desktop publishing). The newspaper is printed with a copying machine and delivered to the tents in the morning. Figure 1 provides an illustration of the press group's operating facilities.

FIGURE 1

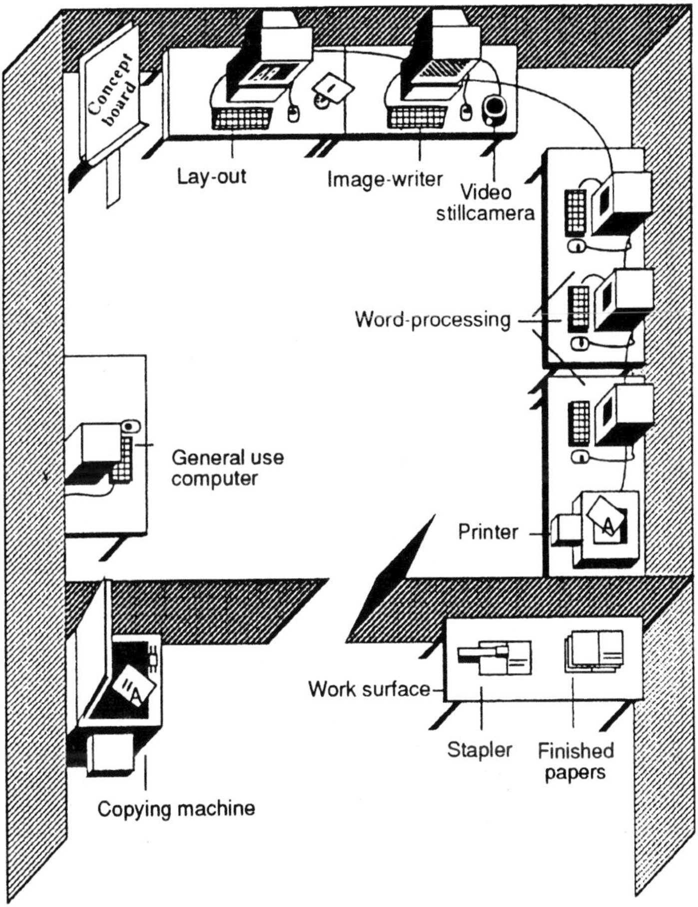

The Video Group

The aim in the video group is to let the children and young people know, at least in principle, how television programmes are made and to teach the camp the elements. The task of the group is to produce the news and a play or some other programme to be broadcast (narrowcast!) in the evenings.

The Radio Group

The aim of the radio group is to practice using microphones and recorders to do interviews and to put a radio programme together as joint projects. The camp becomes familiar with how radio programmes are made in practice.

Telecommunications Activities

The aim is to familiarize the children with different ways to use communication equipment, including the new methods of communication. During the camp telecommunications and data processing activities either assist and support other group activities or are used on their own. Children learn what kinds of communication networks can be built and what types of message transmission they make possible.

The Catering Group

People can not live only on interaction and being together, the physical body needs nourishment! The task of the catering group is to prepare food for the camp. And so the children prepare their own meals and market them to other campers via camp radio, newspapers and ads. They work out the menus and send fax messages to the baker and the shop. The next morning everything arrives ready packed for the camp. The main idea is to learn to use information technology in everyday life.

THE THEORY BEHIND THE ACTIVITIES

Communication is not only about the use of certain tools through which people communicate with each other, but also about experiencing community. (An overview of the camp community is provided in Figure 2.) Society is possible as a network of relationships of varied meaning, but not without them. Being closely together at the media camp, technologies

FIGURE 2

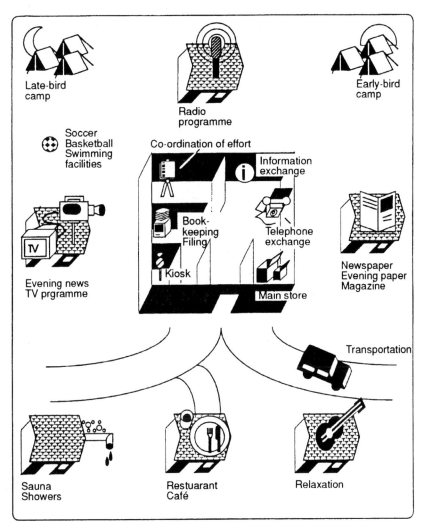

work first of all as tools of interaction. Interactive communication is essential and should honor both the sender as well as the receiver.

New information technology and new ways to communicate can create new interaction where hierarchy is not needed. The camp is very real. The children know that adults take them seriously. The camp stimulates the children's thinking and activates them to do something that is needed, something which is not simulation. The adults are on hand if the children need help; not as teachers always wanting to give advice. Everyone is allowed to try and to succeed and the results come fast. If you succeed everybody is delighted. If the result is less than good you can always try again and maybe next time you will succeed. Younger campers do what they can, older campers are junior leaders. The learning atmosphere at the camp is positive, relaxing and "easy-going," non-authoritative.

There may be a close link between information technologies and cultural change. At the camp we produce our own media culture, not the culture of someone else. Children pick up their own interests. We give the children advice *"to examine all and select what is good."* The exploration takes account of the changes facing the media environment. Only some years ago, few people were in a position to communicate with the world outside their cultural sphere other than by being on the receiving side, whereas now we are heading towards a time when the everyday life of ordinary people will require contacts outside their own community and culture, even on a global scale. Computerisation and information technology have made the world smaller. In today's world and even more so in the future people with different world views will find themselves having to work together. Different world views cover a variety of outlooks on life and codes of ethics. What skills are required for people of different cultures to work together? What knowledge and skills are required for one to understand and interpret others? The camp is one of looking for answers to these questions. It is one view and one statement in the international debate on the future which must be addressed now. We try to *"act locally, think globally."*

The camp believes in democracy: everyone must have equal rights and opportunities to communicate. When knowledge becomes a commodity, it changes. It can happen that only they who have money possess information. Five to ten corporations could be in control of most of the world's broadcast stations, magazines, and newspapers by the end of this century. If present trends continue, those few companies will control not only what we read, watch and play, but also major parts of our interaction; they are also setting out cultural, social and political values. In that sense the concept of global development is a misleading one. The scope for technology transfer is, in part, a matter of will. The demand for justice emphasizes the idea that everyone must have the right to express themselves to an audience. It is just to build the world on the basis of common conversations and resolutions, together with those who know the technicals and those who know the contents; girls and boys together . . . At the camp we examine stages in technology transfer, from a human, cultural point of view, put them into the context of the new culture and study the possible effects. The human process and social consequences which need to be considered in a technology transfer activity are extensive.

Externally the camps are not luxurious: we live in tents and fix food in the middle of the forest if necessary . . . The center, where we keep the equipment, has been an old school. Internally the camps are luxurious: here you can express your opinions on everything in all possible ways, with any communication medium or without any equipment, just as you like. The basic autonomous values are *"having, loving and being"*–we care for all three.

The campers master traditional literacy. The most advanced readers construct personal philosophies by synthesizing information and accepting or rejecting points of view. Knowing the facts is only the beginning. Being able to link them together, to discard one in favor of another, to synthesize them into a personal philosophy–that is the ultimate measure of literacy. But, with the changing media landscape, the concept of literacy is expanding towards what is currently known as media literacy. Traditional literacy is no longer enough, one should also be able to read and write different media texts, whether verbal, visual, oral, auditive, digital, iconographic or any combinations of these. As integration of technology is true, so too is the need for skills to read and write integrated media texts.

Only a hundred years ago we were offered world events in small, neat rations. Today the rations are excessive. The communication flood brings conflicting information and experiences and makes us insecure. How can I mould this shapeless mass into something manageable, something I can live with? Am I in control of my own life? At the camp we are the active builders of the future. Knowledge, skills, values and standards are transferred from generation to generation. The object of media education is to provide the young with the material they need to build a view of the world and actions. It is every individual's inbuilt programme. These are the main goals of the communications camps, but how have the goals been reached?

SOME OUTCOMES

We have made some case studies on the camps and the main results refer to high activity and motivation among the children and young ones. Some junior leaders are so competent that they visit schools as teacher's aids to implement a camp as school work. They have also helped some associations to organize camps of their own. Summer campers seem to be most active pupils in their own schools: they have published a book of their own, *How to improve the school* and made many video and radio programmes, etc. Some quotes from yet unpublished research data on answers of twelve-year-old pupils tell the essential:

- *At the camp it was the best that you could work so independently and learn by doing.*
- *I learned to use all kind of technology and I was allowed to use equipment by myself.*
- *The best was that you were not to do things you don't want to do.*

Experiences of adults at the camp are positive as well:

- *Creative work has been best.*
- *Children had that much responsibility.*
- *With children I learnt new communication skills, co-operation was excellent!*

EPILOGUE

What tools should the young be given to enable them to modernize the attitudes of the previous generation? Could children be educated to become initiators of change? In order to act as individuals and members of the community in the future media society, people should have new skills to send, receive and interpret messages and the ability to estimate and evaluate the means and structures of media and telecommunications, their nature, and their place and meaning in everyday life–at both the national and international level.

We may talk about communicative competence in the future society: children are provided with information on basic tools of communication (knowledge for thinking), basic skills in using and developing communication (will to act) and possibilities to create and evaluate communication content (emotions for feeling). These three factors—cognition, affection, will–are all involved in developing the idea of summer media camps. We work for a better interactively-communicative future. We concentrate on the three basic existential needs: to organize your environment, to join your community and to learn by experience.

REFERENCE

Luokola, T. (1991). "The Story of the Communications Camp," Communications Education Society, Helsinki.

Using Advanced Communications and Multimedia Applications to Provide Real Life Benefits to Remote Rural Areas: BARBARA

Jenny Brogden
Cara Williams

SUMMARY. The Barbara Project is an exciting project which is designing and implementing interactive, multimedia technology to improve the quality of council and other services delivered to rural communities. The rural communities involved in the project are in: Scotland, Ireland, Greece, Germany. The full range of multimedia

Jenny Brogden is Project Leader for the Barbara Project in Scotland and the European Project Socrates, a six month concertation exercise for RACE. Jenny has worked in community development and adult education for 19 years and she studied community development at Reading and received further education at Southampton University.

Cara Williams was Researcher on the Barbara Project, which is being conducted by the Information Technology Department of Highland Regional Council. Currently she is working as Research Officer in the Development and Planning Service of the Central Regional Council, Scotland. Cara's background is in geography; she has studied at Portsmouth Polytechnic (UK), West Virginia (USA) and Clark University (USA).

Address correspondence to: Jenny Brogden, Highland Regional Council, 88 High Street, Nairn, Highland Region IV12 4SG, Scotland.

[Haworth co-indexing entry note]: "Using Advanced Communications and Multimedia Applications to Provide Real Life Benefits to Remote Rural Areas: BARBARA." Brogden, Jenny, and Cara Williams. Co-published simultaneously in *Computers in Human Services* (The Haworth Press, Inc.) Vol. 12, No. 1/2, 1995, pp. 141-150; and: *Human Services in the Information Age* (ed: Jackie Rafferty, Jan Steyaert, and David Colombi) The Haworth Press, Inc., 1995, pp. 141-150. Single or multiple copies of this article are available from The Haworth Document Delivery Service [1-800-342-9678, 9:00 a.m. - 5:00 p.m. (EST)].

will be used to support the service, such as simultaneous: voice, video, data (text and image). The main emphasis of the project is in user-involvement from an early stage, so that technology is not foisted upon rural communities and so the whole project is user-led rather than technology-led. To enable this to happen a continuous process of consultation and review has been instigated to allow for the participant communities to be involved in deciding what services are to be delivered and in which ways the service will be presented on the unit. This paper describes the scope of the Barbara Project and the initial findings of the research. *[Article copies available from The Haworth Document Delivery Service: 1-800-342-9678.]*

INTRODUCTION

Throughout Europe the services and facilities available to people in urban areas are generally far superior to those in the rural areas. The gap between these areas is continually widening with the consequent movement of more and more people from the rural areas into the towns. This drift increases the strain on already overloaded services and infrastructures. Advanced communications could, if concentrated in the cities and within large businesses, further encourage this trend. The BARBARA (Broad Range of Community Based Telecommunications Applications in Rural Areas) Project is about trying to reverse some of these trends and to improve the quality of life of people in the remote areas of the Highlands.

The project has set out to provide a wide range of practical applications which will be of benefit to remote rural areas and to provide services and applications that local people wanted rather than those thought to be needed by providers of services such as local authorities. The project is about meeting the needs of real users living and working in remote rural communities, so a major part of the project has been concerned with research into the requirements of the users and providers of the service in the rural communities. The objective of the research has been to determine the services which will be of practical value and which could be realistically provided using multimedia and advanced telecommunications. The success or failure of the project will be judged on the extent to which it delivers services which the rural communities use.

The Barbara Project is a European funded project under the RACE (Research and Development in Advanced Communications for Europe) programme. The project has partners in Ireland, Greece and Germany, who will be co-operating to develop a single multimedia tele-unit to carry services out to rural communities and the aim of this paper is to describe the research with the user communities, looking particularly at the style of research, the feedback received so far from the communities and the ways in which this feedback has been used to guide the development of the tele-unit. The project is important to the Highland Regional Council not just because of the migration of people to urban areas but because it is the largest local government administrative unit in Europe, almost the size of Belgium, and the Council needs to find a way to ensure that its services and information reaches the scattered rural population of just over 200,000 in the most effective way. Through this improvement of access to services and information it hopes to also encourage and enable people to live and work in the rural areas.

ADVANCED TELECOMMUNICATIONS

Advanced telecommunications with the capacity for real-time (concurrent) face-to-face links through video, sound and data transfer, allow for "meetings" to take place across long distances. The costs of meetings by videophone calls over the networks are justified by the savings in travelling time and expenses. These are benefits which multinational companies have been quick to recognise and to exploit.

The increased use of advanced telecommunications by business has led to outsourcing of work and to the creation of work outside of the office environment. The economic arguments for promoting teleworking are strong: teleworking could increase productivity to an average 45% per person and save approximately £3,000 (@ $4,500) per car on company cars used for commuting. The economic arguments for teleworking are supported by environmental gains whereby if 15% of the working force teleworked there would be a saving of 2.7 million gallons (UK) of fuel every day. Beyond the temples of large scale business enterprise there is a slower but increasing awareness of the benefits of advanced telecommunications. Tele-cottages are being set up to take advantage of the new advances in telecommunications to make technology available to individuals and small business as well as importing work to rural or less-developed areas.

From a telecommunications perspective, the involvement in the project by the Highland Regional Council was facilitated by the ISDN (Integrated Services Digital Network) which has been installed in the region and is capable of carrying simultaneous video/voice and data traffic. The aim of the European programme from which Barbara initiated was to support the advance of broadband telecommunications. However, the cost of installing broadband is prohibitive in rural areas, where the return from use by local small business does not justify the investment in the infrastructure. The option for using ISDN as the communications network to support multimedia was therefore a practical solution in the Highland Region.

THE BARBARA TELE-UNIT

The tele-unit will be an interactive, multimedia computer that will allow users easy access to the information and services of the council and other organisations. The unit is being developed through research in the community and with the service providers. The idea is to develop a unit which is easy to use, uses the full range of multimedia, and meets the service needs of both the communities in remote rural areas and the service providers in urban centres.

The concept of the tele-unit, though using similar communications infrastructure and technology, is different from ideas such as the tele-cottages as the aim of the tele-unit is not to carry work to the remote communities, but to provide services for and to them. The technology is being used to give an enhanced "face-to-face" type service to remote communities and to open opportunities for such things as distance training and education. At this early stage, the unit will be free of charge to the users and is not required to generate income. Currently the Barbara unit is in its early prototype stage and is being taken out to the communities for testing, but the following are some of the features of the multimedia unit. The unit will be accessed in several ways–

- simple touch screen with icons of the services which can be touched to lead the person onto the next stage
- a standard keyboard with marked keys for simple procedures such as a help key
- use of a mouse or roller ball to direct the cursor/pointer on the screen
- dialling for help and assistance from a receptionist via the videophone.

The user will be able to use the videophone to talk to an official who can help the user with any aspect of the service: access information, get advice, search library catalogues, reserve books from the library, book appointments and hold face-to-face meetings with officials and elected members. However, the user will also be able to access these services directly on the tele-unit.

The units in the selected communities across the region will be linked so that groups and individuals can conference with each other. This will enable the extension of the distance learning systems, with the added bonus of the videophone facility. The way in which the unit is constructed and its user interface configured will as much as possible reflect the users' needs.

METHOD OF RESEARCH

As already stated one of the major objectives of the project was that it should be user-led rather than technology-led. To achieve this the style of research could not follow the lines of market research or along the lines of just using questionnaires. The project and the technology it was introducing was innovatory and needed people to be involved in a way that enabled their true participation in an equal partnership with the researchers and developers. To this end we used participative research methods.

Participative research allows a researcher to enter a community group with certain hypotheses and theories, but through communication and reflexive thought, to adjust preconceived notions. Through this process the researcher can approach what is being *understood* by the individuals in the community (Outhwaite, 1975; Spradley, 1980; Evans, 1988). This is a dialectical approach to research which presumes that research is not done in isolation from the cultural, economic, social and political context and that social science, indeed science, is not value-free. Attitudinal research moves into the psychological realm, which encompasses feelings, emotions, culture, and bias and so meanings have to be understood by both the researcher and the researched through increased dialogue, so that the researcher *understands* the communities terms of reference.

The initial contact with the communities focused upon information dissemination. Group discussions with the communities allowed a free-flow form of attitudinal research which didn't restrict community members to the structured ideas of the project workers. The reasons for adopting this strategy of participative research were–

- That the community's knowledge of their circumstances and their understanding of their needs for services vary from one community to another. Open discussions allow these differences in service needs to become clear. Only this way can clear user-driven needs be identified.
- That a high proportion of the individuals in the community have very little exposure to new technology and so a lot of ground work has to be done in terms of developing people's perception of multimedia and what technical facilities the Barbara unit will have. Once the technological capabilities of multimedia are understood, it allows the communities to put forward suggestions for services.
- That the community's understanding of what services are available is not comprehensive and so the possibilities need to be raised and discussed.

FIGURE 1. Involving the community in the development of the project.

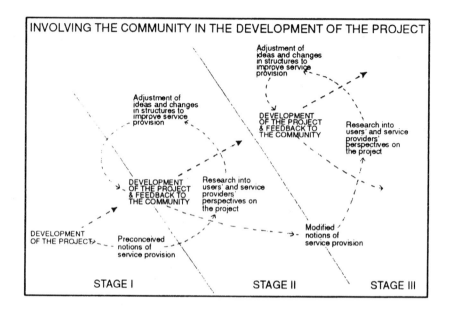

A combination of inductive, group discussion work with the support of more structured questioning was used to research into users' service requirements. Questionnaires used in isolation from less structured forms of questioning in the initial stages of the project risked reflection of the researcher's bias rather than the ideas extant in the community. The approach taken to information gathering in the project is an iterative process, building upon previous work and giving an informed background to structured questioning. This is in contrast to the snap-shot style of research, asking questions once in one place. The research will be participative, feeding knowledge back into the research process (see Figure 1). Participative research also allows local communities to feel involved in the whole project from the beginning so that local people can have a real input into the type of information and services and their style of presentation on the tele-unit.

RESEARCH INTO USER REQUIREMENTS

The users of the tele-unit in the Highlands are the end-users in the community and the service providers working for the public administration and other public services. Contact was made with both groups to determine the user requirements in terms of services and facilities on the tele-unit. At the outset of the project, contact was made with service providers, both within the Regional Council and with other organisations (for example Aberdeen University and the Benefits Agency). When the list of potential sites was decided, contacts were made with the "users" in the test sites. Initial contact was made with Community Councils, local Head teachers, Community Education Workers and through these contacts other individuals were networked.

The aims of the initial meetings were:

- to promote the idea of Barbara as a Region-wide pilot in tele-communications
- to identify the types of services that could be provided over the Barbara unit
- to identify the service providers who are interested in providing a service through the Barbara terminal
- to assess local needs in terms of services, and to determine how Barbara could meet some of those needs
- to open lines of communication between the project workers and the community so that there is a constant dialogue during the development, installation, monitoring and evaluation stages of the project
- to set up a local platform of users which will act as the forum for comments from the community and for the project workers to disseminate information to the local community.

RESULTS

The following are the initial results from the questionnaires distributed to the community group meetings. The tele-unit questionnaire was designed to assess how community members contacted the Regional Council and what services they would be most interested in using through the tele-unit. The respondents to the tele-unit questionnaire, ranked the following services as being the most useful (from the most useful down):

1. Information on welfare benefits
2. Distance learning (including training of unemployed people)

3. Access to community education for community groups
4. Access to library catalogues for both leisure and study
5. General and personalised information on the newly introduced council tax
6. Advertising Highland Region Council job vacancies
7. Face-to-face meetings with Divisional Council Officials (i.e., Planning)
8. Out of office hours emergency contacts
9. Conferencing facilities
10. Access to museum information.

Information on welfare benefits is the highest ranked service, identified by 93% (N = 59) of the respondents as being very useful. Distance-learning and training are the second most useful facilities, attracting positive responses from 86% (N = 59) of the respondents. Other positive responses to services include: access to library catalogues (78%); quicker access to library books (71%); general and personalised access to council tax information (75%); advertising of jobs (76%); meetings with development officers on business development and grants (75%); access to information for community groups (76%); and conferencing facilities for remote staff and community groups (70%).

SERVICES

Details of the services which could be offered by the Regional Council Departments were collected through a questionnaire and through meetings with central and divisional officers. Although the Highland Regional Council is providing the bulk of the facilities for Barbara, there are other services which have been requested by community members and could be made available through the unit:

• Benefits Agency
• District Council services
• Housing officers
• Environmental health
• Access to Aberdeen University library catalogue
• Access to distance-learning courses, through organisations such as the Open University and Aberdeen University
• Community information and bulletin board of local events
• Tourist information
• A facility to connect community groups across the Region using audio-visual links

TELE-UNIT

The tele-unit questionnaire was designed to assess how people felt about the prototype technology that was being demonstrated in the community meetings, and how they would feel about using this technology to access council services. An early prototype tele-unit was taken to a couple of community group meetings, and the different facilities were demonstrated, so that people who were inexperienced in terms of computers and technology could have the opportunity to comment on the ease of use of the equipment, but also so that they could become more familiar with the different technology.

CONCLUSION

It has become apparent that the remote communities are very interested in education, distance-learning and training for employment. Related to the interest in education is a desire for better access to library services and to distance-learning networks such as the Aberdeen University network. Welfare benefits information also ranked very high for community members. People needing benefits often do not know where to get the information and do not like to approach other community members for the information because of the fear of divulging their financial status to the community, and this was often given as a reason for wanting more anonymous contact with officials through the tele-unit.

In most cases the communities asked for services and information that could be made available through the tele-unit. Limitations were set by technical capabilities and cost implications. Taking a simulator of the tele-unit out to communities raised a great deal of interest. A high percentage of the community liked the idea of seeing an official on the videophone, although a number of respondents were less happy about being seen by the official over the videophone. Features such as options for: enlarged text, detailed explanations on screen, a panic or "help" button and a "cancel" command, were found to be desirable on the tele-unit, although detailed explanation by tape-recorded voice was not as popular.

Of the group of community members who tested the equipment, only one third used a computer every day, while just under a half used them "sometimes." From the research on the tele-unit simulator, it was found that despite initial fears from some community members about the difficulties of working with technology, after the demonstration of the equipment and what it could achieve, many of the fears were replaced by cautious interest. For those community members who were more familiar with computer technology, there was active interest in what could be achieved through the technology, especially in terms of services which could be accessed through the tele-unit, even beyond the remit of the original tele-counter.

REFERENCES

Bruyn, S.T. (1966). *"The human perspective: the methodology of participant observation,"* Prentice Hall, Englewood Cliffs, New Jersey.

Evans, M. (1988). "Participant observation: the researcher as a research tool" in Eyles, J. and Smith D.M. (eds.) *"Qualitative methods in Human Geography,"* p197-218, Polity Press.

Jacobs, G. (ed) (1970). *"The Participant Observer,"* George Braziller, New York.

Outhwaite, N. (1975). *"Understanding social life: the method called 'Verstehen,'"* Allen and Unwin, London.

Sack, R.D. (1980). *"Conceptions of Space in Social Thought: A Geographic Perspective,"* Macmillan Press, New York.

Sellitz, C., Jahoda, M., Deutsch, M. and Cook, S. (1959). *"Research Methods in Social Relations,"* Holt, Reinhart and Winston, New York.

Silverman, D. (1986). "Six rules of qualitative methods" in J. Eyles (ed), *"Qualitative approaches in social and geographical research,"* Queen Mary College, Dept of Geography and Earth Science, Occasional Paper 26.

Spradley, J.P. (1980). *"Participant Observation,"* Holt, Reinhart and Winston, New York.

Computer Access for People with Special Needs

Harald Weber
Gerhard Zimmermann
Klaus Zink

SUMMARY. To maximize the accessibility of computers for people with special needs (such as people with handicaps), fundamental changes in the design of the user-computer interface are necessary. The support of user-adapted input devices or techniques and of a multi-sensitive communication embedded in the computer's operating system will be presented. For this, basic models will be shown to describe the user-computer-software system. An analysis of the

---

Harald Weber (dipl.-Inform.) is a member of the Research Institute for Technology and Work in Germany and works at the University of Kaiserslautern. His main fields of professional interest are in vocational rehabilitation and computer-supported (basic) communication.

Gerhard Zimmermann (Prof. Dr. rer.nat.) holds the Chair of VLSI-Design and Architecture at the University of Kaiserslautern. His main fields of research interests are in special purpose computer architectures, high-level synthesis (he developed MIMOLA), layout synthesis, hierarchical design methodologies and in CAD frameworks.

Klaus Zink (Prof. Dr. habil.) holds the Chair for Industrial Management and Human Factors at the University of Kaiserslautern. His main fields of interest are in new forms of work organization (work structuring, organizational development), ergonomic aspects of new technologies, and Quality Management.

Address correspondence to: Harald Weber, Forschungsstelle Technologie und Arbeit, Univerisitaet Kaiserslautern, Gottlieb-Daimler Str., 67663 Kaiserslautern, Germany.

[Haworth co-indexing entry note]: "Computer Access for People with Special Needs." Weber, Harald, Gerhard Zimmermann, and Klaus Zink. Co-published simultaneously in *Computers in Human Services* (The Haworth Press, Inc.) Vol. 12, No. 1/2, 1995, pp. 151-168; and: *Human Services in the Information Age* (ed: Jackie Rafferty, Jan Steyaert, and David Colombi) The Haworth Press, Inc., 1995, pp. 151-168. Single or multiple copies of this article are available from The Haworth Document Delivery Service [1-800-342-9678, 9:00 a.m. - 5:00 p.m. (EST)].

151

user's capabilities and the requirements of both software and devices leads to supporting tools that will be implemented by an installation unit. This package of tools will act as an intermediary between the operating system and every application. *[Article copies available from The Haworth Document Delivery Service: 1-800-342-9678.]*

INTRODUCTION

The influence of computers in private life and in public situations or workplaces as an important tool is continuously growing. Major efforts were made by developers to develop user friendly software, but most of the results are still based on an assumed *standard user*. Individual needs of users are not incorporated. So many potential users will be excluded from the use of computers because of some mental, physical, or other limitation. This group of users is called *people with special needs* (especially people with disabilities and elderly people).

In contrast to the standard user, who is using computers to solve problems more efficiently, the value of computer support for elderly or handicapped people is of another dimension. Limited capabilities can be supplemented or lost capabilities can be replaced by soft- and hardware tools. The user gains from having more independence and greater opportunity to create an individual life. Moreover people with an adequate technological support would have better vocational opportunities, one of the most important steps to physical and economic independence, as well as a positive influence on the user's self-esteem.

The increase in the number of computers used in public life enforces the improvement of accessibility to computer supported services. While computer use in private life is based on everyone's own decision, its use in public places is becoming common and inevitable because of a steady decrease of personal services. This causes a loss of independence if those services are not accessible for all target groups. Existing software solutions often lack a concept to cover the entire use of computers instead of just one single aspect. Some of these disadvantages are–

- the need for support to start applications from a standard user operating system
- inefficient use of resources (specially adapted computers) because of inaccessibility to other, differently-abled users.
- no, or less, support of interaction with other software
- stigmatising of users because of implemented "special" software.

In the following we present a concept based on a user-model which incorporates skills and capabilities of a person. The entities are the guidelines during implementation of tools to support other I/O (in/out) devices (other than screen, mouse and keyboard), to support the handling of these devices, and to support people with different skills and needs.

ACCESSIBLE DESIGN

Accessible design describes the process that leads to or improves accessibility. In former times it was just focused on access to buildings. Today it is transferred to topics like access to information, services, products, or social categories. To avoid inaccessibility of products it is necessary to follow some basic rules during the design process " . . . to include people who, because of personal characteristics or environmental conditions, find themselves on the low end of some dimension of performance (e.g., seeing, hearing, reaching, manipulating) . . . " (Vanderheiden, 1992; see also Thorén, 1993).

Besides opportunities to modify products or to provide extensions, *direct* access through design changes seems to be the preferable way. Especially for software products, a change in design causes no, or small, additional expenses for the producer but may enlarge the group of possible users. These products even stay accessible in situations where no modification or connection of external supporting tools is possible (such as computers at public places). Another very important reason to pursue direct access is the avoidance of stigmatization because of the supporting tool's implementation as a standard option of the product. In this paper we will pay attention to the special needs of people with handicaps, elderly people and sick people.

- *People with handicaps* should be subdivided into the groups of people with physical, cognitive or sensitive impairments. People with *physical impairments* will have most problems in handling input devices or removable storage media. *Blind* or *visually-impaired people* often cannot recognize the computer's output. The wide spread of pointing devices for input excludes more and more visually-impaired people from the use of computers. People with *hearing impairments* or who are *deaf* have less problems. The provision of audio signals in a visual presentation seems to be sufficient. Last, some people are extremely *sensitive to visual, auditive or tactile irritation*; for example frequencies of flashing light between 10 and 25 Hertz can cause severe irritation. People with *cognitive limitations* or who are *learning disabled* have problems with understanding the software itself or with the labelling of keys. It seems not to be sufficient to support these people just with additional software tools, a whole change in the application's concept is inevitable.

- *Elderly people* may have some physical limitations or learning disabilities. They may profit from those tools which are implemented for people with handicaps. Avoidance of stigmatization seems to be a very important aspect for elderly people.
- People may have *accidents or diseases* and as a result of that they may be limited in some important function. To continue their job or other tasks where computers are needed, similar supporting techniques as for physically handicapped persons are required.

The knowledge of the special needs of these additional target groups lead to some basic design rules for software and hardware. Once again we will distinguish between physical, sensory, and cognitive aspects (Vanderheiden, 1992).

Physical Aspects

To handle a computer with its input and output devices and its storage media it is important to–

- design adjustable timed actions
- provide sequential alternatives to simultaneous actions
- provide techniques to simulate keyboard or pointing device inputs
- provide techniques to distinguish unintentional inputs from inputs made on purpose
- design important switches that are accessible (position, form and usage)
- provide soft- and hardware connection points for use of specially adapted I/O devices.

Sensory Aspects

To recognize the computer's output, to handle input devices, or to avoid seizures it is important to–

- enable enlargement of visual or amplification of audio output
- transform visual output to an audio form and reverse
- provide alternatives to eye dependant input devices
- make display colours adjustable

- provide software and hardware connection points for use of specially adapted output devices
- avoid some audio and visual frequencies during output.

Cognitive Aspects

To enable an understanding of the use of computers and software products it is important to–

- provide clear and simple, non-cryptic outputs
- allow intuitive actions, which invoke corresponding operations
- not overload the user's short-term memory
- emphasize important information
- provide an undo-mechanism for all operations
- organise menus in a way that often-used items can be reached in a few steps and rarely used items in more steps
- provide information in different forms at a time, so that each channel of presentation supports the understanding of the output's meaning
- provide clear helping instructions.

Not all of these cognitive aspects can be measured, so evidence is relative. The main goal is to progressively lower the cognitive level of the software–to provide easy handling techniques and to support understanding. It should be noted that none of the above lists is complete, but they give some basic guidelines.

MODELLING THE HUMAN COMPUTER SYSTEM

In the following we identify software tools that support the users in accessing standard software even if they cannot handle a keyboard or a mouse or cannot see the visual output. For this we have to create a model of the user, of the I/O devices, and of the software. A complete description of the models and its structure can be found in Weber (1993, pp. 24-46).

User-Model

The user-model tries to quantify physical, sensory or cognitive aspects of a user. Obviously it is impossible to make this description complete so that it describes all aspects of a person. We will try to build the model complete in respect to the handling of human-computer systems. The measure of aspects which result in numbers should be done by a program, all other aspects by the person himself or herself or by a care person. The results will be used to identify tendencies such as hearing impairments or slow reaction. The model is divided into the description of physical, sensory and cognitive capabilities.

Physical capabilities. To handle an input device a certain workspace is needed. Every position inside this workspace should be reachable by the user without major effort. These positions called targets can be connected with special functions (such as keys of a keyboard). Every target has to be reachable to generate input codes. To measure the precision and range of a user the sizes of the workspace and the target area have to be analysed. The fine-movement is quantified by measuring how many steady different states can be held. The model incorporates minimal times to distinguish an unintentionally caused state (such as key press) from another state activated on purpose. Some sequences of action have to happen in a certain time. The maximum time duration to carry out such a sequence will also be fixed in the model and this shows the speed of reaction. The capability to articulate–independent of its understandability to a human being–will also be noticed.

Sensitive capabilities. Computer outputs can use human input channels (eyes, ears or feel) for communication. Visual capabilities can be separated into three parts: the capability to distinguish colours, light and dark, and to perceive shapes. *Limitations in hearing* and preferred frequency intervals describe the audio capabilities. Next to that *tactile sensibility* to read Braille or the capability to feel tactile graphics will be identified in the model.

Cognitive capabilities. It is almost impossible to quantify human capabilities in the field of cognition. Two groups of capabilities can be distinguished: general intellectual skills and the actual training level. *General intellectual skills* include the knowledge of common symbols, knowledge of foreign languages, understanding of audio or written messages, or the capability to follow instructions. The *actual training level* is characterized by the knowledge how to handle I/O media, the ability to undertake a session or to use different displayed objects (menus, objects, controls).

Device-Model

Dynamic properties. Devices for input or output have to be handled by the user. We try to model every step of this action for automatic analysis and implementation of supporting techniques to enable these steps. The whole input and output process can be expressed by a *flowchart* that describes every single step.

Static properties. Next to these dynamic aspects there are static properties of input and output devices. These properties describe aspects of perception, movement, timing and basic action in more detail. Input devices can be distinguished into several sorts of keyboards, pointing devices and speech recognition tools. Values for the extension of working and target areas are correlated with how the target area is perceived (visual, audio, tactile). Static properties are the extent of code, the hardware interface or the nature of feedback to users. For *output devices* the main criteria is the sensory channel used. Several ways to present information are marked for every channel (such as visual output: alpha-numeric, pictures, colours).

Software-Model

Dynamic properties. Every standard software has a similar basic concept which can be described as an input-execute-output loop ("read-evaluate-print"). During program execution it may be very helpful for the user to know what the actual state of loop–whether the computer is waiting for an input or whether an evaluation or output operation is in process.

Static properties. Most software products can be classified by their goals. Software is available to communicate, to work, to organize, to simulate, to demonstrate, to train, to entertain, or to support. A program may fit into different classes, but no statement about its quality or level of difficulty is made. We also try to classify software by its level of difficulty.

Low claim	Institutional use (computer controlled session). Example: simple games
Moderate claim	Knowledge of basic handling techniques, rules, and courses (computer controlled session). Example: simple training software
Medium claim	Capability to plan a session (user controlled session). Example: training software, simple word processing
Raised claim	Creativity; capability to plan a complex session (user controlled session). Example: complex word and graphic processing
High claim	Wide background knowledge about computers; creativity; capability to plan a complex session (user controlled session). Example: authoring systems, programming environments

SUPPORTING TECHNIQUES

Human-Computer Interface

Today's standard *hardware configuration* of a computer system includes a keyboard and a mouse, trackerball, or joystick for input, a monitor with a built-in loudspeaker for output, and the computer itself. Most software supports just these input and output devices. Certain requirements to the skills of a user are connected with this configuration.

Input requirements. To handle a keyboard, a user has to be able to hit one or more keys at a time without a tremble and with a high precision because of small keys. Also the user has to recognize the keyboard status–the status of the SHIFT-, SCROLL- or NUM LOCK-key (often provided in a visual form). The use of a mouse demands even more precision to place or move it. The capability to recognize the visual feedback of the pointer on the screen is necessary. Next to the movement there are one or more keys on the mouse to launch several operations on displayed objects. To use these keys similar skills are required as for the use of keys on a keyboard–high precision without any tremble. The double-click action–a sequence of two key operations in a certain time–requires a precise and timed control of movements.

Output requirements. The screen as a visual output media requires the capability to see the displayed information. The tendency to overload screen outputs decreases the size of characters and symbols more and more. To read written outputs it is necessary to have normal vision. Different colours are often used to point out important information. The user has to be able to distinguish those colours to avoid missing important messages. Loudspeakers are often used to produce certain signals to make the user notice some input faults, events, or results. The capability to hear these signals is necessary if no other indication (in a visual presentation) is provided. Next to these physical and sensitive aspects there are cognitive requirements. The user has to know the order of input actions (set pointer, type command, acknowledge with ENTER), the required input format (numbers, characters, commands), or the dependence between mouse moves and the movement of the screen pointer. The requirements during output depend on its complexity, the ability to read and understand.

Two goals should be followed in designing the *software interface* (Balzert, 1987, pp. 477-488). First, support of communication between the user and the computer should be achieved. Possible ways are to offer similar or well-known communication factors (such as desktops with files, pencils and waste-paper-baskets) or considering the user's intuition (for example moving a file on the waste-paper-basket will delete the file). Second, supporting human information processing should be taken into account. This means not overloading short-term memory, providing different perspectives of the same information, preferably in a multi-sensory format, or providing helpful instructions to maintain the user's awareness. These goals can only be achieved by changing software concepts.

Support is required at different levels of input and output actions. First, the simulation of keyboard and mouse input needs software support, if no alternative hardware realization is available. This level is called *device support*. Second, depending on the skills of a person, devices may be unusable because of some limitation. These limitations could be supplemented with so called *handling support* techniques. Third, a level of *user support* techniques speed up, simplify, or explain input and output actions. Figure 1 illustrates the three levels of support.

The two bottom levels (device and handling support) are sufficient to reach our goal called "direct access" for people with physical or sensitive limitations. The user support level contains additional features to avoid tedious input actions or to speed up input. As noted earlier it is nearly impossible to support people with mental disabilities without changing software concepts. Nevertheless, some supporting techniques could be implemented in the user support level next to provide help mechanisms for inexperienced computer users. In the following we describe some general techniques for every level, separated into input and output aspects.

INPUT

Device Support

Scanner. A scanner displays a field of keys on a screen or presents it in an audio form. Keys can represent standard keys on a keyboard, whole input actions, predefined strings, or pseudo-commands to control other support tools or output formats. The scanning technique is used to simulate a standard keyboard via an input media with a small extent of code. The user selects a key using any input device or acknowledges a suggestion (highlighted key) made by the scanner (Figure 2).

Conversion table. This kind of tool is a standard feature of every computer, because input codes have to be translated into standard codes (e.g., ASCII). We will extend this translation technique from a plain code-to-code translation into the translation from code into

a. codes (as before)
b. macros (often-used commands can be abbreviated)
c. scanner commands (for movement of the selection cursor)

d. output commands (loudness, enlargement factor)
e. commands to change the state of the input device (e.g., upper-case).

Speech recognition tool. The problems of speech recognition can be handled by software and by hardware. Most tools have an existing spelling function which is sufficient for keyboard simulation. The training phase can be used to connect spoken words with characters, words, sequences of actions, or pseudo-commands (similar to the conversion table).

FIGURE 1: Levels of support.

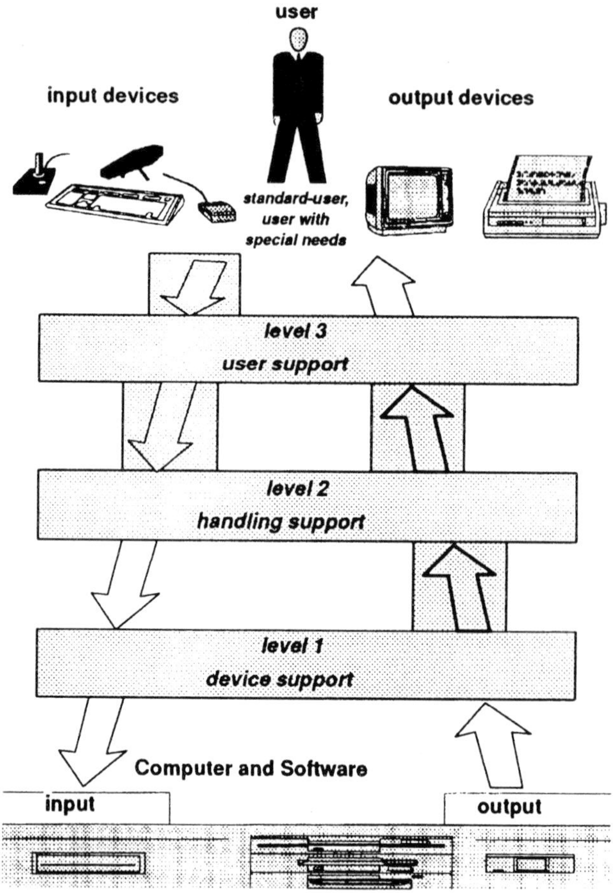

FIGURE 2: Scanner display (block selection technique).

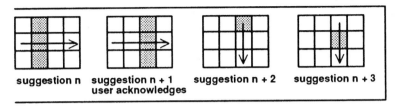

suggestion n   **suggestion n + 1**   **suggestion n + 2**   **suggestion n + 3**
                user acknowledges

Handling Support

Keyboard handling. Despite the general ability to push buttons a user may not be able to use a keyboard in all aspects. To generate all possible codes it is necessary to be able to push more than one key at a time. For those users who cannot realize this simultaneous action, software support is necessary to push buttons sequentially (see Novak et al., 1992; *Sticky-Keys*). If the user has problems in hitting a key precisely, some keys may be unintentionally pressed on the way to the target area. An unintentionally pressed key can be separated from the desired key by its depressed time (see Novak et al., 1992; *SlowKeys*).

If a user trembles, many inputs can be produced instead of just one. This unintentional input can be avoided by using a minimum time between the input of equal codes inside a filter (see Novak et al., 1992; *Bounce-Keys*). If the user has slow reaction a key may be pressed for a longer time. This may invoke the auto-repeat function, that repeats the input code until the button is released. To avoid these unintentional produced codes the auto-repeat function should be switched off or its time until invocation should be adjustable (see Novak et al., 1992; *Repeatkeys*). As noted earlier keyboards may have different states displayed in a visual form. One way to allow non-visual access is to produce different sounds when using modifying keys, for example a rising sound to indicate active states and a deepening sound to indicate inactive states (see Novak et al., 1992; *ToggleKeys*).

Mouse handling. Depending on the user's capabilities or the connected input device the mouse keys may be unusable. For this we have to provide a mechanism to simulate–

- a single key operation (*"click"*)
- a double key operation (*"double click"*)
- a press, move and release sequence (*"dragging"*).

A certain field for every operation should be displayed on the screen. If the user moves the pointer into one of these fields and remains there for a minimum time, the function will be enabled. Then, the user has to move the pointer to the desired location and remain there for another time, until the operation will be executed. In case of dragging, another move of the pointer and remaining is necessary.

User Support

Predictor. Scanner input may be very time consuming compared with standard keyboard input. Also, if the user has to make major physical efforts to produce input codes, some speeding mechanism is desirable. Predictors are very helpful to complete unfinished inputs using a vocabulary created during earlier sessions. Words will be suggested that were used most often previously.

Object-finder. Graphic user interfaces often depend on the intensive use of pointing devices. If those devices have to be simulated the result is not satisfying because of a pixel-oriented movement support. In many situations high-precision movement is unnecessary because only a few objects on the screen can be used. For example, the operating system interface displays windows, menus, controls and objects (Figure 3). The object-finder places the pointer at every symbol controlled by one or more input codes. This scanning method speeds up the choice and relieves the user from tedious input sequences. For blind users this method allows access to graphic inter-

FIGURE 3: Object-finder.

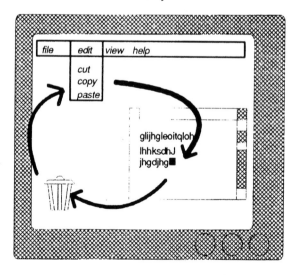

faces if, next to this scanning, the name of the symbol is provided in an audio form.

Input control. For inexperienced computer users, often it is not obvious when inputs are expected or whether the computer is busy with a lengthy operation. Incomplete inputs make the user believe everything is done, whereas the computer is waiting for completion. To distinguish this waiting state from a busy state it is helpful to indicate it to the user.

Display alternatives. This tool assembles possible actions as a menu, i.e., it provides actions, even if its invocation depends on pointing device inputs, in a textual form. The display of alternatives has two main goals. First, the strong link between input actions and pointing devices will be weakened. (What is looking like a step back in development may enable better access for visually-impaired people to computers.) Second, it is possible to hide an operation behind this menu by not taking it up into the menu's item list. This allows us to assemble a user- or task-adapted selection of operations.

OUTPUT

Device Support

Device support is necessary only where other non-visual sensory channels are used. If alongside audio hints, speech is used for output, a text-to-speech converter is necessary. The transformation is a simple 1:1 link possibly extended by some additional information about the format (such as style, start of paragraph). Similarly a text-to-Braille converter is needed, if a Braille line as output media is used. Different kinds of Braille allow incorporation of additional information about the style of each character.

Handling Support

As every different output media may require its own handling support techniques, a general discussion is not possible. Both tools which are explained are focused only on screen outputs. People with visual impairments may be able to recognise a screen output, if its content is enlarged. A great variety of screen-enlarger hardware is available but we plead for software solutions because of lower costs and easier handling. The user just has to change into enlargement mode, all further movements on the screen are controlled by movements of the pointing device. To support people with problems in distinguishing colours, a tool to access and change colour registers is necessary. Through changes in the brightness of colours, the user can adapt the output to their own needs.

User Support

Two supporting tools help the user to over"see" the content of the screen even if he or she is visually-impaired or blind. If Braille lines are used, some method to navigate through a screen page should be provided, for example different keys to scroll a line, paragraph, or page in any direction. Audio output also requires feedback for navigation with provision of *Play, Stop,* or *Rewind* functions, similar to a tape recorder. To support human information processing, information should be provided in different perspectives and in multi-sensory formats. Information can be presented in different formats inside one sensory channel (Table 1).

Control Unit

The problem of enabling access to computers can be divided into sub-problems. The question has to be answered how the system builds up an

TABLE 1: Information formats.

channel of sense	presentation	comment
visual	text	
	numbers	
	pictures	incl. animation, videos, etc.
audio	noise	
	music	
	speech	
tactile	pressure	only used to indicate binary states
	temperature	not used
	voltage	not used
	vibration	indication similar to audio signals
	shape	not used except for Braille output

actual configuration (a set of support tools with parameters) from given information. The separation of the configuration process into two general steps is shown in Figure 4. The *installation phase* assembles the support tools using the user- and device-model. The flow-chart of every device determines each step of transformation from the given data into software routines. At the end of this phase, a global configuration is created and the program code of the installation module is removed from memory just as soon as the runtime module that it created starts.

The second phase is called *runtime phase*. Its parameters are the soft-

FIGURE 4: Steps of configuration.

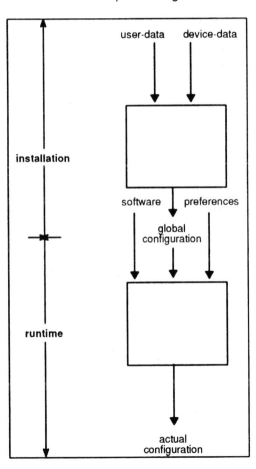

ware-model, user parameters (such as preferences created by output commands) and the global configuration. The former two input streams are variable during runtime, so they cannot be moved to the installation phase. The result of the runtime phase is the actual configuration. It changes with every newly started or finished program or every change of user defined parameters. The program code of the runtime unit remains in memory during the whole session.

Installation Unit

In this section we describe in general terms what happens during the installation phase. The first step is to analyse which input and output devices are connected. For each, a device-model must be available, which will be loaded. Next the user-model has to be loaded into memory. There are several ways to store and to identify the appropriate user-model depending on the context in which the computer will be used–if the computer is used by only a single person or if used by different (abled) persons.

The dynamic properties flowchart of the device-model controls the installation process. Every simple state can be attached to a module, which compares the requirements of the devices with the user's capabilities. Because every simple state of the flowchart was chosen out of a limited set of given states during the design of the device-models, this attachment is clear. Each module generates its own code as a part of the runtime process. In cases of several alternatives (which lead to the same goal) a weighting technique to calculate priorities will be implemented into each module. Preferences, capabilities, or special needs, marked in the user-model, influence the parameters of every module. The executable code for every selected tool will be taken from a tool-library and assembled and incorporated into a code frame. As a result this set of supporting tools and the code frame build up the executable runtime unit. After the code-generation is finished, the runtime unit has to be started and as its first action the installation unit program code has to be removed from memory.

Runtime Unit

One of the first actions after removal of the installation unit's code is to load the software-model of the operating system and to configure internal parameters, because the operating system is the first program the user will be in touch with (except auto-executing programs installed). Furthermore some user preferences recorded during former sessions will be loaded. These preferences will modify some input and output format parameters.

After this initiation phase the runtime unit will work as an intermediate piece between user and computer as described in Figure 5. Besides transformation of input and output signals, the change of some parameters (such as enlargement and colour set) during runtime will also be supported.

Following the guidelines of *direct access,* the whole concept must not be implemented as a "black box." Rather, many connection points in software should be provided for interaction between applications and supporting tools. This can be understood as an operating system extension that provides some general and some specific routines to allow access for people with special needs.

CONCLUSION

This work introduced concepts of how to enable or improve computer access for people with special needs. The basic idea to reach this goal was to model the user's capabilities and the requirements of the I/O devices and of the software. The matching of capabilities with requirements, as it happens in an installation unit, detects deficits and generates code that supplements functions which may be limited. In the case of lost functions, the system tries to change given actions for input and output in a way that the user's remaining capabilities will replace the lost function.

FIGURE 5: Communication model with an implemented runtime unit.

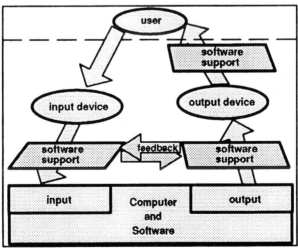

The above described concept is still theory. Some problems during implementation may occur where further inquiries have to be done: the installation process may lead to no result, the result may not please users because of tedious handling or unpleasant appearance, co-operation with operating system developers is necessary or other problems can arise. In difference to other supporting tools, this concept, based at an operating system level, will enable or improve access to software that was designed for the so called standard-user. This widening of the scope from just one program to the whole variety of available software gives an individual with special needs equal opportunities in relation to others.

During design of the user-model we tried to emphasize people's capabilities instead of description of people's incapabilities. *Incapability* is a matter of definition depending on the environment. Changes in the structure of the environment may enable actions that were impossible so far–incapabilities are not permanent properties, but general capabilities are.

The way in which this new concept should be implemented can be described as a modification at the operating system level. Existing operating systems are very powerful, but still lack accessing techniques for people with special needs. This situation of inaccessibility can be weakened via introduction of this concept and in many cases even be removed. However it still remains a long-range goal to change the concepts of operating systems and interfacing techniques. Its central statement is to allow multi-sensory access and to simplify computer handling in all aspects to make it a simple and powerful tool for everyone.

REFERENCES

Balzert, H. (1987). Gestaltungsziele der Software-Ergonomie. In Schoenpflug, W., & Wittstock, M. (Ed.), *Software-Ergonomie* (pp. 477-488). (in German)

Novak, M., Schauer, J., & Vanderheiden, G. (1992). *Access Pack for Microsoft Windows-User Guide* Revision 2.0 (pp. 6-13). The Trace Research and Development Center Madison, WI.

Thorén, C. (Ed.) (1993). *Nordic Guidelines for Computer Accessibility.* Nordiska Nämnden För Handikappfrågor: Stockholm.

Vanderheiden, G. C., & Vanderheiden, K. R. (1992). *Accessible Design of Consumer Products; Guidelines for the Design of Consumer Products to increase their Accessibility to People with Disabilities or who are Aging.* (Working Draft 1.7). University of Wisconsin-Madison.

Weber, H. (1993). *Computerzugang für Menschen mit besonderen Bedürfnissen-Entwurf eines Realisierungskonzeptes auf Softwarebasis* (pp. 24-46). Diploma thesis: Dept. of computer sciences, University of Kaiserslautern (in German).

The Evergreen, Software
for Planning Services for the Elderly

Marja Vaarama

SUMMARY. The Evergreen is a microsimulation computer program intended for strategic planning of welfare and health services for the elderly. The Evergreen software consists of a main file of about 200 variables (databank of services for the elderly), with four planning models added (the laissez-faire, normative, humanistic and economist model), together with a correcting and updating program. The program enables systematization of different policy strategies and their consequences in terms of the number of clients, the resources required for the service system in personnel, funds and room as well as in terms of costs both in total and per head. Primarily it is suited for local and national-level planning, but is also applicable to regional planning. The Evergreen is operable in IBM-compatible microcomputers with the absolute prerequisite of a hard disk with at least 5.9 megabytes of free memory for software files and operation. *[Article copies available from The Haworth Document Delivery Service: 1-800-342-9678.]*

WHAT IS THE EVERGREEN?

The Evergreen may be defined as computer software which produces information for planning at the trend level and renders possible creating

---

Marja Vaarama is Senior Planning Officer at the National Research and Development Centre for Welfare and Health (STAKES) in Helsinki.

[Haworth co-indexing entry note]: "The Evergreen, Software for Planning Services for The Elderly." Vaarama, Marja. Co-published simultaneously in *Computers in Human Services* (The Haworth Press, Inc.) Vol. 12, No. 1/2, 1995, pp. 169-178; and: *Human Services in the Information Age* (ed: Jackie Rafferty, Jan Steyaert, and David Colombi) The Haworth Press, Inc., 1995, pp. 169-178. Single or multiple copies of this article are available from The Haworth Document Delivery Service [1-800-342-9678, 9:00 a.m. - 5:00 p.m. (EST)].

169

alternative scenarios for service systems, with their respective logical development paths. In the area of welfare services for the elderly, the scope of this planning instrument is the total service needs. In the area of health services, the program enables planning of long-term in-patient as well as out-patient care in the primary health care sector, e.g., care in nursing homes, supervised home nursing and care in day hospitals.

The program enables systemization of different strategies for care policy and their consequences in terms of the number of clients, the resources required for the services system in personnel, funds and accommodation as well as in terms of costs both in total and per head. Primarily it is suited for local and national-level planning, but is also applicable to regional planning. So far fifty municipalities and eleven Provincial Boards in Finland have tested and used the program. According to their experiences, the planning philosophy of the Evergreen seems to be lasting, even if the practical application needs further developmental work.

BACKGROUND FOR DEVELOPING THE EVERGREEN

Before taking a closer look at this planning program, let us take a quick view on the Finnish policy for elderly care and at the forthcoming changes in it, which served as the basis for developing the program. Finland is a Scandinavian welfare state with a population of five million, 14% of whom are people aged over 65. Even if this proportion of elderly people is not yet particularly high when compared with other developed countries, there are remarkable differences among municipalities (ranging from 6% to 28%). During the next decades the proportion of elderly will rise very rapidly. It is estimated that in the year 2010 a fifth, and in 2030 a quarter of the country's population will have passed the age of 65 (CSO, 1989). According to these estimations, the number of persons aged over 80 years is going to increase about 200% between the years 1990 and 2030. Even if the process is not a linear one, ageing of the population will tend to increase the need and demand for welfare and health services.

Finland's planning and regulating mechanisms have recently undergone a widespread change and state control has been dismantled. The responsibility for providing welfare and health services has been devolved further to the municipalities. The state still has the most powerful regulating tool, the state subsidies system, but from the beginning of 1993, the municipal authorities have both the power and the duty to make decisions about how to use the state subsidies. Services for senior citizens are regulated by a legal framework with extensive powers for the municipal authorities to determine practical details of the services. Until recently the public sector has been the principal body providing both services for the elderly and the funding of these services from tax revenues. At present there is a tendency to reorganize the municipality's role from that of a provider of services to that of a provider of funds, as well as the tendency towards introduction of market forces into welfare and health services.

The average scope and standard of welfare and health services for the elderly has until recently been regarded to be at quite a reasonable level, but demands for changing the institution-based care system are strong. According to research, elderly people themselves want to live at their own homes as long as possible, supported by community care if necessary (e.g., Sihvo, 1991). Furthermore almost half of all elderly persons now in institutions would do well in a more open type of care or even at home, provided services were available (Vaarama, 1992). Also the present economic recession in the country places economic limits in continuing the institution-based service policy in the care of the elderly (Ministry of Social Affairs and Health, 1992; Vaarama, 1993).

Thus, both the planning of services for the elderly and the balance of care are in need of restructuring. In this process the local decision-makers will need better judgement than previously when using the diminishing resources to maintain a stable policy for elderly care in the long-term. Local planning practices and especially attitudes in elderly policy ought to change towards increased awareness of the needs of the elderly and the efficiency of the servicing system. A passive approach to planning needs to be replaced by goal-orientated and creative planning involving not only the "planners" and decision making bodies, but also the welfare and health professionals as well as elderly people themselves.

These developments made the basis for the previous National Board of Welfare in Finland, now STAKES, initiating a wide-scope elderly policy project in collaboration with thirty-seven municipalities and eleven Provincial Boards. This project, implemented from 1989 to 1992, aimed at finding solutions and strategic approaches applicable to the changing situations. One of the achievements of this very project was the Evergreen, a planning software.

THE PLANNING PHILOSOPHY OF THE EVERGREEN

The main task of the Evergreen was to support the performance of the elderly policy project by making it possible to draw up quantitative scenarios for future policies of the care of the aged. It aimed also at improving the information basis and methods of planning by correcting the shortcomings below, which were identified at the beginning of the project:

- information existed, but it was dispersed and not easily available
- data relating to client or age groups or costs were difficult to find
- planning of elderly services was based more on the needs of the system than on those of the clients
- planning was mostly on a one-year basis, lacking creative and active elements
- quantitative and qualitative planning were separated from each other
- coordination of service planning, even within welfare and health sectors, was lacking
- clients and mostly also employees, were not participating in the planning procedure at all

It can be said that the Evergreen arose from a vision which was both practical and ideological. It was practical in wishing to develop the existing incoherent and awkward planning apparatus, to endow it with new types of instruments which also might motivate a systematic gathering of data, seeking alternatives and improving cooperation between welfare and health fields.

Its idealistic side was the attempt to introduce into planning activities a new kind of philosophy: dynamism, openness, debate about values, goals and needs. The Evergreen aimed at making human needs, subjective factors and alternatives in planning visible. It aimed at diminishing the concealed subjectivity in planning by bringing into the open definitions and basic presumptions of each model, exposing them to debate and criticism. It also aimed at encouraging efforts towards cooperation and creativity by revealing the different results from different choices, and by reminding of possibilities to influence the future by means of planning. Consequently, the Evergreen represents a voluntaristic idea of the future: this is not driftwood but the result of conscious human choices (cf. Cole, 1976; Wilson, 1978).

In planning services, problems arise mainly in defining needs and in measuring these. Usually we refer to normative, experienced, expressed and comparative needs, which in part are overlapping (Bradshaw, 1977). In the Evergreen the concept of need is viewed also from other standpoints than using the definitions of expressed or normative needs traditional to public planning. Thus, each of the four planning models in the software represents a different approach to the client's needs, rendering possible choosing the approach most convenient to the planner's own attitudes or to the collective standpoint for planning services for the elderly in the respective state, region, municipality, planning office, etc.

EQUIPMENT REQUIREMENTS OF THE EVERGREEN

The Evergreen is operable in IBM-compatible microcomputers, preferably equipped with 286, 386 or 486 central processing units. There has to be a DOS 3.0 operating system or a higher version, and the computer has to possess 640 kilobytes of random access memory (RAM). An absolute prerequisite is a hard disk with at least 5.9 megabytes (MB) of free memory for software files and operation. The software with files take 5.3 megabytes of hard disk memory, and furthermore about 900 kilobytes are used as paging memory during operation. In addition, the models recorded take 10-15 kilobytes of memory each, and the output files recorded 20-40 kilobytes each. Thus, at least 6.8 megabytes of free memory have to be available on the hard disk for the installation and operation of the Evergreen, if using the whole volume of the basic file in the planning (national, regional, local). If using the Evergreen only in planning of one municipality, the capacity needed is much less.

Performing output or graphics on paper is done using other software in the work station, and output equipment. For this purpose, in output modes the software uses one of the three common recording softwares, ASCII, Lotus or Excel. Implementation of the software has been made using the APL*PLUS application generator of the STSC. However the user does not need any skills in APL when using the program.

THE MAIN FILE AND THE UPDATING PROGRAM

The main file consists of data considered essential for planning the welfare and health services for the elderly at the national/regional/municipal macro level. These include data on the population age structure based on population projections of the CSO, and data on the present services system such as the use of services, numbers of personnel and available beds, and expenses incurred. These are summarized data from municipal databases. It is also possible to feed a municipality's own population projections into the main file. The main file serves both as an independent key file for reporting and analyzing the state of art of the services for the elderly, and as a file for the use of the planning models.

Data is recorded in the main file by use of the correcting and updating program. The basic data in a display has been received from the annual report system of the state. In this program segment, the stored data can be corrected, and one's own population projections as well as a new data recorded.

THE PLANNING MODELS

The software includes four planning models for the planning of services for the elderly: the laissez-faire model, the normative model, the humanist model, and the economist model. All these models are operating by use of the same concepts: needs, resources, services, costs. The laissez-faire model and the normative model are based on the existing services system, the humanist model is proceeding from needs, and the economic model from available resources.

The laissez-faire model and the normative model are deterministic, linear planning models. In these, the decisive factor is the development of the number of elderly persons. The humanist model and the economic one are dynamic models, which offer ample prospects for creation of alternative services systems. These two are open models in which the user defines almost all the factors: needs, services system, resources, costs, and policy regarding to the charges. Because it is just the user with his/her planning team who determines the data to be fed into these models, the humanist and economic models are the most challenging ones in the Evergreen. The use of these two planning models presupposes high expertise in elderly care, as also willingness to put in planning more efforts than the small trouble of "pushing a button."

The laissez-faire model (or the driftwood model) is based on the logic of expressed needs of services, e.g., on the statistics of the service utilization. The model describes the future development of clients, room, personnel and costs if only the change in the number of elderly persons is taken into account. The service structure and the utilization rate for services are kept on the current level and cannot be influenced. Thus, this model is a tool for a tendency planning.

The normative model is based on the logic of normative needs, e.g., the needs determined by the experts, politicians or researchers. In this model the services system will be given target values according to the above need definitions. The software makes annual linear transformations to the effect that the values will reach the given rate of targets at the predetermined year. Thus, this model is a tool for a normative planning.

The humanist model is characterized as humanistic because it proceeds from wide understanding of needs and aims to build up the model of elderly care, fitting best to the needs existing in different groups of elderly people with different dependency rates.

In defining needs the starting point is the age structure of elderly population. Proceeding from this, the total is divided into smaller units by determining percentages of elderly people needing help round-the-clock, part-day, weekly and occasionally. On basis of the above, services system will be determined. Each separate group will receive its own services combination composed of percentages indicating the proportions of different service types satisfying the group's needs. After that the resources needed and the average unit costs in each service form are to be determined. When these development paths are defined, results such as future expenditure costs can be observed and further changes can be made. A prepared model can be stored and subsequently altered. Thus, this model is a tool for need-orientated planning.

This model is the most dynamic of all models discussed here, as all its factors can be changed. Using this model the user can construct alternative services system models and speculate about different need developments and respective service systems, policies regarding to the charges, cost trends, efficiency of service production, etc. There are innumerable possibilities to develop different alternatives, which is why this model is most challenging to its user. The best results are achieved when using this model stepwise in a collaborative process involving the planning team consisting of welfare and health professionals as well as politicians and service users.

The model does not indicate the proportions of public and private sectors. The model only aims at very carefully defining the existing needs and the best suited respective services system, without taking a stand on the mode of services production. The model anyhow classifies persons needing services in a primary and a secondary group. Consequently, considerations of action strategies on the basis of this model might also take a stand on questions like division of service production between the public, the private and the voluntary sectors. This can be simulated by use of the economic model.

The economic model proceeds from the total of resources which make the marginal conditions of future development. According to the model idea, the user defines at the very outset the framework of available resources. On this basis the software then calculates the amount of needs for services which can be satisfied by these resources, and also the expenses to be incurred.

Using the economic model it is possible to seek and find a services system alternative with an appropriate level of needs satisfaction possible in the limits of available resources. This model enables the same types of speculation as the humanist model. Because the basis of an economic model is always the previously constructed humanist model, the model also renders possible coming out of the numbers of those in need excluded from services in different alternatives. This, understandably, is most important for the follow-up analyses.

The program enables also "the game for an active planner," as it is called. This "game" is aimed at an optimization of available resources in relation to existing needs. The usual way to "play this game" is to start with using the humanist model to build up an ideal model. On this, the economic model will be applied with the view of constructing a practical action model based on the limited resources available. Thus, this model can be labelled as a tool for resource-orientated, dynamic planning.

THE CALCULATION PRINCIPLES OF THE SOFTWARE

On the basis of the data recorded in the main file, the software calculates proportioning of services to population, to number of available beds, and other parameters. The years in the planning term have to be the same as the years of the population projections. Up to 2000 any year may be selected. From the year 2000 models can be constructed on a five-year basis.

The calculation rules in laissez-faire and normative models include presumptions of utilization intensity (number of clients/place/year) of different places, enabling use of these values in calculating numbers of clients. In humanist's and economic's models the user defines these values. Overlapping use has not been reduced from the number of clients, as this would be most difficult, lacking reliable research results. Consequently, numbers of clients indicate the total "servicing capacity" or the total activity volume of the respective services system.

The software cost calculation gives the trend of cost development in each separate model. In the laissez-faire model the cost calculation is performed on the basis of the present situation, while in other models it is done by the use of average costs per unit (home help hour, care day, operation day, investment costs/place). The effects of under-utilization are not taken into account in cost calculations. Even if this makes the cost calculations very rough, it is simple for the user.

Laissez-faire and normative models give the costs in today's money values. Alterations in money value or in labour costs are not taken into account. Humanist and economic models enable speculation with these alterations, by means of including them in costs per unit. Increase in the number of places affects the numbers of places in planning years, as these latter include all places needed (the previously existing and the new). Investment costs affect the planning years in a cumulative manner, as a planning year is always compared with the presently existing situation. A result falling below zero means a decrease in the need for places and, thus, projected economic savings. Crucial points in the increase of need for places enables planning of investment periods and of the sizes of units needed.

At the end of each model the program writes out summary tables indicating the number of clients in each model. Clients are classified separately as institutional and "open care" clients (in the community), shown as a proportion of the number of elderly persons. It shows the number of personnel in institutional and domiciliary care, in proportion to the total population and also indicates total costs and costs per head. The summary tables enable making of comparisons between different models on the basis of client numbers, need for personnel, and costs. These tables can also be utilized in presenting models to decision-making bodies.

EXPERIENCES FROM THE EVERGREEN

Those who have tested the Evergreen agree that it improves the information basis of services planning, increases cooperation in the field and promotes know-how in the development work. In the project municipalities, the Evergreen was considered as a planning instrument which opens a totally new period, enabling the combination of quantitative and qualitative planning, and new possibilities to the strategic management of the care of the elderly on the municipal level. Simultaneously, when based on the team work, the Evergreen has increased the possibilities of both social and health professionals and users to participate in decisions concerning the plans. It seems also, that by doing this, the Evergreen has opened debate about the contradictions in values and other factors related to the planning process. This applies especially to the humanist model.

However, the municipalities were not as pleased with the operative qualities of the software, and wishes for increased user-friendliness were expressed. The main file was considered too detailed, as compiling such an amount of basic data is a heavy task. However, at the same time the program is too narrow concerning the health sector. In some municipalities the humanist and the economic models were considered too open and difficult models, as numerous details were left to the discretion of the user.

The Evergreen is now undergoing further developments. Its operational qualities are being improved, the main file will be restructured and diminished to about 50-70 variables, missing health data is being included in the main file, and further processing prospects for outputs are being developed. Version 2.0 is planned to be ready before the end of 1994. Also a European working group under the umbrella of the EU-project "Ageing and Technology" is evaluating the possibilities of developing the planning program usable in all European countries and whether the Evergreen can form a base for this.

REFERENCES

Bradshaw, J. (1977). "The Concept of Social Need," Gilbert, N. & Specht, H. (Eds.), *Planning for Social Welfare*. New Jersey.

Central Statistical Office of Finland. (1989). *Population Projection by Municipalities 1988-2010*. Helsinki.

Cole, S. (1976). "Long-term Forecasting Methods: Emphasis and Institutions," *Futures* 1976, vol. 4, 316.

Luoma, K., Hintikka, R. & Vaarama, M. (1991). *Cost Variation in the Care of Elderly among Finnish Municipalities*. Paper presented at the 4th International Conference Systed 91 on Systems Science in Health-Social Services for the Elderly and the Disabled, 10-14 June 1991, Barcelona.

Ministry of Social Affairs and Health. (1992). *Development alternatives in Finland's Social and Health Policies to the Year 2030*. Helsinki.

Sihvo, T. (1991). *The Finnish Population and Social Welfare. Information and Results of a Nationwide Population Survey of Social Welfare*. National Agency for Welfare and Health, Research Report 4/1991. Helsinki.

Vaarama, M. (1993). *Present Problems and Development Strategies of Welfare and Health Services for the Elderly in the 1990's and the First Decades of the 2000's. A Summary of the Results of the Elderly Policy Project*. STAKES. Helsinki.

Wilson, I. H. (1978). "Scenarios" in Fowles, J. (ed.) *Handbook of Futures Research*. Greenwood Press, Westport, Connecticut.

Towards Consensus
in Human Services Computer Networking

Thomas Hanna

SUMMARY. Human services providers have not taken quickly to the idea of using computers to expand their networks for solving problems. Recently, the technical and external barriers to human services networking have been lowered. Networking specialists involved with Human Services Information Technology Applications meetings (HUSITA) worked as a consortium to build a set of connected networks operating under the banner of HumanServe on the Institute for Global Communications computers in San Francisco, California. In the broader world of computer networking, connectivity continues to be a key concern, and the Internet backbone seems to hold the solution. The HumanServe experiment was accompanied by two years of cooperation among human services network coordinators. The climate for connectivity and accessibility are more favorable now than at any time, but networks are proliferating with only few subscribers and weak information resources. The new challenge is to organize and network the knowledge base. The field of child abuse and neglect, with its interdisciplinary nature and its critical in-

---

Thomas Hanna began exploring the potential of computer networks in solving problems in the field of child abuse in 1985. He is the facilitator of HumanServe on the networks for the Institute for Global Communication, and is host of the Child Abuse Forum on America Online. He is co-editor, with Richard Reinoehl, of "Computer Literacy in Human Services," Haworth Press, 1990. He coordinates development and leads information technology initiatives for the Family Life Development Centre, Cornell University.

Address correspondence to: Thomas Hanna, Family Life Development Centre, Cornell University, G20 MVR Hall, Ithaca, New York, NY 14853-4401.

[Haworth co-indexing entry note]: "Towards Consensus in Human Services Computer Networking." Hanna, Thomas. Co-published simultaneously in Computers in Human Services (The Haworth Press, Inc.) Vol. 12, No. 1/2, 1995, pp. 179-194; and: Human Services in the Information Age (ed: Jackie Rafferty, Jan Steyaert, and David Colombi) The Haworth Press, Inc., 1995, pp. 179-194. Single or multiple copies of this article are available from The Haworth Document Delivery Service [1-800-342-9678, 9:00 a.m. - 5:00 p.m. (EST)].

179

formation needs, may be the prime candidate for implementing the new model network.[1] *[Article copies available from The Haworth Document Delivery Service: 1-800-342-9678.]*

INTRODUCTION

Less than ten years ago, using computers to encourage networking in the human services was a novel idea. It was hard to anticipate, at the dawn of the microcomputer age, that a time would come when human service workers would have access to computers, let alone that those computers would be linked in networks. Today, desktop computers are ubiquitous in offices and the electronic meeting places of the world–networks and local bulletin board services–are springing up everywhere. John Quarterman, author of *"The Matrix"* (1992), estimated that five million people were communicating via the worldwide Internet in 1992, and he predicted that the number would double every two years, under which arithmetic assumptions everyone in the world would be on the networks by 2012. Since that prediction, assessments keep climbing. David Goldsmith, staffer of HandsNet estimated in December 1993 (Goldsmith, 1992) that twenty-seven million people were then on networks of all kinds. The Internet World '93 conference in New York City indicated that 150,000 new users join the Internet every week, and the total user base was estimated at thirteen million (Lewis, 1993). Another source provided a range of recent statistics on the Internet, including the fact that a new network is connected to the Internet every 10 minutes (Treese, 1993).

TABLE 1. Selected Statistics about the Internet as of December 16, 1993.

Newspaper and magazine articles about the Internet during the first nine months of 1993:	over 2300
Internet hosts in Norway, per 1000 population:	5
Internet hosts in United States, per 1000 population:	4
Internet hosts in July, 1993:	1,776,000
Countries reachable by electronic mail (approx.):	137
Countries not reachable by electronic mail (approx.):	99
Countries on the Internet:	60

(Hosts are computers set up to provide some sort of information service and to allow network traffic. Electronic mail, for instance, can be sent from a user of any one host to a user of any other host.)

CURRENT PATTERNS IN THE HUMAN SERVICES:
FOCUS ON CHILD ABUSE

With so many network connections and so many people using networks, how does the picture look for human services agencies? A survey
of child abuse agencies across New York State in March 1993, yields some
perspective. A list of 1,000 agencies, compiled as a resource and referral
source by a statewide prevention consortium, was used.[2] These agencies
are all involved in some aspect of child abuse prevention, intervention and
investigation although many have wider human services agendas as well.
A telephone survey of 50 randomly selected agencies showed 45 (90%)
had computers while 20 (40%) had modems for telephone-based computer
networking. It was not clear if agency size was a factor in networking. Of
the twenty agencies with some networking potential, eight had ten or
fewer employees. Of organizations with over fifty employees (12% of the
total sample) six had modems (33% of the total modem group).

Does the source list of 1,000 equal the total universe of child abuse
agencies and programs in the state? It is arguably incomplete. In the
author's home county, twenty-one agencies were represented on the statewide list. However other scans yielded a count of at least thirty-five child
abuse agencies. There are 18,236 children under the age of 18 in this
county (Census Bureau, 1990), so the thirty-five agencies represent one
agency for every 521 of total child population. Extrapolated to the whole
state (child population: 4,259,549) suggests 8,175 agencies statewide–
eight times the number on the survey source list. Readers who find these
numbers to be high should bear in mind that more than three million
children are involved in child abuse reports each year in the USA
(NCPCA, 1993). In 1992, over 227,000 were subjects of reports in New
York State alone where the reporting rate is fifty-three children per thousand children (N.Y.S. Department of Social Services, 1993).

The trial survey and these extrapolations do not represent a scientific
calculation but do suggest that:

• Human Services agencies in the USA seem to be computerized
• A significant percentage have the capacity to use computer tele-com-
  munication services
• There are scores of thousands of agencies nationwide–just in the
  field of child abuse prevention–which already have the technology
  needed to participate in computer networking in the information age.

Despite this potential for an explosion in computer networking in child
abuse and neglect, only a small fraction of human services workers in the

USA have made links to the outside world via computers. Despite many agencies having modems, their presence on networks built for their use is minimal even though many useful networking services are available with a local phone call.

THE "FIT" OF NETWORKING
WITH HUMAN SERVICES WORK

The adoption of the innovation of computer networking lags behind accessibility of the technology. While reasons for slow acceptance have to be examined, the burden on those offering networking services is to remove as many barriers to connecting as possible. Accessibility has to be measured by the perceptions of the user as well as by technical measures of mechanical ease of use and facility in locating the access point. One way to assess such perceptions is to discover if the innovation offered fits with the expectations of potential users. The concern is with ensuring that networking is an accepted idea for human service workers. Some evidence exists that networking is indeed a comfortable concept for human services workers. John Naisbitt (1980) picked networking as the end-state for one of his ten "megatrends." He describes the "old state" as that of the predominance of hierarchical organizations. He comments:

The failure of hierarchies to solve society's problems forced people to talk to one another–and that was the beginning of networks. (p. 191)

Naisbitt cites pioneers Jessica Lipnack and Jeffrey Stamps in their landmark 1980 article in *New Age* (Lipnack & Stamps, 1980) for the key "early" examples of the new trend. It is instructive to review those examples. Two of the four models were human services oriented: a parenting "warm line" in Massachusetts, and the national Women's Health Network. A third was a resource center called TRANET which focused on supporting appropriate technology applications. The final was the Denver Open Network, a computerized listing devoted to linking people with common interests, such as investors and inventors. Naisbitt also noted the use of the word "network" in the names of new organizations; the Consumer Education Resource Network; the National Network on Runaway and Homeless Youth;[3] the California Food Network and the Chicago Rehabilitation Network. Three of these have a human services aspect.

Naisbitt also cites Virginia Hine (1977) to define the origins of networks, summarizing that "networks emerge when people are trying to change society." Again, such a concept is far from alien to human services work. Another way to look at accessibility of networking from the perception of human service workers is to observe what self-help groups do. Madara and Meese list hundreds of self-help groups across the range of human service topics. While these are formed and operated by individuals, not professionals, such groups are often developed with the tacit or explicit support of human service professionals. In the third edition of *The Self-Help Sourcebook,* Madara and Meese (1990) devote a chapter to encouraging and to documenting examples of computer networking in the self-help arena. Among existing networks cited are a number that are linked worldwide through the volunteer FIDOnet system of personal computers. These cover such topics as AIDS, alcoholism, drug abuse, child abuse, diabetes, disabled interests, social services, stress management, and a range of specifically health related topics.

Madara and Meese also note that such networking resources are available at no charge or for the cost of a telephone call, since all their examples are either personal computer bulletin boards or one of the "free nets" developed under the model of the National Public Telecomputing Network (NPTN). In fact the NPTN is leading a national movement in the USA, working to have Free-Nets made available to all communities. The goal of NTPN is to "assist in the development of free open access community computer systems in cities throughout the USA and abroad" (Grundtner, 1990). Hence, it would be reasonable to conclude that (a) networking, with or without computers, is consonant with human services work and (b) availability of accessible computer networks is not a barrier to participation by either human service workers or by their clients.

In Child Abuse Prevention, Where Are the Networks?

The FIDOnet and Free-Net options are the most democratic computer networking environments in the world. The topics representing child abuse and neglect as well as other human services occupy only a minor place in these network pantheons and there, as on Usenet, discussions are dominated not by professional practitioners, but rather by survivors and support groups. In the FIDOnet universe, CUSSnet (Computer Use in Social Services Network) forms the major exception, with probably 200 individuals in practice and in social work schools leading active online discussions on an ongoing basis.

THE HUMANSERVE EXPERIMENT

The not-for-profit network environment provided by the Institute for Global Communications (IGC) which has for fifteen years hosted a family of networks that now includes PeaceNet, EcoNet, ConflictNet, LaborNet and HomeoNet, is linked worldwide through APC, the Association of Progressive Communications (1993) (see Table 2). IGC-APC has 16,000 subscribers worldwide, mostly devoted to environmental and peace initiatives, covered in 750 separate conferences. It also provides access to mail across the Internet, BITNET, FIDOnet and full utilization of the 2,726 conferences (or "newsgroups") of the Unix-based Usenet. Only a couple of dozen of these conference resources reflect human services concerns.[4] They also now offer access to a part of the world-wide data access system called *"Gophers."*[5]

Some of the conferences[6] operating on APC are a result of work by the human services networking Special Interest Group (SIG) of the Human Services Information Technology Applications 1991 meetings (HUSITA-2). With the help of APC, the SIG built a multi-network environment called HumanServe. Besides relevant existing conferences (childnews and child.abuse, for example) IGC has succeeded in linking in a CUSSnet node, the Social Services BITNET list, SocWork at the University of Maryland, and two Internet lists from Cornell University. One of those was especially set up to support the interest group for HUSITA-3, the 1993 international conference at Maastricht, The Netherlands. The other Cornell listserv is devoted to networking child abuse researchers. Altogether, HumanServe taps around 300 human services professionals from several countries.

HumanServe achieved its technical objective, which was to break down the barriers between network environments. These barriers prevent individuals and organizations from linking efforts because of a lack of communication (connectivity) between and among networking environments. In other words, with these barriers, when you join one network, you have little or no access to the people, or the information services of other networks. HumanServe was able to bridge FIDOnet, Bitnet, Internet and IGC networking environments. Without the willingness of IGC to drop its gateway filters, the bridging could not have occurred. And without the support of technical specialists from HUSITA, CUSSnet and Cornell, the linking would never have started in the first place.

The picture of the HumanServe experiment is far from a blazing success. Its strengths are emblematic of what is needed on the technical side; its weaknesses are the classic weaknesses of computer network initiatives. The group of network conferences thus linked have been modestly active, with traffic running around a dozen messages a week. But the total number of people involved has increased only by a few, those being mostly subscribers to the HUSITA-3 list. Only a small handful of users actually

TABLE 2. Association for Progressive Communication Access Information.

Region	APC Network	Telephone/Fax	E-Mail
Brazil, South America	**ALTERNEX IBASE** *Brazil*	Tel: +55 (21) 286-0348 Fax: +55 (21) 286-0541	suporte@ax.apc.org
Uruguay, Paraguay	**CHASQUE** *Uruguay*	Tel: +598 (2) 496-192 Fax:+598 (2) 419-222	apoyo@chasque.apc.org
Germany, Austria Switzerland, Italy Zagreb, Beograd	**COMLINK e.v.** *Germany*	Tel: +49 (511) 350-1573	support@oln.com-link.apc.org
Ecuador	**ECUANEX** *Ecuador*	Tel: +593 (2) 528-716 Fax: +593 (2) 505-073	intercom@ecua-nex.apc.org
Russia, C.I.S.	**GLASNET** *Russia*	Tel: +7 (095) 207-0704	support@glas.apc.org
Europe, UK Africa, Asia	**GREENNET** *England*	Tel: +44 (71) 608-3040 Fax: +44 (71) 253-0801	support@gn.apc.org
USA, Mexico China, Japan Middle East	**IGC–EcoNet/PeaceNet/Conflict/LaborNet** *USA*	Tel: +1 (415) 442-0220 Fax: +1 (415) 546-1794	support@igc.apc.org
Central America Nicaragua, Panama	**NICARAO CRIES** *Nicaragua*	Tel: +505 (2) 621312 Fax: +505 (2) 621244	ayuda@nicarao.apc.org
The Nordic, Baltic St Petersburg reg.	**NORDNET** *Sweden*	Tel: +46 (8) 6000-331 Fax: +46 (8) 6000-443	support@nn.apc.org
Australia, Pacific Islands, SE Asia	**PEGASUS** *Australia*	Tel: +61 (7) 257-1111 Fax: +61 (7) 257-1087	support@peg.apc.org
Southern Africa	**SANGONET** *South Africa*	Tel: +27 (11) 838-6944 Fax: +27 (11) 838-6310	support@wn.apc.org
Argentina	**WAMANICCI** *Argentina*	Tel: +54 (1) 356842	apoyo@wamani.apc.org
Canada, Cuba	**WEB** *Canada*	Tel: +1 (416) 596-0212 Fax: +1 (416) 596-1374	support@web.apc.org

joined IGC under the HumanServe banner, and their use of the network is minimal. In other words, those on "free" network access systems (FIDO-net and university-based Internet users) remain on their home networks; those who paid to participate on IGC also work on other networks. Also, even though HumanServe passed its second birthday in November 1993, few among the 16,000 subscribers to IGC and APC networks have yet "found" the five HumanServe conferences among the 750 conference choices on APC itself. Low utilization is directly related to two factors:

- lack of marketing and active support of new users and existing users on all the participating networks
- lack of active posting of interesting information.

Until substantial paid or volunteer effort is expended on an ongoing basis on these activities, or until significant numbers of users participate, the Human-Serve environment–and perhaps any network–will most likely continue to operate on a minimal basis. The HumanServe experiment has been instruc-tive, however, as a case example of the emerging issues in human services networking. Among the most pertinent are technology issues, user issues, the "fit" between computer networking and the human services, and the important boundary area of accessibility and connectivity.

COMMERCIAL NETWORK SERVICE PROVIDERS

Commercial network service organizations host significant human ser-vices networks in the not-for-profit sector. GTE Educational Services provides the host computers for the Human Services Internet. This is a collaboration of four networks:

- MCHnet–Maternal and Child Health institutes which operate under the auspices of the US Federal Government
- SpecialNet–teachers in the field educating developmentally and physically disabled children in the school setting
- SCAN–one of the oldest networks, dealing with disabled persons in university-affiliated programs
- NACHC–The National Association of Community Health Centers in the USA.

These four affiliated networks (a subscription to one provides access to all) have historically been completely closed. Only in January 1993 did

GTE-ES open up an Internet gateway (or access point) for its users. Interestingly, counter to the industry-wide trend, this gateway is offered only at a premium ($7.50 US per hour). Other commercial providers (such as America Online or CompuServe, both of which have their cadre of human services professionals working online) have made the Internet gateway available at no extra cost to their subscribers.

An important example of a network environment that has some significant representation of the human services in general and child abuse and neglect in particular is CONNECT. Like GTE-ES, a commercial network service provider targeted primarily at the business sector, CONNECT also hosts a number of non-profit networks. Most significantly for the present discussion is HandsNet, a 2,800 subscriber network with extensive forums[7] in the fields of housing, poverty, legal services, nutrition and hunger, community organizing and development, health and child and family services, including child abuse prevention. All the major national child abuse prevention organizations in the USA (governmental and non-governmental) have joined HandsNet with seventy-five significant state and national groups currently subscribed. CONNECT's access to the Internet is limited to electronic mail but subscriptions are available to European users.

Finally, it is important at this point to mention America Online in more detail, since there are two very active human service areas operating and growing there: The Parent Information Network and the Information Network on Mental Health. America Online has committed to provide a full-range Internet gateway in early 1992 at no extra charge. It already has "real-time" chat facilities; it supports sound and graphics; it has over 500,000 subscribers, and it charges $5.95 US per month, which includes 5 hours of usage. Its main limitation is revealed in its name: the network service is currently set up primarily for US consumption.

Hence, a wide range of network options already exists on well developed systems. Yet these human services network initiatives are by no means all that is currently available, but discussion of other existing networks will have to await another time. Adding up the rough numbers available, it is estimated that no more than 500 professionals and organizations use these networks for primarily human services purposes. Within that larger number, several score are particularly focused on using networks to support child abuse prevention. In this latter area, three organizations of national and international scope, NCPCA (The National Committee For Prevention of Child Abuse), ISPCAN (The International Society for Prevention of Child Abuse and Neglect) and FLDC (Cornell University's Family Life Development Center) have made some form of organizational commitment to supporting and promoting networking.

TECHNOLOGY ISSUES

This discussion does not focus on the technicalities–the author is no networking engineer–but discusses the general concepts that frame the coming period of expansion of networking–one in which computer-based telecommunication will be available to all in the same sense that telephones are today. Not that telephony is 100% accessible. The telephone system has been moving to expand capacity and accessibility through the use of new technologies, such as fiber optics, satellite and microwave transmission. These technologies are relevant to transmission of computer data as well. In short, technologies for data transfer and routing have enjoyed considerable attention. It has been a productive search, and we are moving ever closer to the time when the "world will be at our fingertips." Computer networking happens on all continents; new protocols are constantly being developed, and many key building blocks are falling into place. Setting international standards is a major component of this work, and huge investments of time go into the negotiations to allow the networks to expand to meet demand while engineers track research and development for future needs.

Current discussion is about hooking computers to networks for four simple functions: transmission of electronic mail, transfer of electronic files, access of databases, and posting to and reading from electronic bulletin boards. These are based on use of a computer keyboard and/or a mouse. However the future of networking involves very interesting permutations. Already, several networks provide online "chat" capabilities in which groups of individuals carry on "conversations" by typing messages to one another in "real time." Already, sound, pictures and movies can be transmitted and experienced on-screen while one's computer is linked to a host computer that might be anywhere in the world. These capabilities reflect a near future in which similar capabilities will be available to homeowners using their telephones or their televisions. Personal computers are already equipped to break out of the ties to the standard keyboard as well, providing voice and handwriting recognition. These capabilities will also be tied into networking, as will on-screen, real-time transmission of live images.[7]

USER ISSUES

To be sure, technology has advanced far beyond the general human services worker's readiness at this point. For the most part, they are not aware of what is available, let alone what it can do for them. Accessibility, long a major concern, is now much less of a problem. Through technological advances, the burgeoning of network access points and market pressures, there has been a lowering of barriers (including cost barriers) to access by some of the national telecommunication monopolies.

Cost

A modem can cost less than $100 US. The additional cost of connecting to and using a computer network that is set up to be supportive of human service workers is quite modest. Even where access is somewhat limited or unusually influenced by national communication monopolies, access can be available for about the cost of adding a single new telephone line to the agency's communications arsenal. So, for the communications decision-maker within a human service agency, the cost of networking is not in itself a significant barrier, though the opportunity cost may continue to be critical for financially strapped organizations. Still to be dealt with on the user side are the current problems and expectations that potential users have.

Vitality of Information

The technology is present today to allow users adequate access to networking. With a computer in nearly every human service agency with more than ten employees, the opportunity exists. But is the information one can gain from computer networking worth the cost? What does the human service agency get from networking? The two-word answer is: quantum reach. By the simple device of hooking up a modem, the ten-worker agency, currently dependent on the existing interpersonal networks formed by staff, now has access to expertise all over the country, or the world, for that matter, at the cost, normally, of a local phone call.

The network services that provide electronic mail access worldwide already have literally hundreds of professionals who could be of help to any local agency person. And many of those electronic mail connections allow access to hundreds of individuals through the mailing of a single letter to a multi-member list supported on BITNET or Internet. In January 1994, for example, the SocWork list sponsored by the University of Maryland had 350 members. Besides SocWork, many other lists, also available through e-mail, were identified by Ogden Rogers as being of interest.[8]

Human service providers have not flocked to the networking option, but they have adopted the FAX machine. It may be that FAX is a much simpler device to include in an office and its utility may be easier to comprehend. In a metaphorical sense, a FAX machine is just an office copier attached to a telephone. To obtain access to a computer network, one has to attach a computer to a telephone and then do computing. The image is more tenuous, the activity more troublesome. And images have a special power in the decision-making chain.

Accessibility and Ease of Use: The Image of Computer Networking

In the early 1980s it was my experience that when I talked about "computer networks" people would operate according to their existing information set. If they had used online databases through libraries or other means, the assumption they held was entirely based on Boolean searches of archived data. If they had no such experience, the concept was totally novel. Interpersonal communication via the keyboard, across telephone lines, was not an easy concept to grasp. From these discussions I found that the world was made up of two kinds of people, those who prefer to get information primarily through archives, and those who prefer interpersonal communication.

Until very recently, the methods of using computers to network in these two ways were quite distinct. Kreuger (1988), dealing with an individual's use of the microcomputer, attempted to define the phenomenology in a discussion of inter-subjectivity. He points out about interpersonal communication that:

> I am aided by the language which is available to me in everyday life which carries along with it a set of meanings which I employ to understand myself in relation to others. Microcomputer encounters, on the other hand, are solitary endeavors which, for the most part, presume little or no communication with other humans. (ibid)

He is describing what, for him, are the operant rules of communication–what is called meta-communication. That is, we know the rules of talking with each other (whether we use them effectively or not) much as we know what a red light means at an intersection. When he was writing, the meta-communication of microcomputing was less commonly known, and poorly taught. With microcomputing and networking as we now know it, two changes have occurred: microcomputers (and the metaphors they have taught us for their use) are common, and as we experience computer letter-writing and other interactive chores, we begin to treat these as if contact with other humans is implied. Meanwhile, in the world of databases, accessing information is following the new metaphors, so our computer activity with networked databases becomes very similar to our computer activity with networked human beings, strange as that may sound at first.

Several factors in database development, and in creation of the interfaces for accessing such databases has influenced the change. On my Macintosh desktop, when I tap into a database such as ERIC, I experience the old "solitary" experience Kreuger describes. My task is to choose a database from a menu, and then conduct a Boolean search to narrow the information set to my current need. However when I open my *World Access to Information Sources* (WAIS) software–a rather personalized data access system–I use keywords to find sources of information. Variations on this technology exist in the examples of Gopher and Archie. Once the computer tells me what sources may help me, I can choose one or another, and then tell the computer to go wherever that database is anywhere in the world, and it will take me there. Once connected, I can ask for full text files, and I can back out, and go to other sources as well.

This experience is not so different from logging onto a network, looking for my topic of interest in any number of bulletin boards or conferences, and finding full text postings that someone has placed there for my perusal. In Kreuger's terms, both these experiences still meet his criterion of "solitary" work, but in both also, one can easily perceive the personal hand behind the posting of information. In network bulletin boards, the turn-about is for me to provide postings of my own. In WAIS, the turn-about is for me and my colleagues to develop a database on our computer (a WAIS server) and make ourselves a source of useful information.

The World Wide Web (WWW) and its multimedia approach to interactive computing provides an even stronger example of what is now the nature of networking. Hypermedia, including text, movies, still images and sound recordings shape the new data environment. All are created by individuals, seeking to share their information via the network. This is the heart of the networking concept. At one time, I am a consumer of information and expertise, at other times I am a resource to those seeking the knowledge I happen to have. This user-provider relationship is at the core of networking.

CONCLUSION: FROM ACCESSIBILITY TO CONNECTIVITY

Accessibility is no longer a matter of having a local bulletin board one can tap. It is now wedded to the concept of tapping the world's information resources. One of the elegant qualities of the ideal Free-Net is that it is built on a partnership between a community and a local university which has organized libraries of information, networking resources and technical staff, and access to the worldwide telecomputing "superhighway" of the Internet. It is possible to acquire subscriptions to Internet without being connected with a local university; however the advantages of having a university partner are many. The Internet provides an incomparable vehicle for connectivity. Without true connectivity, the goal of having a networking system that is as ubiquitous as the telephone will remain elusive. However the present accessibility of networks to the Internet makes that goal visible nearly everywhere. Many special interest areas have succeeded in beginning to exploit the potential of computer networks. The human services still need to see to the dismantling of a variety of barriers–technical, mental, political, financial, interdisciplinary and marketing–if they are to enjoy the benefits of the new technologies. The HumanServe experiment shows how application of knowledge, on a voluntary basis, and on a non-profit worldwide network service, can also diminish the barriers. Child abuse, social work, and other human service professionals can, at this moment, and from most countries in the world, gain access to the resource made accessible by the lowering of such barriers. But, it must be said, that it takes dedicated effort by both paid and volunteer workers to make computer networking a vital resource.

The current state of affairs is that we have the technology and the expertise, we have substantial latent demand for the kind of resource that only computer networks can provide. We lack very few elements in an overall coherent blueprint for linking new users into existing networks which provide full accessibility. What we lack most is the force of marketing to channel that latent demand into the network systems, particularly through the Internet. We also lack the human resource bank needed to nurture and support the networks that we have. With the technical problem all but completely behind us in most parts of the world, the other major task for the near future is the organization of the knowledge of the field in forms that are appropriate for presentation through computer-facilitated communication technologies. These technologies now span a continuum in computer networking that stretches from interpersonal interaction (including voice and image) out to worldwide access to systematic databases.

Arguably, child abuse and neglect is the prime field of concern in the human services that is most susceptible to successful outcomes from energy invested in the organization of knowledge. Two key considerations: First, child abuse and neglect is by its nature a problem area that depends on a wide range of disciplinary contributions to solve the problems faced by professionals. Second, the problems faced on a day-to-day basis are complex and urgent with local problems tending to persist and local solutions tending to remain local. Implementing a blueprint in the area of child abuse and neglect could provide a model for human services network initiatives everywhere.

NOTES

1. The current version of this paper is considerably altered from the one presented in June 1993 in Maastricht because the networking scene has changed so much in the meantime.
2. The author thanks the New York Federation on Child Abuse and Neglect for access to their agency database which made this pilot study possible.
3. This organization established a computer network, YouthNet, for its affiliates.
4. This count was done on January 6, 1994. When I first explored USEnet on IGC in 1989, there were 365 news groups.
5. A Gopher is a local database, set up on a host and available anywhere in the world, if one owns the client software, and has access to the Internet. Gophers can use specialized search engines, some of which are set up to seek out topics in 10,000 Gophers across the world.
6. Forums and conferences are interchangeable terms, describing places where subscribers post and read documents on a single topic or issue.
7. Cornell' CU-See Me project currently links into computers across the world with real-time interactive visual contact between networkers, including the possibility of several locations (and visual images) online at the same time.
8. Much abbreviated from a list published by Rogers, Ogden (OROGERS@SSW02.AB.UMD.EDU), SocWork, University of Maryland at Baltimore, January 7, 1994.

REFERENCES

Association for Progressive Communication (1993) *About APC*. Institute for Global Communications, Downloaded 12/93.

Census Bureau (1990) *U.S. Census of Population*.

Goldsmith, D. (1993) workshop presentation, *10th National Conference on Child Abuse and Neglect*, December 3, 1993, Pittsburgh, PA.

Grundtner, T.M. (1990) "Community Computing and the National Public Telecomputing Network," the *National Public Telecomputing Network*, Cleveland, OH.

Hine, Virginia (1977) "The Basic Paradigm of a Future Socio-cultural System," in *World Issues*, May-June.

Lewis, P.H. (1993) "A Growing Internet Is Trying to Take Care of Business," *The New York Times*, p. F7, Sunday, December 12, 1993.

Lipnack, J. & Stamps, J. (1980) "Networking" in *New Age*.

Kreuger, Larry W. (1988) "Encountering Microcomputers: A Phenomenological Analysis," *Computers in Human Services*, Vol. 3, 3/4, p. 77. Haworth Press, New York, 1988.

Madara, E.J. & Meese A. (1990) *The Self-Help Sourcebook*. St. Clair-Riverside Medical Center, Denville, NJ.

Naisbitt, J. (1980) *Megatrends*. Warner Books, New York.

NCPCA (1993) *NCPCA Annual Report*. National Committee to Prevent Child Abuse, Chicago, IL 1993.

N.Y.S. Department of Social Services (1993) *State Central Register Reporting Highlights, 1974-1992.* Albany, NY.

Quarterman, J. (1990) *The Matrix: Computer Networks and Conferencing Systems Worldwide.* Bedford, MA: Digital Press.

Quarterman, J. (1992) *The Future of the Internet.* Paper presented at the Networking Services Conference, Pisa, Italy, November 1992.

Treese, W. (1993) Excerpted from "The Internet Index," posted on Communet Digital Equipment Corporation, December 16, 1993.

ASSESSMENT AND PROVISION OF SERVICES

Introduction

David Colombi

The use of computers for assessment and for direct provision of human services presents a series of tensions, contradictions, and dilemmas for developers and practitioners alike. Many of these contradictions are apparent in the contributions in this section. There is the contradiction of an established history and proven efficacy of the computer as an assessment tool compared with the frustratingly slow development of new systems. There is the tension between those who see the computer as a threat to their professional role and expertise and those who welcome and seek out its potential for help and support in their work. There is the dilemma for software developers of whether to switch to easier and less controversial tasks such as compiling new databanks to inform and assist practice and education. The continuing demand for education courseware also draws the attention of developers away from the needs of practice.

Much has to do with the imprecise nature of social work practice, what Joe Ravetz memorably described as "ill-defined domains" (Ravetz, 1991).

David Colombi is Information Manager of West Sussex Probation Service, UK.

[Haworth co-indexing entry note]: "Introduction." Colombi, David. Co-published simultaneously in *Computers in Human Services* (The Haworth Press, Inc.) Vol. 12, No. 3/4, 1995, pp. 195-201; and: *Human Services in the Information Age* (ed: Jackie Rafferty, Jan Steyaert, and David Colombi) The Haworth Press, Inc., 1995, pp. 195-201. Single or multiple copies of this article are available from The Haworth Document Delivery Service [1-800-342-9678, 9:00 a.m. - 5:00 p.m. (EST)].

195

For Expert Systems, this limits the use of traditional rule-based systems. Alternative and less precise approaches based on probability theory, heuristics, and normative analyses must be used. Such was the frustration of some who embarked on ambitious expert systems that their focus switched from actual development to the more fertile area of writing and lecturing on the problems involved. However, this is neither a full explanation, nor does it do justice to the progress that has been made in established areas and in new developments. Expert systems are only a part of the picture. The limited development and use of computers as tools to support professional social work practice is not simply a function of the complexity of the task. Any explanation has to take into account a complex interaction between management and practitioner attitudes and priorities. This interaction is set in the context of funding and development polices within agencies locally and at a regional and national level.

As always the changing technological environment is crucial, which brings new opportunities for developers as well as further dilemmas. The most dramatic for now is the tension between using "traditional" DOS-based systems and the opportunities created by graphics environments (Windows) and multi-media systems. The former approach provides applications that run on systems to which practitioners and clients have greater access. Many of these are "hand me down" computers, as managers and administrators move on to technology of ever higher specification and sophistication. However, new Windows-based software tools enable developers to create more professional and higher quality products, even if these take longer to filter through to impact onto practice.

As noted elsewhere HUSITA 3 was a time for consolidation and realism. The contributions in this section are primarily important either as the application of existing approaches in new social contexts or as development of existing work to new levels. They could be categorised in a variety of ways, each of them valid. One such way would be based on the stage in the helping process (assessment/treatment/disposal). Another way would be on the agency focus (psychiatry/disability/unemployment/home care). A third way might be according to the application type (social databank/expert system/decision support) or degree of sophistication. However, the distinction adopted here is between, firstly, those arising within a particular agency according to needs and pressures identified within the agency. Secondly, there are those that are part of a planned geographically wider intervention across a particular area of social intervention.

In the first category, Mary Howard and Mike Ferriter present very different aspects of work in response to needs in particular local psychiatric settings. In contrast Jana Hanclova and Eric Verkaar describe systems planned and being implemented regionally or nationally, whilst Dorit Barak et al. and John Vafeas describe prototypes or models of systems for wider development at a later stage.

The importance of this distinction is the increasing emphasis on "macro" approaches which marks a growing confidence about use of the technology in the human services. However, this carries with it greater threats about systems not being responsive to local needs. They may not feel "owned" by those who have to use them and processes of introduction can become routine, with both beneficial and negative consequences. For each contribution in this section, interest lies in part in the specific application of the technology but equally, or more so, in the human dimensions to the work and the complex business of managing change.

In Mary Howard's work the focus is on information about community resources and the process of referring patients to these on discharge from hospital. This is a complex task at the best of times, but recession made it not the best of times. Economic factors affected the increased demand (pressure from insurers), the shrinking supply of resources, and the consequent demand for greater social worker productivity. What is striking about this paper is the lively analysis of the process and the clear presentation of the social, cultural, technical and political dimensions to introducing the changes. The paper shows how these dimensions were mediated by personal interactions. It also shows how a planned, sensitive and responsive approach avoided many of the potential pitfalls of introducing change. This was despite the unpromising background of changes being driven by economic pressures rather than quality concerns. It was a transition Howard describes as "the rich lore of social workers would be translated from an oral to a computer medium." While the proposals started from a basis of mistrust and doubt, the combination of enthusiastic leadership and working with the fears of those most affected seems to have been critical. There were deft touches, such as having a "Social Workers Against Tedium" (SWAT) team leading the changes. All in all, this is a compelling account that deserves to be read widely for its contribution to understanding the human aspects introducing new technology.

Another contribution from a psychiatric social work setting, but again with a wider relevance, is Mike Ferriter's "Automated Report Writing." Here the focus is on the application itself and the paper takes forward work originally presented at the HUSITA 2 conference in 1991. His work is with relatives of patients at Rampton Hospital in England, a high security forensic psychiatric hospital. It started from a comparative analysis of structured and un-structured interviewing and developed on to a sophisticated application of technology to "get the best of both worlds." The resulting prototype system provides narrative reports through the interaction of the interviewing package with word-processing. As the author notes, this has a much wider potential than the specific and highly specialised setting within which the author works. This potential includes other areas of psychiatry. It also includes probation work which works with, and reports on, similar and overlapping aspects of human behaviour. However, all the human services depend on collection of data and translating that into useable information. It is the contribution that Ferriter has to make to that process that lends wider force to his work.

In the work by Dorit Barak, Dina Alon and Magi Amara, the focus is on use of a decision support system in a prototype disability centre for a national development program within Israel. There is the central issue of the contribution the system has to make to the lives of disabled people. However, particular features of interest are: (1) the way in which the growing literature on expert and decision support systems shaped the process, (2) the use of a *group* decision support system (GDSS), and (3) the implications and experience of this. Additionally, the paper deals with the impact on the practice and reactions of the professionals involved and the focus within the system itself on evaluating interventions. These factors combine to make it a stimulating and valuable contribution at an intellectual and practical level. There is evidence, not only of efficacy goals achieved, but also of widespread acceptance by social workers involved. As with Mary Howard's work, much of its success lies with careful planning and with working with the concerns of social workers in the prototype setting. A key question for all macro-level developments is how much of that work is transferable to new settings and how much has to be re-experienced in each new centre.

Also in the area of vocational rehabilitation, John Vafeas describes a model of a training scheme in North America for physically challenged individuals. The training is in computer-related occupations, particularly in computer programming. Here the whole focus is on the training process and its demands on people rather than on any computerised system of help. This distinguishes it from other papers in this section, although there are common threads about people interacting with technology in the workplace. It shares concerns as well about the influence of economic factors, issues of prejudice and the importance of partnerships between academic, human service agency, and commercial worlds. Since only a minority of people will have the aptitude or inclination for this type of work, it is a notable development. There is the important and all too rare dimension here of enabling people to break down the barrier between professional and client. The author's conclusion of the relevance of the model to other stigmatized groups within society is one that deserves to be heard. It involves a fundamental shift from perceiving clients as bundles of problems to helping them develop their potential as valuable human resources. Shifting the focus back to unemployment, Jana Hanclova's paper is on an expert system for assessing unemployment compensation in the North Moravian Region of the Czech Republic. It is an important contribution in its own right, as well as extending the spread of HUSITA contributions into Eastern Europe. It shares with the final paper in this section a focus not just on change within a single agency, but within a specific aspect of social intervention across a whole region of a country. As with other contributions, the human dimensions are vital. Here they are focused at a macro level on the impact of massive economic and political changes within the Czech Republic. These changes followed the development of a market economy and the splitting up of the old Czechoslovakia. As befits Hanclova's background in economics and management, the paper begins with a clear analysis of the demographic, fiscal, and economic factors that impact on unemployment. It goes on to identify contemporary problems in managing unemployment. This provides a framework for the task of "improving the process for finding suitable jobs" which led to the expert system described in this paper.

The process of defining characteristics of decision making processes identified a rules-based expert system as a viable solution. This is complemented by establishing principles for its use. The hurdles encountered of a lack of established software expertise and of finance for hardware and technology support makes the development work pioneering. However, these factors inhibit its implementation across the Moravian Region. The paper ends tantalisingly at the stage of testing the prototype system, based on sixty-five rules and thirty-eight qualifiers. Many aspects of this general picture will sound familiar to many human services practitioners in western countries. The wealth and the expertise remain concentrated in commercial organisations or within the management hierarchies of agencies rather than at a practitioner level.

Finally in this section, we have Eric Verkaar's paper on the ambitious and far-reaching system for computerising information in home care in the Netherlands. This scheme is firmly at the level of implementing social policy. It followed from a process of merging a wide variety of home nursing and family care organisations to provide a "completely integrated system of home care." The most important single characteristic of this program is that the computer system developed, called GIRST, is "designed as a tool to facilitate the provision of care: it is not focused upon managerial issues but on information needs and issues of those who actually provide care." Later it is noted that "Support of the primary process, the direct provision of care is the focus of concern."

There is of course little new in developing and implementing new computer systems as an integral part of organisational change within social welfare and other organisations. The two processes are often intertwined as cause and effect. However, such organisational changes are invariably the opportunity to introduce new systems for managing and controlling the new organisational structures. What makes GIRST remarkable is the conscious rejection of this approach as the primary and immediate concern in favour of the direct focus on the needs of practice. In this important decision, a key factor was locating responsibility for the system with the Netherlands Institute of Care and Welfare (NISW) and accepting their professional development goals and values.

Verkaar's paper describes in some detail the four stages of care coordination, care allocation, care in practice, and evaluation that shape the modular structure of GIRST. The tensions between different situational demands necessitated considerable flexibility in the program. This aspect of a total approach to computerising the care process is another important dimension to this work. It contrasts with processes that focus on a single stage or assessment, as with Ferriter's assessment and report work, or Howard's work on information resources for discharge and rehabilitation. There are, however, shared themes with other papers as in the role of partnerships between NISW, agencies, and commercial developers. This has parallels, for example, with the situation described by Vafeas in vocational rehabilitation in the USA. There are also interesting technical features in the prototyping model of development of the system. These include the development of programming tools and the planned use of lap-tops and of DPAs (Personal Digital Assistants). The latter extend the more familiar scenario of mainframe- or PC-based solutions.

Inevitably with a project of this type, the paper leaves us at a critical point of development and the question for the future is how effectively the ambitious plans can translate into effective practice. This is both in terms of the quality of care offered and the impact on professional freedom and judgement of care professionals. The innovative approach, the focus on practice needs, the nationwide application to a whole area of changing social care, and emphasis on the whole process of care are all factors that make this work of international interest and importance. The Netherlands is a country with an enlightened track record of commitment to the idea of using information technology to support social work and social care. Here we see those ideas being put into practice.

This is perhaps an appropriately optimistic point to bring this introduction to a close. In looking back on the classification used it would be wrong to draw conclusions about the merits of local developments in response to local needs, as against planned programs of social change. It is a rather a reflection on the growing maturity of this work that the larger scale plans are possible. However, they have only become possible through small scale pioneering initiatives, which are the "seed-corn" for future developments. A fundamental issue for any organisation involved in developing use of information technology is not just about the purposes for which it is used. It is about handling the tensions between encouraging local initiatives for local needs against the economies of scale available in larger projects, particularly in development costs.

From Oral Tradition to Computerization: A Case Study of a Social Work Department

Mary D. Howard

SUMMARY. Demands for increased productivity of social workers in a suburban psychiatric hospital were buffered by developing a computerized information and referral system of community aftercare resources. The development and implementation of the system are discussed with the administrative, technical, and social-psychological problems encountered in the first three years. *[Article copies available from The Haworth Document Delivery Service: 1-800-342-9678.]*

INTRODUCTION

This is a chronicle of the development of a computer-based information and referral (I&R) system and its introduction into a hospital social work

Mary D. Howard, MSW, PhD, coordinates the social work sequence at Brooklyn College. From 1991 to 1993 she developed a computerized information and referral system of community mental health resources for the Social Work Department of New York Hospital, Cornell Medical Center, Westchester Division, White Plains, NY.

Address correspondence to: Mary D. Howard, MSW, PhD, Department of Sociology, Brooklyn College, Bedford Avenue and Avenue H, Brooklyn, NY 11201, USA.

The author wishes to thank Lynne Heilbrunn, MSW, and Judith Sokol, MSW, for their comments on an earlier version of this paper, and Fran Thurston, MSW, for sharing her knowledge of the follow-up studies of psychiatric patients.

[Haworth co-indexing entry note]: "From Oral Tradition to Computerization: A Case Study of a Social Work Department." Howard, Mary D. Co-published simultaneously in *Computers in Human Services* (The Haworth Press, Inc.) Vol. 12, No. 3/4, 1995, pp. 203-219; and: *Human Services in the Information Age* (ed: Jackie Rafferty, Jan Steyaert, and David Colombi) The Haworth Press, Inc., 1995, pp. 203-219. Single or multiple copies of this article are available from The Haworth Document Delivery Service [1-800-342-9678, 9:00 a.m. - 5:00 p.m. (EST)].

203

department. The setting is a 50-member social work department in a 300-bed teaching psychiatric hospital servicing a metropolitan area encompassing parts of three states, two dozen counties, and over 3,000 community-based, mental health services (clinics, programs, and residences).

The immediate precipitant for the I&R system was the insistence of insurers that hospital stays be limited in favor of less expensive outpatient treatments. At the same time the economic downturn was forcing the closing of outpatient services and service reductions in those still open. Patients were competing for a shrinking pool of aftercare resources; and, social workers were spending more and more time searching for appropriate services. This was time they would have preferred spending with patients and families, educating them about mental illness and preparing them for the patient's return to the community. The better prepared a patient is for the return to community life the better the patient's adjustment (Vernon & Bigelow, 1974). In this hospital social workers provide the psychoeducation of the mental illness (etiology, signs and symptoms, management) for patients and their families. They coordinate the discharge plan as well. The aftercare plan or discharge plan is individualized according to the patient's needs. The ideal plan builds on the patient's strengths and supports areas of weakness. The discharge plan reflects the input of the multidisciplinary treatment team (psychiatry, social work, nursing, and therapeutic activities), the social worker's knowledge of community-based aftercare resources, and the preferences of the patient and family.

The social worker's responsibility is to coordinate these separate pieces. It is a complicated process. There may be differences within the team as to the degree or types of supports needed. And, locating appropriate community resources that have an opening is a problem. Finally, the patient and/or family may disagree with some aspect of the plan. The social worker must mediate among the parties. Mutschler (1990) describes the social worker's role as one of integrating the hospital, family, and community resources. The best discharge plan is useless if not followed by the patient. Hence, the role of the social worker is critical (Cooley 1989; Thornicroft & Bebbington, 1989).

Noncompliance with the discharge plan is a frequent reason for a patient's decompensation and re-hospitalization. Re-hospitalization is seen as a failure for the patient; and, statistically, makes subsequent hospitalizations more likely (Geller, 1986; Sandler & Jakoet, 1985). It is also a problem for the hospital. Should re-hospitalization occur within 60 days of discharge, the hospital may be penalized by the insurer, i.e., a reduced reimbursement.

In the present study the shortened lengths of stay and constant bed-census (95%) and the hospital's refusal to hire additional staff amounted to a work speed up. In Figure 1 admissions are shown rising 15% from 1990 to 1992. The impact on the staff was dramatic. Depending on the unit,[1] social workers were processing from one-third to two-thirds as many patients in 1992 compared to 1990. The threat of a "performance gap" loomed large. Social workers were at risk for failing management's expectations for patient psychoeducation, a timely discharge to waiting community supports, and an aftercare plan accepted by the patient, family and the treatment team.

PROPOSED SOLUTIONS

In the face of pressures for increased productivity, some social workers favored turning over searches for community resource providers to clerical workers, reserving for themselves decisions as to which of the found services most suited the patient. In a limited way, this was implemented. As might be expected the clerical workers were unhappy with their increased workload. But the social workers were also frustrated. The clerical workers' lack of understanding of the organization of aftercare resources and ignorance of search strategies generated noticeable inefficiency (which improved when social workers were able to provide supervision). They also lacked the know-how to negotiate with the service providers and this could not be remedied through supervision. On another front the department director took steps to streamline the paperwork in patient charting and referrals to aftercare providers; and, she was effective in reducing the number of staff meetings hospital-wide.

Taking yet a different approach, the author lobbied for the development of a computer database of the 3,000-plus community mental health services.[2] Each service site was to be researched as to address, telephone, hours, cost, insurances accepted, client eligibility, application procedures,[3] name of intake worker and program/facility director, languages spoken by the staff, physical appearance of the facility and environs, availability of transportation. The plan was to use listings obtained from the licensing agencies (such as the department of mental health and social services department) in the belief that this would insure the completeness of each service inventory. (This proved to be a naive assumption as will be seen.) Finally facilities and programs were to be annotated from the reports of social workers who had made site visits and whose patients had used them. The rich lore of the social workers would be translated from an oral to a computer medium.

Thus the shrinking pool of aftercare services might be offset if all

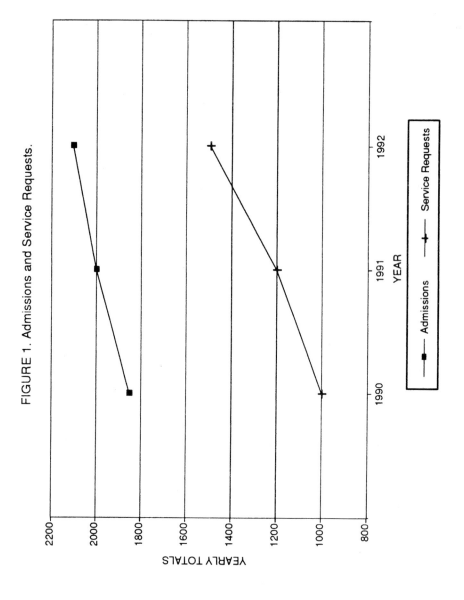

FIGURE 1. Admissions and Service Requests.

206

existing services could be identified. Each social worker could be given a roster of thoroughly researched and amply documented services several times greater than those previously known to any one of them. When services changed, as they frequently did, the computerized listing would allow for easy updating. Until each social worker would have a computer networked with the I&R system, the data could be downloaded as a directory and distributed to the staff. Periodic updates would keep the directory fairly current.

Initial estimates were for the total project to require about 500 hours spread over eight months. Interruptions, data problems, and staff cuts stretched it to three years and twice the number of hours.

It is a truism that every solution begets its own problems. This was no exception. The hurdles encountered were of three kinds: administrative, technical, and social-psychological. Furthermore, these areas were interconnected such that an administrative decision impacted on technical and social-psychological issues; and, vice-versa. A systems approach helps capture the complex interactions that produced the I&R system.

A SYSTEMS APPROACH

The value of a systems perspective is that it directs attention to subsystems of the hospital (administrative, technical, social, for example) whose intra-and inter-connections shaped the life course of the innovation, the I&R system. The application of systems theory to organizational innovation is an adaptation of Ogburn's (1922) classic work on culture lag. He theorized that change originated in the technological sector and worked its way through society, in the process enveloping social relationships, customs, norms, values and beliefs. While the process was under way there was confusion and conflict owing to the uneven rate of change, and for this Ogburn coined the expression "culture lag." The direction of change and the disruptions attending it has been researched by several organizational theorists.

In a study of the computerization of public libraries, Damanpour and Evan (1984) attempted to identify the origin of innovations in either the administrative, technical or social subsystems and then track the responses of the others. They found (in distinction to Ogburn) that administrative innovations tended to trigger technical innovations. Yet, regardless of where change began, if all parts of the organization were adaptive, disruption was minimized.

Beyond the research on organizations as systems, the course of an innovation has been found to owe much to the characteristics of staff and leadership. Kimberly and Evanisko's (1981) study of technological innovations in hospitals found them to be responsive to the staff's educational background and cosmopolitanism. They also looked at the organizational involvement of the leaders. Those whose management style was more hands-on were likely to accommodate technical innovations more easily because boundaries between the technical and administrative spheres were more permeable. These variables figure prominently in the present case study and help to account for the relatively frictionless assimilation of the I&R program by the social workers.

In libraries as in hospitals and social work departments, technical innovations are often the result of adopting technology, e.g., hardware and software, developed in another field and applying it to one's own. Envisioning how these tools might be used in a hospital social work department and then doing so are complex processes involving at one time or another the technical, administrative and social-psychological subsystems within the Social Work Department, the hospital's administrative and budgetary subsystems, and the external environment, especially mental health service delivery systems and reimbursement policies. In the following paragraphs, the administrative, technical and social systems of the Social Work Department are reviewed with an eye to their role in the evolution of the I&R system.

The administrative problems involved re-structuring the department's budget to include the necessary hardware and software; and, selling the idea to the hospital's Computer Committee. A second challenge was to re-allocate tasks among social workers so as to permit a long-term commitment to this project without negatively impacting the day-to-day productivity of the department. To those on the units, this meant being asked to continue at their under-staffed level while staff (who might have assisted on the units) were working on the I&R project. Furthermore, there were no precedents for such a data bank in the mental health field and despite considerable interest expressed by other psychiatric hospitals,[4] social workers were dubious as to the project's chances of success and uncertain as to its payoffs for them.

The technical decisions would be critical to the success of the project. Unless grounded in an understanding of the user's needs, the mental health and social services delivery systems, and state and hospital rules and regulations governing discharge planning, the I&R system would fail its mission. Furthermore, mental health and social service systems are dynamic. They alter their programs and eligibility requirements, facilities and programs close, and others open. The technical infrastructure of the I&R system would have to allow for these changes or its half-life would be short. The choice of software and of programming techniques would do well to be guided by the convenience with which changes could be made to the finished product; the hardware should be of sufficient speed and capacity to permit the database to grow; and, important, but often lost in the pressures of time, a detailed documentation of the computer program should accompany the finished product.

Finally, there were interesting social-psychological issues having to do with the role of social work in the hospital. Social workers were anxious about the changes taking place hospital-wide, such as staff cutbacks in nursing, psychiatry, therapeutic activities; and the scaling back of services, and the meaning of these changes for their jobs and for social work as they knew it.

To assist the discussion that follows, Figure 2 shows a time line for the project. The critical events are indicated in the order in which they occurred. The subsequent discussion elaborates upon these events, attempting to capture the intra- and inter-system dynamics even when it means sacrificing a chronological account.

STAFF INPUT

Approval for the project was needed from the department director and, of course, the staff had to accept it. The director was immediately favorable to the plan, though alert to the obstacles, mainly personnel and equipment, that could not be overcome without the cooperation of the hospital administration. It helped that the director was a computer user and familiar with various software packages. Known for her interest in discharge planning, she often taught the seminar in discharge planning to the interns. Her leadership style was noted for her hands-on approach. She welcomed social workers who brought her their "unsolvable cases." It was common to see her pouring over directories, searching for an obscure resource. Some years back she had developed the Resource Center, stocked it with service directories, and staffed it with two half-time people. The Center offered support for social workers unfamiliar with a procedure or in need of an appropriate referral. The I&R system would eventually be housed in the Center–the next generation Resource Center.

In the Fall of 1990, the director proposed relocating the Center from a remote corridor of the hospital to the main social work office complex where the secretaries, mail boxes, and supplies were housed. Social workers stopped in the main office several times a day. Within seven months the relocation became a reality and the Center became instantly more visible.

FIGURE 2. I&R Project Time Line.

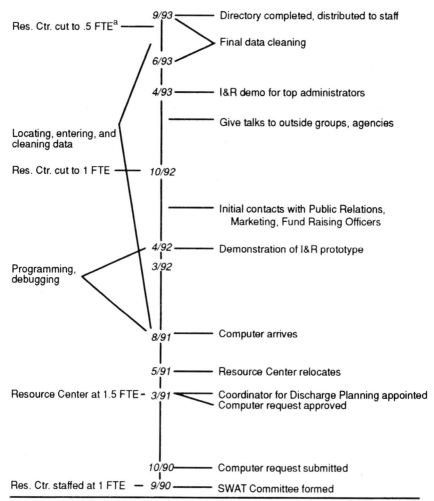

[a]FTE refers to *full-time equivalent.* 1 FTE equals the equivalent of one full-time person.

Due to strategic initiatives by the Center staff, utilization increased dramatically.

Sensitive to the latent messages conveyed by spatial arrangements (Gutheil, 1992), the Resource Center staff reorganized their space. Bookshelves were mounted on the walls and filled with directories grouped by geographic area and target population–children, geriatrics, substance abuse–

and so forth. Shelves were prominently labelled as to their contents. The traditional office desks were discarded in favor of desk-height counter top that ran the perimeter of the room. This made for a fluid workspace that could accommodate several people. The center of the room was left open to give a sense of space. Two large windows afforded good light and with a few plants and artwork, the Center was functional and inviting. The door was left open to give the message that staff were welcome anytime. Figure 1 shows that the number of requests coming into the Center rose by 48% from 1990 to 1992. Though data was not kept on the number of staff who came to the Center to research their own requests, the impression is that it grew even faster.

Around the same time, the director gave a green light to the I&R project, but not before she assembled a committee of administrators and staff and charged them with identifying obstacles to discharge planning. They dubbed themselves the SWAT Committee–Social Workers Against Tedium. They were unanimous in citing the locating of resources as one of the major sources of frustration. They agreed that housing seemed to be the most difficult resource to come by and the key around which the rest of the discharge plan (clinic, day program, etc.) had to be fitted.

The author attended SWAT meetings and it was here that the broad outlines of the project began to take shape. The computer literacy of SWAT members was superfluous because their mission was to describe the workers' needs. The division of labor and assignment of tasks reflected the skills of each committee member. The process was short (SWAT met but half a dozen times), and the participants professed to enjoy the work. Once the priorities were agreed, the SWAT Committee recessed with the understanding that they would be called upon individually to review different phases of the project's development.

SOME RESERVATIONS

There were social workers who voiced fears that the computer-based I&R system would eventually take over the job of matching resources to patients, and professional standards would be compromised. Social workers were concerned for their patients, but also for themselves. They felt their professional role was being challenged. Peter Plant finds a similar feeling among guidance counsellors in Denmark who feared loss of their "information monopoly" and reduction of their role to that of a "facilitating networker" (Plant, 1991).

Opposition within the department to the computerized I&R project might have been expected given an average age of 40 (Pardeck et al.,

1987; Shye & Elizier, 1976). Most workers had completed their MSWs (Master of Social Work) before microprocessors were incorporated into the curriculum. Yet, the department holds its own in this research-oriented hospital as measured by grants, professional papers given, and articles published. Twenty percent of the staff were working on doctorates or already had them. Despite the reservations already noted, the prevailing reaction was not of an "alien encounter," social worker versus computer, about which Geiss and Viswanathan (1986) have written.

ADMINISTRATIVE INITIATIVES

Following the SWAT Committee, work on the database began in earnest. However it was a personnel change that breathed life into the project. The director shifted her discharge planning functions to a new post, Discharge Planning Coordinator, to which she appointed one of her administrators. The Resource Center and its I&R project then reported to the new Discharge Planning Coordinator. The Coordinator was an experienced psychiatric outpatient social worker, firmly committed to the importance of discharge planning. She had no computer background and perhaps because of this she worked tirelessly to insure that the data was accurate and that the system was user friendly. Furthermore, her association with the project signalled its legitimacy.

Though the department director remained a powerful and effective ally of the Resource Center and the project, because of her broad responsibilities she was not able to give them her undivided attention and energy. The Coordinator however, had fewer competing claims on her time and was able to give the Center and the project the scrutiny they required.

THE HARDWARE

The director lobbied the hospital's Computer Committee over several months for a computer and laser printer. This would be the first computer allocated to a social worker in the hospital. The Computer Committee took some convincing.[5] It helped that social work gained a spot on the Committee and asked the author to represent the department. When it became clear that social work would assume responsibility for the development of the I&R system and would not burden the Computer Department, the committee became more amenable. At this point, the committee member from the Computer Department insisted that the hardware proposed was excessive. After some back and forth there was a compromise. From the initial request to the arrival of the equipment, ten months passed.

The Social Work Department urged the committee to adopt a single database program for use throughout the hospital. Economies could be achieved through a site license; users could be trained as a group, and with multiple users informal technical support would be at hand. When no agreement was forthcoming, the author chose Paradox by Borland. Paradox is a relational file system with a versatile programming language. It has a system for rapidly prototyping an application. It is fast, its files are convertible for use by other leading databases and spreadsheets, it is moderately priced, and Borland offers technical support. Six months later the committee chose FoxPro by Microsoft. FoxPro can import Paradox data though the I&R system will need to be re-programmed in the FoxPro language. While awaiting the hardware, attention turned to a classification scheme for the database.

THE TAXONOMY

It came as a surprise to learn that there were no taxonomies available for mental health resources. (There are several for social service resources, United Way of Greater New York being one of the better known.) The taxonomy that the author developed flowed from the four questions that drive the discharge plan:

1. Where will the patient live after discharge?
2. Where will the patient receive psychiatric treatment?
3. How will the patient spend each day?
4. How will this plan be paid for?

The I&R system translates these questions into a series of hierarchical menus. The top level menu has four options:

Housing (question 1)
Community Treatment (questions 2 and 3)
Updates (for making changes to records)
Exit (for exiting from the I&R system)

Each of these menu items opens to a series of additional choices. For example, Housing opens to: adult homes, community residences, nursing homes, therapeutic communities, etc. Each second tier option leads to a third tier menu which permits three choices: location by zip code, by name or by county. The funding sources (Question 4) for the various services are covered in the description of each nursing home, clinic, etc.

LOCATING, LOADING AND UPDATING

Locating accurate information proved to be unexpectedly difficult. Licensing agencies' lists were hopelessly out of date and even so, contained information on sponsors but not the service sites. Telephone calls to service sites proved of limited value when the director was not available. Agency intake workers and occasionally directors, too, were unable to give full and accurate information. To compensate, information was cross checked among several sources. Initial estimates for this phase greatly underestimated the 24 months and 600 hours that were eventually spent on the data gathering, checking and cleaning.

When it came to loading the information into the database, fields were masked where possible to preclude the entering of obviously incorrect information. "Help and fill" options were built-in to cut down on typing and reduce errors. All data were reviewed by social workers familiar with the services.

The Center staff did most of the data work in between their other tasks, though volunteers from the community and an outpatient who wanted an internship as preparation for paid employment contributed about 10% of the total effort. The author handled the data entry training. This yielded valuable feedback for debugging and fine-tuning the system.

As soon as there were enough data in the I&R system to "play with," a demonstration was given for a top administrator whose influence might help spare the project in the event of future budget cuts. A latent effect of this presentation was to force project staff to look at the project from an outsider's perspective and to address the question of why anyone beyond the Social Work Department should be interested. The Computer Committee had been asking how a computerized database contributed to the hospital's mission; now the question was being repeated.

Following the success of this initial demonstration, the Resource Center began thinking about marketing the database. It seemed that if other hospitals were willing to buy the I&R system, this would be tangible evidence of its value. Such reveries were short-lived as pressures from the acute units mounted and the director deployed a half-time person from the Center to the units. The Center then operated with a half-time Coordinator, the author at 1/5 time, and 30% of a clerk.

The Coordinator, sensing that more budget cuts were likely and that the project needed outside funding to insure its completion, contacted the hospital's public relations officer who agreed to do an article for the hospital's newsletter that had a large external circulation. The fund raising officer, marketing director, and public relation's officer formed a loose advisory group. Their message was clear. The project would not find funding without publicizing its relevance to individuals and organizations that had money to give, e.g., computer manufacturers, banks, insurance companies. Furthermore, several potential donors would have to be courted over time to increase the chances that at least one might come through.

Without additional staff it was not possible to both complete the database and pitch it to potential donors. While the fund raiser identified possible donors, the author took the message on the road. Talks were given at a hospital, a school of social work, and to social work field supervisors from local agencies. Each of these audiences had a somewhat different interest in the database and the presentations varied. As the system was not ready for market, these talks served to generate interest and provide feedback. In the Spring of 1993 a large group of administrators from the hospital was invited to the launch of the database. By then the presentation was polished.

At about this time, a prototype of a directory was printed and distributed to SWAT members who used it for several weeks and then critiqued it. Comments ranged from suggestions for clearer wording to requests to include additional information. Most suggestions were useful and were implemented. The final version of the directory was issued to staff in September 1993, almost three years to the day that SWAT was formed.

To keep the database current staff were issued "update" forms on which to indicate any discrepancies between a directory listing and feedback from the facilities and programs. The form is turned into the Center where staff verify the information and update the database. Updating of records is done through the maintenance module which is password protected and accessible only by selected Center staff. Updating a record captures the date of the change as well. Eventually, records that have not been updated within the past year will be downloaded and followed up by telephone. Annual editions of the directory are planned. Time will tell whether this "rolling" approach keeps the data acceptably current.

Staff training on the I&R system was done individually in 15-minute intervals. Each orientation began with how to turn on the computer and stepped through the process of locating information and printing the results. Social workers were encouraged to come with actual resource questions and to use the training session to find the answers. Trainees sat at the computer and with verbal encouragement as needed, followed the instructions on the screen. The most frequently voiced fear was that they might do something that would cause the data to be lost. Debunking this fear involved reframing it. The trainee was told that the data were protected from accidental erasure; however, the program might act up. And if the program still had bugs, it was important to find them. The trainee would not be causing trouble, but rather would make a contribution. The most timid neophytes ended the session with the answers to their resource questions and volunteered assurances that they would make use of the system on their own.

LESSONS FOR THE FUTURE

From the outset social work was asked to justify its request for hardware. Would this investment in technology make money for the hospital? Perhaps it would save money? Social work has not attended to such questions. Like other helping professions, it has relied on client satisfaction as its primary measure of effectiveness (Gerber et al., 1986). In good times no one pays much attention. But in an era of "bottom line fever" it is vital that social work be able to "make its case," to clearly demonstrate that the hospital's objectives are more reachable given a social work presence. Inexperience in evaluation research and lack of empirical outcome measures is a handicap and requires attention in MSW and DSW curricula.

The department's response to such queries was to utilize outcome measures that the hospital already tracked, selecting those for which it could be plausibly argued that social work played an important role. One example is patient compliance with the discharge plan. All patients are contacted two-weeks post-discharge and queried as to whether they are adhering to the plan. Research has found that the more personalized the plan (accomplished by the social worker's involving the patient and family or significant others) the greater the likelihood of adherence and the lower the risk of readmission (Boone et al., 1981; Vernon & Bigelow, 1974). Tracking compliance over three years (from before the I&R system through the early use of the system) shows an increasing compliance rate even in the face of the growing workload on social workers. Figure 3 confirms this.

Ensuring a project's success requires balancing direct work on the project with the indirect work of publicizing and fund raising. Interestingly, these forays into the "outer world" served to keep the staff from closing in on itself, of succumbing to the "bubble effect" and the "group think" that can develop when a small group is wedded to an idea that is struggling for its life. Inside the bubble all that matters is what the devotees believe and they and the project become more and more divorced from reality. Down that path lies irrelevancy and failure.

CONCLUSION

This has been a case study of three hectic years in the life of a large social work department in a teaching psychiatric hospital manoeuvreing to

FIGURE 3. Patient Compliance with Discharge Plan.

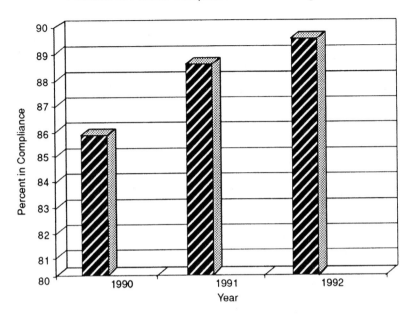

accommodate demands for shortened patient stays, growing sanctions on hospitals whose patients are prematurely re-hospitalized, budget cut backs, staff layoffs, and a hiring freeze. Crisis can be the catalyst for change and so it was here. The proposal to develop a computerized database found support in the department due to the cosmopolitan, hands-on leadership style of the director, an informed, responsive staff, a strategic personnel change and the presence of the requisite computer skills within the department. Had the Social Work Department not been self-sufficient it seems unlikely that the hospital would have underwritten this project.

Unlike other studies that have identified a definite route taken by innovations as they travel through organizations, the present case study reveals a constant interaction among the Social Work Department's several subsystems. This is due to the permeability of their boundaries. And this also accounts for the successful management of tension and the relative lack of disharmony despite the growing pressures on the department.

In a budget-conscious era social work departments can expect to be asked to account for their contribution to the bottom line; social workers need to be prepared with facts and figures. This requires a willingness of social workers to examine their practice and experiment with new technology or develop it when necessary. Increased efficiency in discharge planning need not be at the cost of patient care. In the present case increased efficiency led to improved patient outcomes. Management, however, must be willing to invest in social work departments to make self-study possible and underwrite the changes these studies recommend.

NOTES

1. Each unit houses around 21 patients. Units are either acute (average stay of 29 days), intermediate (average stay of 55 days); or, long term (average stay of 320 days).

2. The hospital planned to computerize the patient chart and install a network which would make every intervention from medication changes to family contacts accessible to all disciplines. The proposed database could become an integral part of this.

3. Each county had its own eligibility rules and application procedures specific to each type of service.

4. Psychiatric hospitals expressed interest in the I&R project though none were willing to participate due to pressures of time and lack of funds and staff.

5. The spread of computers within the hospital followed the pattern identified by Mutschler & Hasenfeld (1986). Structured, routine, and repetitive tasks were computerized early on. Inpatient billing was first. Secretaries soon followed, while psychiatrists bought PCs out of their research grants. The outpatient departments then computerized billing.

REFERENCES

Boone, C.H., Coulton, C., & Keller, S.H. (1985). "The effect of early and comprehensive social work services on length of stay." *Social Work in Health Care, 7*, 65-71.

Cooley, K. D. (1989). "Social work cost benefit within the Veterans Administration." In B.S. Vourlekis & C.G. Leukefeld (Ed.), *Making our case: A resource book of selected materials for social workers in health care.* Silver Spring, Md: NASW, Technical Assistance Report.

Damanpour, F. & Evan, W.M. (1984). "Organizational innovation and performance: The problem of 'Organizational Lag.'" *Administrative Science Quarterly, 29*, 392-409.

Geiss, G. R. and Viswanathan, N. (1986). *The human edge: Information technology and helping people.* New York: The Haworth Press, Inc.

Geller, J. (1986). "In again, out again: Preliminary evaluation of a state hospital's worst recidivists." *Hospital and Community Psychiatry, 37*, 386-389.

Gerber, L., Brenner, S., & Litwin, D. (1986). "A survey of patient and family satisfaction with social work services." *Social Work in Health Care, 11*, 13-23.

Gutheil, I. A. (1992). "Considering the physical environment: An essential component of good practice." *Social Work, 37*, 391-396.

Kimberly, J. R. & Evanisko, M.J. (1981). "Organizational innovation: The influence of individual, organizational, and contextual factors on hospital adoption of technological and administrative innovations." *Academy of Management Journal, 21*, 689-713.

Mutschler, E. (1990). "Computerized information systems for social workers in health care." *Social Work, 15*, 191-196.

Mutschler, E. & Hasenfeld, Y. (1986). "Integrated information systems for social work practice." *Social Work, 31*, 345-349.

Ogburn, W. F. (1922). *Social Change.* New York: Viking.

Pardeck, J.T., Umfress, K.C. & Murphy, J.W. (1987). "The use and perception of computers by professional social workers." *Family Therapy, 11*, 1-8.

Plant, P. (1991). "Vikings on the Seine: Policy challenges confronting career guidance counsellors in Denmark." *British Journal of Guidance and Counselling, 19*, 258-266.

Sandler, R. & Jakoet, A. (1985). "Outcome after discharge from a psychiatric hospital: A retrospective study evaluating demographic factors as predictors of risk of readmission." *South African Medical Journal, 66*, 470-472.

Shye, S. & Elizier, D. (1976). "Worries about deprivation of job rewards following computerization: A partial order scalogram analysis." *Human Relations, 29*, 63-71.

Thornicroft, G. & Bebbington, P. (1989). "Deinstitutionalization-from hospital closure to service development." *British Journal of Psychiatry, 155*, 739-753.

Vernon, D. & Bigelow, D. (1974). "Effect of information about a potentially stressful situation on responses to stress impact." *Journal of Personality and Social Psychology, 29*, 50-59.

Automated Report Writing

Mike Ferriter

SUMMARY. This paper describes the development of a prototype computerised psychiatric social history system that provided both statistics and a draft narrative report in word processed form. Using this prototype system roughly halved the production time for the final report. The paper then goes on to describe a user-friendly shell system developed from the prototype that allows new systems, based on user defined interviewing schedules to be developed with relative ease. This system, called R-Quest©, allows the user to construct libraries of questions, tables and lists which can be drawn upon to construct new questionnaires. *[Article copies available from The Haworth Document Delivery Service: 1-800-342-9678.]*

THE PROBLEM

Within the human services, both researchers and managers have a need for quantifiable data for statements about populations and subpopulations and data that have been collected consistently. Social work practice, in

---

Mike Ferriter is currently Senior Social Worker with special responsibility for information technology at Rampton Hospital, a high security forensic psychiatric hospital in the United Kingdom. He is also a Visiting Research Fellow at University College, Swansea. He carried out research on computer aided interviewing for his M.Phil. degree and is currently carrying out a doctoral research project on blame, guilt and the parents of schizophrenics, also at University College, Swansea. He worked in the computer industry before gaining a degree in psychology at Sheffield University. He qualified in social work in 1980.

Address correspondence to: Mike Ferriter, Social Work Department, Rampton Hospital, Woodbeck, Nottinghamshire, DN22 0PD, England.

[Haworth co-indexing entry note]: "Automated Report Writing." Ferriter, Mike. Co-published simultaneously in *Computers in Human Services* (The Haworth Press, Inc.) Vol. 12, No. 3/4, 1995, pp. 221-228; and: *Human Services in the Information Age* (ed: Jackie Rafferty, Jan Steyaert, and David Colombi) The Haworth Press, Inc., 1995, pp. 221-228. Single or multiple copies of this article are available from The Haworth Document Delivery Service [1-800-342-9678, 9:00 a.m. - 5:00 p.m. (EST)].

221

contrast, makes a virtue out of the individual and the unique in the individual. At times, the collection of consistent information for large groups of clients may seem opposed to the philosophy of social work itself. Social workers may also protest that to adopt a too rigid and structured approach to information gathering may result in important information being lost and result in questions being failed to be asked.

Sometimes this view is merely an excuse for "reaction;" particularly where the imposition of consistent data collection is linked with information technology, but in other instances this view seems to have some force. In a research project carried out by the author (see Ferriter, 1993) the contents of interviews, carried out under three conditions with parents of psychiatric patients for the purposes of gaining information for psychiatric social histories, were compared. The three conditions were: the traditional unstructured approach, a structured interview using a multiple choice questionnaire and the same questionnaire delivered by computer.

It was found that structured interviewing collected more information than unstructured interviewing. There was also indirect evidence that the subjects were more candid in giving information to a computer than to a human interviewer. This was in line with previous research that showed that patients were more honest when giving information to computers than when giving information to a psychiatrist (see Carr, Ghosh and Ancill, 1983; and Lucas, Mullin, Lunar and McInroy, 1977). All the subjects in the author's research were in their late middle age and despite their lack of previous computer experience found no problem in using the system. Some subjects commented on the thoroughness of the interview compared to previous interviews they had had with social workers and doctors in the past. Human interviewers, of course, often tailor their interviews based on previous information, experience or intuition. The structured interview does not do this but, by its very inflexibility, it can give the appearance of greater thoroughness.

However, the structured interviewing omitted certain areas of questioning that *were* incorporated in the unstructured approach that may have been of vital importance. The author concluded that structured interviewing by itself was superior to unstructured interviewing by itself (and there were clear advantages to using a computerised structured approach where subjects might be more candid with the computer than with the human interviewer) but the best result would be gained by combining the two, by having an interview that had a structured component that would also allow the interviewer to pursue areas or hunches in depth.

The problem then was how to get the best of both worlds and how to convince the practitioner that the solution offered the best of both worlds?

There was the further question of whether information technology had a role to play in this process.

THE PROTOTYPE

A solution to these problems was developed as follows. A structured interviewing schedule was developed, based on the previous research. This schedule consisted of 112 items, mostly multiple choice questions with a limited range of free text responses covering the following topics: family background and family psychiatric history, pre- and post-natal development, health, education, employment, partners and children, hobbies and activities, culture and religion, sexuality and relationships, psychiatric problems, addictive behaviour and substance abuse, behaviour problems, degree of burden to the family and contact with family.

The results of this interview were fed into a database system, initially into a temporary file from which the data was exported in two different formats. The first format was the conventional multiple choice responses, "Y" and "N" etc. and these were added to the main research data-files. Built into the system, were "statistics macros" available from a menu that performed frequency counts on all questions. At two or three keystrokes it was possible to find out how many patients suffered head injuries, how many abused a certain drug and so on. This data file could be relationally linked to the main patient database containing information such as clinical diagnosis, so more sophisticated analysis was possible, for example research into schizophrenia and obstetric complication.

The second form of the data was narrative. Within the database systems were extract routines that assigned appropriate narrative to each multiple choice response and concatenated groups of narrative, with punctuation, into sentences and paragraphs. These, in turn, were exported to a word processor where, using the word processors own macro language, the final construction into the finished report with headings, date, name of author took place (see Figure 1). The report was automatically saved on disk and printed. The information on the database could be amended, in the case of error, by clerical staff. The individual social worker retained full editorial control, amending, deleting, qualifying and expanding on the word processed version of the data. The whole process was so automated, using the database and word processor macro languages, that all the above took place immediately after the last response to the last question was entered. No further effort was required from the operator.

What were the benefits of the system? Although the complete system was available to the whole department it would be management and those

FIGURE 1

RAMPTON HOSPITAL

SOCIAL WORK DEPARTMENT

SOCIAL HISTORY REPORT

Name: JOSEPH ANDREW SMITH

Surname at Birth: SMITH

Known as: Joe

Date of Birth: 12/12/63

Date of Interview: 12/12/92

Present at Interview

Name	Relationship
Mrs Smith	Mother
Joanne Smith	Sister

Family Structure

Name	Relation	Age	L	Occupation
Mrs Smith	Mother	58	L	Shop assistant
Mr Smith	Father		D	Engineer
Mrs Simmons	M/Gmother	79	L	Pensioner
Mr Simmons	M/Gfather	83	L	Pensioner
Joanne Smith	Sister	27	L	Nurse

L = Living D = Dead

Family Psychiatric History

There is a family histroy of nervous problems on the father's side.

Birth Details

---

engaged in research who would gain most benefit from the core database with its statistics routines of data collected in a standardised form. What the practitioner got out of this, at the cost of incorporating a structured component to their pre-existing working practice (and many social workers found the schedule a useful aide memoir), was a file on disk and hard copy that became the first draft of a psychiatric social history report. Production time for the final social history report was cut by about half.

R-QUEST©

The prototype system generated a great deal of interest within social work and other disciplines but, as it stood, the programming of the system was inextricably linked to the content of the interview. To adapt the system for other use, say to generate a probation Pre-Sentence Report, required a complete rewrite of the system.

The database component of the system was written in a 4GL relational database language called Aspect©, developed by a London-based, software house, Microft Technology Ltd. A series of negotiations with Microft on how we could best respond to the interest generated by the prototype system resulted in Microft being commissioned to rewrite the prototype system as a "shell" provisionally called R-Quest©. This takes full advantage of Aspect's relational nature. The important difference between R-Quest© and the prototype system is that R-Quest© stores questions, answers and associated narrative, as well as responses to individual questions as items of data in a series of data files and not, as in the case of the prototype, programmed into the system itself. It stores the questions as displayed on the computer screen (e.g., *"Have you ever felt you ought to cut down on your drinking?"*, multiple choice responses ("Y" or "N," etc.), the actual values of those responses ("Yes" or "No," etc.) and the text to be placed within the word processed environment for a given response ("FAMILIAR NAME has felt that he/she ought to cut down on his/her drinking") in various data files.

R-Quest© also allows for system variables and certain conventions. Provided the questionnaire begins with a list (See Figure 2) that also includes "familiar name" and "sex" of the interview subject/interviewee the first sentence in any section can be configured to start with the familiar name and subsequent sentences with "He" or "She" as appropriate, simulating a natural English style. Use of a gender field will also assign the appropriate possessive pronoun. Figure 3 shows the input screen for setting a response to a multiple choice question.

R-Quest© also allows for the construction of up to four column tables of twelve lines depth (Figure 4).

From the libraries of questions, tables and lists the user may define questionnaires, and may also utilise questions, tables and lists developed for previous questionnaires. The questionnaires developed are then stored in another library. The user can then run a questionnaire, input the results

FIGURE 2

```
Display for Data List SHQ

                                        PSYCHIATRIC SOCIAL HISTORY
            Hospital number:

                  Surname:

            First Names:

            Familiar name:

                      Sex:

Notes




F2 = jump to start,  F3 = jump back,  F4 = resume,  F5 = jump to end
Action     F = forward    B = back    C = choose    X = exit
```

FIGURE 3

```
Question Definition File Input Screen - Question Details

Question reference 12
Description           Drinking Problem Question 1
Question text         Have you ever felt that you ought to cut down on
your drinking?

                 Answer Details

Answer seq. no     1 Type * to select
Answer character Y
Answer text        Yes

Report text        %FAM has felt that %SUB ought to cut down
                   on %POS drinking.

Last updated       09/11/93 13:47    by John Smith
F2 = jump to start,  F3 = jump back,  F4 = resume,  F5 = jump to end
Action : U=update  F=forward  B=back    C=choose
          X=Exit    D=delete                    U=update M = menu
```

FIGURE 4

```
Data Table Family 1
         Members of the Family

   ┌──────┬──────────────┬──────┬──────────────┐
   │Name  │ Relationship │ Age  │ Occupation   │
   ├──────┼──────────────┼──────┼──────────────┤
   │      │              │      │              │
   │      │              │      │              │
   │      │              │      │              │
   │      │              │      │              │
   │      │              │      │              │
   └──────┴──────────────┴──────┴──────────────┘

   Notes


F2=jump to start, F3=jump back, F4=resume, F5=jump to end
Action      F=forward   B=back    C=choose   X=exit
```

of interviews and finally generate a narrative based report, either displayed on the screen, printed in ASCII format or exported to a Word Processing environment. Other features of the system include the ability to "step" where appropriate. One might, for example, ask if the subject took drugs followed by a checklist of types of drugs. If the answer to the first question is "No," R-Quest© can be made to branch around the other drug related questions. Each question automatically includes three lines (of sixty character length) of notes that, if used, will be incorporated in the exported narrative for that particular question. Within the questionnaire, questions lists and tables are grouped into sections with section headings. Where there are a number of multiple choice questions in a section, R-Quest© can report the appropriate narrative for each question as sentences or phrases and the section itself, as a complete paragraph.

Currently, we are negotiating an arrangement with Microft Technology by which R-Quest© will be commercially available. It requires a limited degree of development, including the availability of a user-friendly statistics routine. A manual is still to be written and production organised. At the time of writing no price has been decided.

R-Quest© is very easy to use. A social work student with no previous computer experience developed a thirty item questionnaire in three hours.

We see R-Quest© as being of use in any situation in which an interview has a structured component, where the final report should be in narrative form but where the interviewer must have editorial control over the content of the final report. As such although R-Quest© is an obviously useful tool within social work and probation it could also prove useful in a much wider range of professions and areas of work.

REFERENCES

Carr, A., Ghosh, A., and Ancill, R. (1983). "Can a Computer Take a Psychiatric History?" *Psychological Medicine.* Vol 13, pp 151-158.
Ferriter, M. (1993). "Computer Aided Interviewing in Psychiatric Social Work" In *Technology in People Services* edited by Leiderman, Guzetta Struminger and Monnickendam (1993). Haworth, New York.
Lucas, R. W., Mullin, P. J., Lunar, C. X., and McInroy, D. C. (1977). "Psychiatrists and a Computer as Interrogators of Patients with Alcohol Related Illness: A Comparison," *The British Journal of Psychiatry.* Vol 131, pp 160-167.

Decision Support System for Planning and Evaluating Interventions in Vocational Rehabilitation Services for the Disabled

Dorit Barak
Dina Alon
Magi Amara

Ms. Dorit Barak is a Doctoral Student and Teacher at the Paul Baerwald School of Social Work of the Hebrew University of Jerusalem, Israel. She holds an MSW in Social Work. Ms. Barak is the overall project coordinator, and serves as the principal researcher and developer of the Decision Support System.

Ms. Dina Alon, holds a BSW and is completing her MSW in Social Work. She is Coordinator/Supervisor of all social workers in the Vocational Rehabilitation Center of Ashkelon, Israel and is head of the development team of the system in the Vocational Rehabilitation Center.

Ms. Magi Amara, holds a BSW and is completing her MSW in Educational Counselling. She is the Evaluation Supervisor in the Vocational Rehabilitation Center of Ashkelon, Israel and is the developer of the Evaluation Sub-System.

Address correspondence to Dorit Barak, Social Work Dept., Hebrew University, Yosef Haim 4, PO Box 1266, Mevasseret-Zion, 90805, Israel.

The authors wish to acknowledge the cooperation of the Joint Distribution Committee of Israel, who funded the project's development; the Israeli Vocational Rehabilitation Fund; the Rehabilitation Unit of the Israeli Ministry of Labor and Social Affairs; and the Paul Baerwald School of Social Work of the Hebrew University, who have aided the project's ongoing development. Also, the authors wish to recognize the ongoing participation of the employees of the rehabilitation center in the city of Ashkelon, Israel, which has been designated as the experimental center for the system's development. Thanks also to Ms. Debby Salan who provided numerous valuable suggestions in preparing the article in its English version.

[Haworth co-indexing entry note]: "Decision Support System for Planning and Evaluating Interventions in Vocational Rehabilitation Services for the Disabled." Barak, Dorit, Dina Alon, and Magi Amara. Co-published simultaneously in *Computers in Human Services* (The Haworth Press, Inc.) Vol. 12, No. 3/4, 1995, pp. 229-241; and: *Human Services in the Information Age* (ed: Jackie Rafferty, Jan Steyaert, and David Colombi) The Haworth Press, Inc., 1995, pp. 229-241. Single or multiple copies of this article are available from The Haworth Document Delivery Service [1-800-342-9678, 9:00 a.m. - 5:00 p.m. (EST)].

229

SUMMARY. This paper presents a Group Decision Support System (GDSS) for planning and evaluating interventions in the area of vocational rehabilitation of disabled people. On the basis of the conceptual framework of planned, systematic social work, the workers' current practice knowledge was mapped out and a model for planning and evaluating interventions was developed. This model served as the basis for developing the system's prototype. This system has been designed with the full cooperation of the workers, who, following a two-year implementation period, concluded that the system contributes to their professional decision making and interventions. *[Article copies available from The Haworth Document Delivery Service: 1-800-342-9678.]*

INTRODUCTION

The overall goal of this project is the development of a Group Decision Support System (GDSS) for planning and evaluating interventions in the area of vocational rehabilitation of disabled people. The first priority of this system is to support the professional workers in order to improve the treatment they give to their clients. The system concentrates on the individual clients. It offers a guiding model of decision making to practitioners such as social workers, evaluation workers and the workshop counsellors. This model concerns the planning of the rehabilitation process. The system follows all stages of the rehabilitation process: for each location in the process a sub-system has been developed which matches its special needs.

Decision support systems (DSS) are designed to support cognitive, rational processes, such as drawing conclusions from facts, predicting on the basis of past operations or making decisions about a plan of action (Markus, 1984). Keen (1986) claimed that DSS are designed to improve the effectiveness and productivity of managers and professionals, yet they cannot replace human judgement. Their main function is to support the intuitive and unstructured parts of the decision making process. A special kind of DSS is Group DSS (GDSS). This is a system which supports decisions that are made by a group of decision makers, who work together as a team. According to DeSanctis & Gallupe (1986), GDSS is directed to encourage active cooperation between the team members, resulting in improved communication and collaboration.

At the core of a DSS is an abstract model. A good model can capture the important parts of the situation, and disregard irrelevant details (Emery, 1987). Markus (1984) differentiates between three categories of DSS systems, according to the model each one uses: she calls the first two kinds, expert systems, since they simulate the expert's analysis and recommend decision options to fit the data. Those systems are based on descriptive models, which simulate processes in the real world: the first type of expert system relies on past data analysis, with the application of a statistical model to those data. The second type of expert system includes models which are based on systems of "if-then" deductive logic. These deductive models are based on artificial intelligence, and simulate human experts' cognitive processes. In addition to the expert systems, Markus has designated a third category of decision support systems: those systems which are designed for situations that do not fit any other descriptive model. There are at least four possible explanations for this other group of systems:

1. There are no results of past analysis of research data, thus making it impossible to fit a model to the problem.
2. The required data are not available.
3. That relevant assumptions related to the decision options are unknown.
4. There is no expert whose decision processes can be observed in order to build a model upon them. For those cases, it is possible to build DSS systems which help people analyze the available data.

Those systems are based on normative, prescriptive models of decision making, specifying how the decision is to be made and which information is required (Keen & Scott Morton, 1978; Markus, 1984). The aim of this type of DSS is to support decision making by improving both the process by which the user learns about the problem, and the cognitive activities utilized by the user in reaching solutions. These systems intend to force structure on the activities of planning and decision making. There are only a few examples of systems of that type in the literature (Markus, 1984; Preece, 1990; Jagodzinski et al., 1990). Further, all of those systems were described while they were in trial implementation. Our DSS belongs to this third category: a decision support system that gives support to the processes of decision making.

The guiding theoretical base in the development of this DSS system is anchored in approaches which emphasize the need for systematization and evaluation in Social Work. Planned, systematic practice is primarily meant to be a process which will insure choosing the most appropriate goals of intervention and the attainment of the desired change for the client. The conceptual framework which guides the development of this system has been proposed by Rosen, Proctor, Livne, and others (Rosen et al., 1985; Rosen, 1993). This conceptual framework refers to the practitioner's cognitive organization of his/her future actions, within the context of the client's problems, during the entire therapeutic process. On the basis of the conceptual framework, the workers' current practice knowledge is mapped out by identifying and creating formulations for frequently encountered problems, desired outcomes, and possible interventions. The "mapping out" of the process served as a basis for developing the system's prototype. The system provides the practitioners with a model for planning treatment decisions, and for evaluating their interventions. The model specifies the types of problems frequently encountered by the rehabilitation center, the outcomes which are possible to attain, and a variety of interventions which may be employed in order to achieve the desired outcome. The practitioner can choose amongst the alternatives, according to the needs of the client. One of the features of the developing system is that clients undergoing rehabilitation will be partners in planning their own rehabilitation programs, and in the on-going evaluation of the outcomes.

This Group Decision System (GDSS) has three main sub-systems (subsys): the social worker sub-sys, the evaluation sub-sys, and the workshop sub-sys. The social worker sub-sys has two functions: one is to support the social worker's direct practice with the client and the other is to help plan and monitor his/her duties as a case manager. The evaluation sub-sys accompanies the entire process of assessing the client's abilities, professional inclinations and ambitions. The workshop sub-sys deals with the client's rehabilitation process, during the vocational training phase. As it is a GDSS, a substantial portion of the information and decisions is a result of the inter-disciplinary team's working process.

ILLUSTRATION OF THE SUB-SYSTEMS

In order to clarify the operating principles of the sub-systems, the social worker sub-sys will be presented as a detailed example; the other two sub-systems will be summarized.

The Social Worker Sub-System

This sub-system accompanies the treatment process from the intake stage until the treatment is terminated. During the intake stage the social worker collects information about the client from various sources, with as much input from the client as possible. Next, the social worker defines the client's problems and strengths, by identifying the client's general and the specific problems (see Screens 1 and 2).

The next step is to evaluate the severity of each problem, and offer explanations for each definition, illustrated in Screen 3.

SCREEN 1. Frequently Encountered Problem Areas by Clients in a Vocational Rehabilitation Center

GENERAL PROBLEMS

- [ ] Means of Support
- [ ] Liesure Activities
- [x] Disability
- [ ] Difficulties in Adapting to the Rehab. Center
- [x] Unknown Abilities, Aptitudes and Interests
- [x] Behavioral Difficulties Related to Voc. Rehab.
- [ ] Gap Between Client's Expectations & Abilities
- [ ] Independent Functioning
- [ ] Clients Stigmatic Appraisal of Voc. Rehab Center
- [ ] Psycho-Social Problems
- [x] Cultural Adaptation

SCREEN 2. Example of Specification of Behavioral Difficulties Related to Vocational Rehabilitation

SPECIFIC PROBLEMS

- [ ] Other Obligations Which Prevent Employment
- [ ] Using the Disability as an Explanation for Unemployment
- [✓] Lateness: At Starting Times and After Breaks
- [✓] Lack of Persistence in Focusing on Work Tasks
- [ ] Lack of Cooperation with Authority Figures
- [ ] Organizing Tasks at the Work Station
- [ ] Unable to Work in Closed Places
- [ ] Inappropriate Dress
- [ ] Inappropriate Workplace Behavior
- [ ] Difficulty in Coping with Stressfull Situations
- [ ] Either Lack of or Excess Initiative in Problem Solving
- [ ] Difficulty in Cooperation with Co-Workers
- [ ] Difficulty in Accepting Criticism From Supervisors
- [ ] Lack of Motivation

PROBLEMS & STRENGTHS

Client: Dan

Explanation of: Vocational Disability

From the Client's Perspective:	From the Professional's Perspective:
Since becoming an amputee (arm) I can't do any kind of work.	As a result of becoming an amputee it is necessary to match certain kinds of work to the client's ability.

Strengh

Not Problematic

Very Problematic

| Disability: Vocational | Disability: Family | Unknown Abilities Aptitudes Interests | Behavioral: Lack of Persistence | Behavioral: Lateness | Cultural Adaptation |

Next, the social worker specifies ranked priority ordering for treating each problem. Subsequently, he or she determines the desired outcomes for each problem. There are two types of outcomes: ultimate outcomes and intermediate outcomes. Ultimate outcomes represent a significant change in the client's situation, leading to his or her placement in the open market, or change which will enable placement in a sheltered work situation, or securing alternative resources which will compensate for the disability. In order to reach each ultimate outcome, a continuum of intermediate outcomes is needed. In contrast to ultimate outcomes, there is no pre-defined content for intermediate outcomes or interventions. The desired intermediate outcomes are determined by the social worker, often with the active participation of the client. Next, the social worker decides which interventions are most appropriate for attaining each one of the intermediate outcomes, and how the tasks will be distributed amongst the team members. It is the social worker who determines which team member will implement each one of the interventions, and what the time framework will be (see Screen 4).

The system generates a concentrated graphic summary of individual rehabilitation plans for each client. In addition the system also provides the worker with an aggregate of all individual plans which serves as the social worker's "daily work sheet" and task planner. These products assist the worker in implementing the plan and in evaluating the level of outcome attainment at each stage of the treatment. This helps the social worker to follow the specific evaluation procedure for each case, as required by the system.

The system is dynamic. Throughout the entire rehabilitation process, the social worker and the members of the inter-disciplinary team evaluate the client's problems and strengths and update the treatment plan accordingly. Inputs from the other sub-systems enable the social worker to monitor and validate his/her evaluations and decisions. The system enables the workers to compile summary reports which provide knowledge-based details about the client's problems. The reports include the treatment plan and an evaluation of outcome attainment.

The Evaluation Sub-System

The computerized evaluation system accompanies the evaluation stage by collecting, weighting and summarizing the client's evaluation data by means of graphic profiles. The system generates an evaluation summary report which includes recommendations about the rehabilitation process and possible placement options. These recommendations are incorporated into the other sub-systems, where they can subsequently influence their decisions. The main advantages of the computerized evaluation sys are:

SCREEN 4

TREATMENT OUTLINE ▶

◼️◻️◼️

Client: Dan

Disability: Vocational

INTERMEDIATE OUTCOMES:

| Information on the Arm's ability, and on the possibility of using a prothesis | Inf' on skills, inclinations, and learning abilities | Acquires work skills according to inf' about disability skills and inclinations | Works at job which is compatible with abilities and limitations |

INTERVENTIONS:

| 1) Consultation with physician 2) Interviews with the client in order to collect info' | 1) Assessment via observational workshop and simulated tasks 2) Assessment summary meeting | Rehabilitation proces in vocational workshop at the center | Vocational placement committee and placement process |

🕐 10/6/93   🕐 10/7/93   🕐 10/8/93   🕐 10/12/93

INTAKE   ❓   COPY   🔙   🔨

1. It provides an immediate ranking for the "work samples." That is to say, a ranking of the various evaluation tools and vocational simulation situations.
2. It enables comparison between the results generated by the evaluation examinations.
3. It generates an immediate profile of abilities.
4. It provides summaries.
5. It implements the technical component of the evaluation, thereby allowing the practitioner to plan, observe and draw conclusions.

The Rehabilitation (Workshop) and Placement Sub-System

The main feature of the rehabilitation workshop and placement sub-sys, which differentiates it from the social worker sub-sys is its high level of specification. Many of the treatment components can be quantitatively measured. The rehabilitation process is accompanied by a detailed treatment plan, which is made together with the client. The plan defines the problem areas and the specific outcomes and interventions for each problem that the practitioner and the client want to solve. Further, each intervention is specified along with a timetable for the attainment of each outcome. (This timetable also serves as a predictor of the pace of the treatment's progress).

Treatment plan decisions are always coordinated by the social worker, who is the case manager, and with other inter-disciplinary team members, if necessary. The treatment plan's implementation is accompanied by ongoing evaluation of the client's progress in every area which was defined, at each and every stage of the rehabilitation process. The evaluations are made by the counsellor, the social worker, and the client. The evaluations serve as mechanisms of monitoring and accountability, as support and encouragement for the client, and as a basis for clarifying and making decisions within the context of the rehabilitation process.

THE EXPECTED CONTRIBUTION OF THE SYSTEM

It is expected that the system will contribute to the efficiency and to the effectiveness of treatment in several areas:

1. Clarifying and improving professional decision making processes of the workers both as individuals and as a team.
2. Ensuring the accountability of all members of the system.
3. Involving the clients in the planning and evaluation of their rehabilitation programs.

4. Improving the coordination of activity and cooperation between the inter-disciplinary team members.
5. Processing and presenting accumulated data, thus serving decision making needs at the organizational level. These accumulated data will serve both as a management information system and as a clinical information system (Benbenishty, 1993).

THE APPROACH TO DEVELOPMENT

System development is carried out by means of prototyping, an approach which has evolved in recent years (Monnickendam, 1988). A prototype is not a complete picture of a future situation: it is an initial conceptualization which is sufficient for its analysis in real situations. The prototype allows the examination of concepts, the clarification of expectations, decision and data trials, while helping to define efficient and user-friendly interface. The system is being developed together with its future users stage by stage: the development of each stage is based on the implications from the previous stage. The prototyping approach is unique for system development, since it integrates analysis, construction, and implementation into one process. The approach emphasizes expedient initial development, continuing on to expansion, coordination and construction, while receiving ongoing feedback from the users, until the completion of final product.

In order to design a usable and useful tool, this system is being designed with full cooperation of the workers themselves. The workers were required, through the entire development process, to express their ideas and their attitudes towards every feature of the system. In addition, they were asked to try and retry every screen and every process, and to suggest ideas for improvements. They were asked again and again to consider the system from the users' perspective, which means to answer two questions: Is the system useful for planning their decision making, and will they use it?

SOME RESULTS FROM THE TRIAL IMPLEMENTATION

This system has been implemented on a trial basis for almost two years. Our conclusions are divided into two groups: first, conclusions from routine implementation and second, conclusions which have been reached by non-routine, trial implementation. The first group refers to the evaluation sub-sys, which has been implemented routinely during the past two years, with most of the clients in the Ashkelon Rehabilitation Center. The workers have already made 400 computerized evaluations. Their overall findings show that the evaluation sub-sys is reaching its expected goals, and contributes to the efficiency of the evaluation process. The workers claim that they would not agree to return to non-computer assisted evaluation. The second group of conclusions refers to the social work sub-sys and to the workshop sub-sys, which were implemented only on a trial basis. Six social workers and two counsellors used the system with almost eighty clients. One of their main findings is that the system helps them to focus their professional efforts on the important aspects of the rehabilitation process, both on the level of planning and intervention. Further, the workers concluded that the system improves the decision making process amongst the team members, and contributes to collaboration between them. Most of the workers are satisfied with the system and want to participate in the completion of the development process.

The main weak point in the system is that it creates a situation where the professional must face exposing his or her decision making processes, which were not previously placed under scrutiny. This may be threatening to the workers, possibly leading to resistance. We tried to include elements aimed at minimizing these threatening factors. It is important that workers feel legitimation of their practice, and support for their decisions, without being observed by a critical "big brother." For example, the system may threaten the worker because it directly structures his or her job performance, yet on the other hand it supports the implementation of work tasks by offering decision options. Another way of giving the workers a feeling of support is by sharing responsibility for decision making between the team members. Further, the system ensures the rehabilitation process is visible and accountable. Following trial implementations, the evidence is showing that most of the workers do not feel threatened by the system and that their attitudes towards it are very positive.

HARDWARE AND SOFTWARE TOOLS

The original program was developed, and is being used, on an Apple Macintosh computer, using the HyperCard software system. Due to implementation problems and the high cost of hardware and software development on the Macintosh platform, a revised program is currently being developed on PC compatible platform under the DOS operating system and the Windows environment.

REFERENCES

Benbenishty, R. (1993). *Clinical Information Systems for Human Services.* Jerusalem: The Magnes Press, The Hebrew University. (Hebrew)

Desanctis, G. & Gallupe, B. (1986). "Group Decision Support Systems: A New Frontier" in R.H. Sprague, & H.J. Watson (eds). *Decision Support Systems.* (pp.190-201). Englewood Cliffs, New Jersey: Prentice-Hall.

Emery, J.C. (1987). *Managing Management Information Systems.* New York: Oxford University Press.

Jagodzinski, P., Holmes, S., & Dennis, I. (1990). "User-Acceptance of Knowledge-Based System For the Management of Child Abuse Cases." In: D. Berry, & A. Hart (eds). *Expert Systems: Human Issues.* (pp. 48-64). Cambridge, Massachusetts: MIT Press.

Keen, P.G.W. (1986). "Value Analysis: Justifying Decision Support Systems." In: R.H. Sprague, & H.J. Watson (eds). *Decision Support Systems.* (pp. 190-201). Englewood Cliffs, New Jersey: Prentice-Hall.

Keen, P.G.W., & Scott-Morton, M.S. (1978). *Decision Support Systems: An Organizational Perspective.* Reading, Mass: Addison-Wesley.

Markus, M.L. (1984). *Systems in Organizations: Bugs and Features.* Cambridge, Mass: Harper & Row.

Monnickendam, M. (1988). *The Prototype Approach-A Preferred Development Approach for Computerizing Human Services.* Society & Welfare, 9(2), pp. 173-184. (Hebrew)

Preece, A.D. (1990). "DISPLAN: Designing a Usable Medical Expert System." In: D. Berry, & A. Hart (eds). *Expert Systems: Human Issues.* (pp. 48-64). Cambridge, Mass.: MIT Press.

Rosen, A. (1993). "Systematic Planned Practice." *Social Service Review,* 67(1), pp. 84-100.

Rosen, A., Proctor, E. K., & Livne, S. (1985). "Planning and Direct Practice." *Social Service Review,* 59, pp. 161-177.

Training
in Computer Related Occupations:
An Opportunity
for Vocational Rehabilitation
of Physically Challenged Individuals

John Vafeas

SUMMARY. The need for qualified computer professionals world-wide is presenting physically challenged individuals with unique employment opportunities. This paper presents a model for initiating and operating training programs in computer related occupations. Emphasis is placed on admission and selection procedures, the computer curriculum and professional behavior training, as well as on placement activities. The special partnership between industry, the vocational rehabilitation system, and educational institutions is examined. Attention is given to the role of social work in initiating and maintaining this partnership and implementing the professional behavior training aspect of the program. *[Article copies available from The Haworth Document Delivery Service: 1-800-342-9678.]*

Dr. Vafeas is Assistant Professor of social work at Kutztown University in Pennsylvania. He has worked for ten years as a social worker in the field of vocational rehabilitation of physically challenged individuals, training them for computer related careers. Dr Vafeas holds a doctorate and a masters degree in social work from the University of Pennsylvania and is also a consultant and software developer for human service agencies.

Address correspondence to Dr. John Vafeas, Social Work Dept., Kutztown University, Kutztown, Pennsylvania, PA 19530, USA.

[Haworth co-indexing entry note]: "Training in Computer Related Occupations: An Opportunity for Vocational Rehabilitation of Physically Challenged Individuals." Vafeas, John. Co-published simultaneously in *Computers in Human Services* (The Haworth Press, Inc.) Vol. 12, No. 3/4, 1995, pp. 243-255; and: *Human Services in the Information Age* (ed: Jackie Rafferty, Jan Steyaert, and David Colombi) The Haworth Press, Inc., 1995, pp. 243-255. Single or multiple copies of this article are available from The Haworth Document Delivery Service [1-800-342-9678, 9:00 a.m. - 5:00 p.m. (EST)].

INTRODUCTION

Work is extremely important to adults in western societies. Work provides people with satisfaction arising from their sense of competence and a valid psychological identity (Germain, 1991). Often, however, disability may prevent people from meaningful participation in the work world and block the satisfaction and validation that comes from work. Vocational rehabilitation is a way of helping physically challenged individuals develop and maintain the ability to work. This paper presents a model for establishing and implementing a vocational rehabilitation program in computer related occupations for physically challenged individuals. The original model was introduced by IBM in the early 1970s in cooperation with state vocational rehabilitation agencies, industry and colleges and universities. By 1993 IBM helped establish more than thirty-five training programs for physically challenged people in the United States. These programs are free-standing, independent of each other and of IBM. However they are all members of, and exchange information and expertise through, the Association of Rehabilitation Programs in Data Processing (ARPDP).

THE ESSENTIAL INGREDIENTS OF THE MODEL

The need for the establishment of training programs in computer related occupations for people with disabilities stems from three sources. First, a large number of people with physical disabilities experience low labor force participation. In the United States of America there are approximately 11.2 million people of working age with a work disability (Bowe, 1987). Fifty-one percent of these people reported that they were prevented from working altogether (Bureau of the Census, 1982). Second, the computer and information technology industry which is based on the ability of the mind and not the physical ability of the body is rapidly expanding. In 1970 there were 143 thousand people employed in the computer industry; by 1980 the number increased to 784 thousand and it is projected that the industry will employ approximately 1.5 million people by the year 2005 (Statistical Abstract of the US, 1992). Third, legal and social pressures exist to integrate disabled people into the mainstream of the society which includes full participation in the labor market (Americans with Disabilities Act [ADA], 1990).

PREREQUISITES

The essential prerequisites for successfully implementing this model are a long-term funding and referral source, usually a government agency, a long-term involvement of local employers, and an educational institution willing to host the training program.

Funding and Referral Sources

In the USA the state vocational rehabilitation agencies serve as the prime funding and referral sources for vocational training of adults with disabilities. Vocational rehabilitation of physically challenged individuals was first sponsored by the federal government in 1920 with the passage of the first Vocational Rehabilitation Act (Oberman, 1965). The involvement of the federal government in rehabilitation was expanded during the Second World War due to the number of disabled people produced by the war (Whitten, 1977). In 1973 a new Vocational Rehabilitation Act passed which maintained the provision of vocational rehabilitation and training services to disabled individuals of previous legislation but also enforced legislation designed to remove architectural barriers and facilitate employment of disabled individuals by employers receiving government funds (Rehabilitation Act, 1973). It is through this legislation that training expenses, as well as start-up cost, for programs training physically challenged individuals in computer related occupations may be secured. Additional support for disabled people in the labor force came from the most recent government legislation, the Americans with Disabilities Act of 1990 (ADA, 1990).

Long-Term Relationship with Employers

Before a program begins training disabled people in computer related occupations, there must be a strong need for these skills in the local or regional labor market. The need for computer related skills keeps increasing every year because of the new applications that are being developed and the new computer technology that is emerging. Employers are searching for qualified individuals to fill the available positions. A nationally or internationally recognized computer firm, such as IBM or Apple computers, must be involved in calling together local business people to help create a training program. A well-recognized firm lends legitimacy to the program and attracts larger local companies. By involving local industry from the very beginning two broad aims are achieved. First, local companies feel they have a stake/ownership in the product of the program. Second, they become desensitized to disability. Ownership and desensitization are accomplished through the companies' involvement in an advisory board to the program. This is a working advisory board and its members are assigned to various committees. One very important committee is the curriculum committee. The curriculum of the training program is designed to respond to the computer skill needs of the local market. When local computing needs change, so does the curriculum. Based on the prescription of this curriculum, another committee is charged with the development of criteria and standards for admission to the program. A third committee is responsible for mentoring and internship and placement of the graduates. Mentors play a very important role in the professional development of the trainees. Mentors are encouraged to regularly invite trainees to their places of work so that trainees gain a real sense of what work in the field entails.

The relationship with employers is further strengthened by the program staff providing consultation to local firms on issues related to employment of workers with disabilities. Legal issues related to site accommodation, performance evaluation of workers with disabilities, and issues related to employee-supervisor relations often times become troublesome for employers who are unaccustomed to employing workers with disabilities. Technical assistance by professionals working with the program is always welcomed and appreciated by industry.

The program also must employ computer trainers who are experts in the state of the art computer hardware and software. These experts can also provide technical assistance to local companies and help them utilize the latest computing techniques and hardware.

The Training Program

The training program must be associated with an institution of higher education that has "name recognition," at least in the local area. The name of the institution will not only attract students but also employers will know that the educational program is carried out in a respectable institution which provides additional legitimacy to the program. Many colleges and universities consider it their obligation to offer educational opportunities to people with disabilities and are willing to establish programs with proper incentives, such as tuition paid for by a state agency and employers willing to hire and mentor students. In addition to the aforementioned benefits, a university has housing, dining and library services of which trainees can take advantage.

Having a vocational rehabilitation program in an institution of higher education raises some interesting issues. Some universities might find it difficult to justify the existence of a training program that does not fit into their focus of providing broader education to their students. This could certainly be a problem in a university that provides such a training program open to the general public. However, when the program is limited to persons with physical disabilities who fulfil certain intellectual, social and academic qualifications and when the courses offered in this program are of university caliber then this becomes less of a problem. Another issue related to universities offering a specialized course for only disabled individuals is that of mainstreaming disabled students. Of course there are many non-university related computer training programs for non-disabled individuals that could accept disabled candidates. However, the legitimization offered by a university is very helpful especially when additional credentials are needed to offset employer attitudes toward a group that traditionally has not been seen as a part of the professional labor force. Also, a forty-five-year-old intelligent and motivated ex-truck driver who became a quadriplegic due to an accident may not be able to afford to go to a four-year college program while his family needs him to provide financial support for them as soon as possible.

The three-way partnership between a state agency, employers and an academic institution is a mutually beneficial relationship. The state agencies are able to place their clients, employers meet their needs for qualified employees who are selected and trained based on industry needs, and the industry's legal obligations to hire people with disabilities are satisfied. Educational institutions benefit from having a relationship with industry and they too meet their legal and moral obligations to offer access to education to people with disabilities. People with disabilities are the ultimate winners of this arrangement because it increases their participation in the labor force in a field commanding respectable higher financial and social status rewards.

THE ADMISSIONS PROCESS

The admission process starts with an inquiry and an application in which the applicant supplies information about his or her disability, educational background, work experience, and motivation to train and work (see Figure 1). Also, a physical and psychological evaluation is requested to assess the applicant's physical and mental readiness for training. The program is equipped to handle people with a variety of disabilities ranging from musculo-skeletal to blindness and visual impairments and from neurological disorders to head trauma. The nature of physical disability per se is not a factor in the admission decision. Some disabilities, however, such as blindness and visual impairments require the program to make some creative accommodations. With the tremendous advances in speech output devices most of the challenges in this area have been conquered.

FIGURE 1. The Admissions Process.

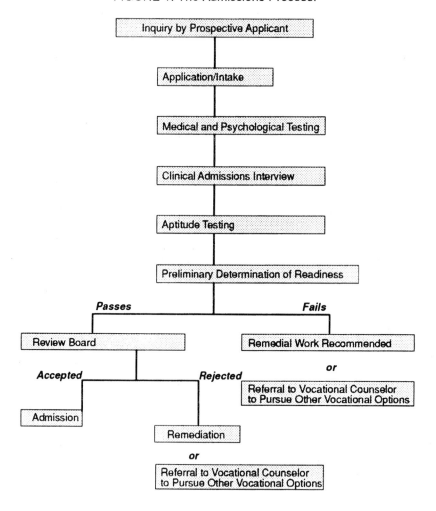

After an application is received, a clinical interview by a social worker is scheduled to review the application information and the medical and psychiatric evaluations and assess motivation and readiness for training. The social worker arranges for testing of the prospective trainee's employability and computer programmer aptitude. Employability is assessed by the *Handicapped Employability Assessment Scale* (HEAS) and the *Handicapped Employability Assessment Profile* (HEAP) (Estes, 1987). HEAS and

HEAP are divided into fourteen areas of employment related qualities, including self-care and mobility skills, previous work history, and motivation. Scoring in each category offers helpful assessment of employability strengths and deficiencies for immediate or future remedial work.

Aptitude for programming is assessed through the use of the *Computer Programmer Aptitude Battery* developed by the Science Research Associates (Palormo, 1974). The SRA test is divided into five sub-tests–Verbal Meaning, Reasoning, Letter Series, Number Ability, and Diagramming.

Verbal Meaning indicates the candidate's ability to understand terms in technical manuals and business environments. Reasoning evaluates ability to translate word problems into simple algebraic equations. Letter series tests abstract reasoning ability and problem solving skills. Number ability assesses ability to make rapid and accurate arithmetic calculations. The diagramming and algorithms sub-test of the SRA evaluates ability to flow chart a problem and follow a logical process to solve a problem. A candidate with a score of sixty percent or above on each of the sub-tests is considered to have the technical potential to be trained. Often times candidates have uneven scores among the sub-tests. Higher scores, however, in the letter series and diagramming sub-tests are considered to be better predictors of a person's ability to do computer work.

Based on the preliminary analysis of the collected data, the social worker forwards the information of the candidate's case to the admissions review board. This board is composed of a representative from industry, a vocational rehabilitation counsellor from the state agency, a representative of the teaching staff and the social worker. The board interviews the candidates who have an opportunity to present their background and their motivation to participate in the program. The criteria guiding the board's decision are motivation, employability, twelfth grade math and reading ability, above average intelligence, high programming aptitude and preferably some post high school work experience. The review board can accept, reject, or recommend that the candidate does some remedial work. Recommendations for remedial work are often associated with either increasing math and reading ability or referral for counselling related to adjustment to disability.

THE TRAINING PROCESS

Candidates who have been recommended for admission by the review board begin the forty-week training program which is divided into five phases–foundation, core curriculum, specialization, internship, and advanced topics seminar phase. The phases vary in duration and course content (Figure 2). The goals of the curricular design of the program are two pronged. On one hand, the program must produce graduates with excellent technical skills; on the other, the students must also learn professional behavior skills which will help them gain and maintain employment and advancement in their field.

The Technical Skill Training

The goals of the technical aspect of the program are guided by the skills required by a computer programmer for business applications (D.O.T.#

FIGURE 2. The Training Process.

PHASE	DURATION	COURSES/CONTENT
Foundation	8 Weeks	Computer Concepts BASIC or C Programming & Logic Programming with Lotus 1-2-3 Intro to DOS Organizational Psychology
Core	8 Weeks	Programming with COBOL Programming with dBASE III+ Principles of Management
Specialization	8 Weeks	Traditional Mainframe
		Advanced COBOL Operating Systems JCL Job Readiness Training
		End User Micro Computer Programming
		Advanced dBASE III+ Multi-user Programming Local Area Networks Programming with Foxbase Programming with Clipper Job Readiness Training
Internship	12 Weeks	Trainees are Placed with Local Firms
Advanced Seminars	4 Weeks	Seminars in Advanced Programmed and Design Topics Intensive Job Search

020.162-014) as defined by the Dictionary of Occupational Titles (D.O.T.) published by the U.S. Department of Labor (D.O.T., 1977). According to this definition the graduates of the program must be able to write detailed logical flow charts, convert these flow charts into a language processable by computer, and provide documentation of the program development and subsequent revisions. They also must be able to analyze, review, and rewrite programs to increase programming efficiency or adapt to new requirements. To accomplish these technical outcomes a comprehensive training program is implemented in five phases.

The foundation phase is eight weeks long. The courses taught during this phase deal with basic computer and information technology concepts, computer logic development using classic programming languages such as BASIC or C, personal computer literacy and intermediate level programming using Lotus 1-2-3.

The second phase, the core curriculum, also lasts eight weeks. Trainees learn business related computer languages for both mainframe and personal computers. Trainees are taught COBOL and dBase III+ and are expected to write programs for business applications. These programs are usually prescribed by the industry advisory board's curriculum committee. At the end of this phase, trainees are expected to make a choice regarding specializing in either mainframe or personal computer oriented applications.

During the specialization phase, which lasts for another eight weeks, trainees either specialize in end-user microcomputer software and applications or traditional mainframe software and applications. In the microcomputer specialization trainees become proficient programmers in Lotus 1-2-3, dBase III+, FoxBase, and Clipper. They develop single and multiple user applications and understand the fundamentals of local area computer networks. Those who specialize in mainframe applications become proficient programmers using advanced COBOL techniques and become familiar with JCL. They also become familiar with the use of COBOL PC. Occasionally a local company will request that a preselected trainee is trained on either a particular programming technique or even another language such as RPG, PL-1, or SAS.

At this stage the trainees are ready to assume a twelve-week internship. During the internship the trainees become members of programming teams or work on specialized assignments and they follow all the work rules, schedules, and procedures of their hosting firm. On completion of the internship trainees return to the program where they participate in advanced topics seminars ranging from telecommunications, to data structures, to designs of local area networks.

The amount of material covered during the program is certainly enormous given the relatively short period of time involved. The rationale behind covering all this material is to expose trainees to the breadth of computer programming but develop high quality skills in the use of at least one computer language for business applications. The students are required to submit a final project. The skills tested by this final project are the same skills found in the D.O.T. for the occupation of computer programmer for business applications (D.O.T. # 020.162-014). Successful completion of this project is a testimony of competence in understanding a business problem, performing a systems analysis and design, charting the system, writing the code and documenting the system.

Professional Behavior Training

Parallel to the computer related course content of the training, the students are expected to adopt behaviors consistent with those of computer professionals in the field. According to the Dictionary of Occupational Titles description of the duties of a computer programmer for business applications (D.O.T. #020.162-014), a programmer must be able to communicate with supervisors and other personnel and translate the informational needs into coherent computer program/system. Dependability, punctuality, and teamwork are some of the professional qualities of computer programmers that graduates must develop. This is often a very challenging aspect of training because of the variety of socio-economic backgrounds, work experiences, and the level of adaptation to disability of the trainees.

Adapting to disability is a major area of concern in the professional behavior training. The level of adaptation a person has made to his or her disability often does not depend on the disability itself. It is rather a combination of a person's effort, the success of the rehabilitation program they participated in, the time length since the onset of disability, and the level of assistance from formal and informal support systems. For example, a person with a C-4 level quadriplegia who has made good progress towards adapting to disability and independence may provide less challenges to professional behavior training than a person with a lower level (less severe) quadriplegia. During training, students are sensitized to the fact that non-disabled peers may have certain prejudices and difficulties accepting, working, and communicating with people with disabilities. The professional behavior training deals with how the physically challenged trainees can handle such situations and how they can turn potential uncomfortable and unproductive professional relationships into positive and fulfilling experiences.

A social worker is charged with overseeing the professional development of the trainees and designs individualized plans to meet their needs. Some of the trainees will need very little intervention and others will need substantial social work effort. The overriding purpose of social work in this setting is to identify, mitigate, circumvent, and eliminate personal and environmental barriers to the employability of physically challenged individuals.

One of the most frequent areas of intervention is in the area of independent living. Accessible housing, transportation, and management of attendants often overwhelm trainees especially when these arrangements have to be made during an intensive training period where time limitations are severe. Time and project management skills are often needed to reduce the stress that is produced by the intensity of the program. The trainees are treated as professionals and they are expected to fulfil the responsibilities of the role. Attendance, punctuality, grooming and hygiene, interpersonal relations, professional communications with supervisors and fellow workers, meeting deadlines and accepting responsibility are some important parameters defining professional behavior.

Trainees have an opportunity to receive instruction and support from others in the area of professional behavior during a regular class in the organizational psychology and management class which meets once a week. In this class, topics such as time and stress management, supervision and employee evaluation, attitudes of disabled and non-disabled people towards each other at work, and career development are covered. This class turns into a job readiness seminar during the third phase of training.

Job readiness training is an essential part in preparing trainees to search, apply, interview, and negotiate offers for employment. During this phase, trainees develop skills in identifying relevant job advertisement sources and advertisements, and develop resume writing and interviewing skills and employment negotiating techniques. Trainees have an opportunity to apply and interview for mock positions prescribed by members of the advisory board who act as interviewers. Interview sessions are videotaped and trainees have an opportunity to view themselves being interviewed and enhance their interviewing skills. Critical to increasing learning are the evaluation and comments of the interviewer to the trainee.

Before the internship phase, the social worker works with internship hosting and individual trainees to make a match between the needs and qualities of a trainee and the learning opportunities offered by a hosting site. This match is very important because it maximizes learning and often hosting firms, if they have a job opening, will offer the position to the person that they spent twelve weeks training to their specifications. During internship, problems requiring the social worker's attention are frequently related to adjustments to the work environment and miscommunication about work expectations. Frequently, however, trainees report that internship is a very satisfying experience that required little adjustment. They also report that internship gave them an opportunity to get an independent validation of their "worth" as professionals. Often times they report that adjusting to the demands of work is easier than adjusting to the demands of training.

When internship is over, the trainees return to the program for four weeks of advanced seminars and independent study projects as well as intensified individualized job search. The job search is monitored by the social worker who assists the trainee in the application process and who is also in touch with employers seeking qualified candidates.

An important element of facilitating placement is a relationship with industry that is based on trust and competence. The social worker communicates frequently with members of the advisory board and helps employers deal with issues of disability at work ranging from accessibility to hiring and firing, and from promoting disabled workers to dealing with the attitudes and fears of non-disabled employees. The social worker must appear to employers as an ally who is there to help them maximize production and satisfaction when they hire a physically challenged individual. The central point of the marketing approach for the social worker is competence of the trainee and not disability. Both physically challenged individuals and industry want to base their relationship not on the base of disability but on the base of competence and contribution.

APPLICATIONS OF THE MODEL WITH OTHER POPULATIONS

This model can apply to other populations who are experiencing chronic employment difficulties, especially members of "stigmatized" groups such as prisoners and welfare recipients. The fact that employers are involved in the curriculum design and the selection of trainees makes them less apprehensive about hiring individuals who have been previously excluded and many times discriminated against. In addition, the fact that the program is sponsored by a recognized college or university adds legitimacy and prestige to the certificate of completion. The need for computer related skills is growing fast creating a shortage of qualified professionals in this field. Technically competent computer professionals will fill this need. It will be a mistake, however, to believe that technical competence is the only necessary set of skills for successful employment in computer related occupations for members of "stigmatized" groups. Work skills and professional behavior training as an integral part of this program should

circumvent many of the non-technical problems experienced by these people.
The spread of computer technology worldwide is making increased demands on local labor markets for qualified computer professionals. As these economies move from industrial base to information base, physical strength and function will not be a major barrier to employment for physically challenged individuals.

REFERENCES

Americans with Disabilities Act of 1990, PL 101-336, 104 Stat.327, (1990).

Bowe, F. (1987). *Disabled adults in America: A statistical report drawn from census bureau data.* Washington, D.C.: The Presidents Committee on Employment of the Handicapped.

Estes, R. (1987). Assessing employability of disabled adults. *Public Welfare,* 45(1), 29-39.

Germain, C. B. (1991). *Human behavior in the social environment.* New York: Columbian University Press.

Oberman, E. (1965). *The history of vocational rehabilitation in America.* Minneapolis: Denison and Company, Inc., 1965.

Palormo, J. M. (1974). *Computer programmer aptitude battery examiner's manual* (2nd ed.). Chicago: Science Research Associates, Inc., 1974.

Rehabilitation Act of 1973, PL 92-112, 87 Stat. 1817, 1973

U.S. Bureau of the Census (1983). *Labor force status and other characteristics of persons with a work disability: 1982.* Washington D.C., U.S. Government Printing Office. This Current Population Reports Special Studies Series P-23 No. 127, was prepared by John McNeil.

U.S. Bureau of the Census (1992). *Statistical abstract of the United States: 1992* (112th edition). Washington, D.C.: U.S. Government Printing Office.

U.S. Department of Labor (1977). *Dictionary of Occupational Titles* (Fourth Edition). Washington, D.C.: U.S. Government Printing Office.

Whitten, E. (1977). Disability and physical handicap: Vocational rehabilitation. In *Encyclopedia of Social Work* (17th ed.) (pp. 268-277). Washington, D.C.: National Association of Social Workers.

Unemployment in the Czech Republic and Development of an Expert System for Assessing Unemployment Compensation

Jana Hanclova

SUMMARY. This paper addresses contemporary problems of unemployment in the Czech Republic (finding optimal alternatives of organizational structures of services of employment agencies). Based on characteristics and knowledge of information flows of the decision making process of claimants of unemployment compensation, a prototype expert system was developed to support this decision making. Results of this research were evaluated from two points of view–the theoretical and practical benefits. *[Article copies available from The Haworth Document Delivery Service: 1-800-342-9678.]*

Mrs. Hanclova is Assistant Professor of economic modelling processes at the Faculty of Economics at the Technical University in Ostrava (Czech Republic). She received her Ing.(M.Sc.) in Mathematical Methods in Economics from the University of Economics in Prague in 1984 and her CSc. (Ph.D.) in Theory of Management and Planning at the Technical University in Ostrava in 1992. Her research interests include Operations research business-oriented applications and implementation of computer based information system for business (especially decision support systems and expert systems). She is a member of the Operations Research Society in Czech Republic and is on their advisory committee.

Address correspondence to: Ing. Jana Hanclova, Faculty of Economics, Technical University, 70221 Ostrava 1, Czech Republic.

[Haworth co-indexing entry note]: "Unemployment in the Czech Republic and Development of an Expert System for Assessing Unemployment Compensation." Hanclova, Jana. Co-published simultaneously in *Computers in Human Services* (The Haworth Press, Inc.) Vol. 12, No. 3/4, 1995, pp. 257-271; and: *Human Services in the Information Age* (ed: Jackie Rafferty, Jan Steyaert, and David Colombi) The Haworth Press, Inc., 1995, pp. 257-271. Single or multiple copies of this article are available from The Haworth Document Delivery Service [1-800-342-9678, 9:00 a.m. - 5:00 p.m. (EST)].

INTRODUCTION

There are six sections in my contribution:

- The development of unemployment in the Czech Republic in 1992.
- Contemporary problems connected with unemployment in the Czech Republic.
- Characteristics of the decision processes leading to employment in job centers in the North Moravia region.
- The contemporary state of information for decision making process of claimants of unemployment compensation.
- The development of a prototype expert system to support decision making and to provide system assessment for the claimants of unemployment compensation.
- The benefits of the prototype expert system.

THE DEVELOPMENT OF UNEMPLOYMENT IN THE CZECH REPUBLIC IN 1992

With the arrival of a market economy in the Czech Republic came the creation of a labor market and increasing problems of unemployment. The advancing transformation of the economy reflects the development of unemployment during 1992. We experienced considerable worker movement with about 400,000 people looking for new jobs in job centers. We did not find the considerable tension expected with the new labour market. Indeed, the rate of unemployment decreased from 4.31% at the end of 1991 to 2.57% at the end of 1992 (Figure 1).

The basic facts, which characterized the development of employment in 1992, can be summarized from the following perspective:

(a) Labour resources (Figure 2)

- growth in the population of productive ages. Starting around 1970, new social conditions provided greater pregnancy benefits, causing an increased birth rate.
- Considerable decline in the employment of those of post productive age (about 50% the result of business management policies and requirements for declaration of income, with resulting higher taxes for pensioners in 1992).

FIGURE 1. Trends in Unemployment.

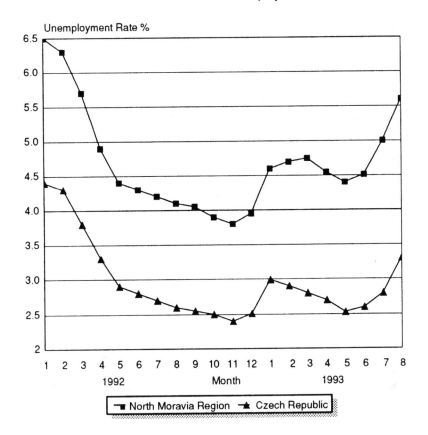

FIGURE 2. Labour Resources (productive activities)–in thousands.

	1991	1992	Difference abs.	%
Total resources from:	6,420	6,348	− 72	98.9
Citizens of productive age	6,090	6,152	+62	101.0
Citizens of post-productive age	294	150	− 144	51.0
Other	36	46	+10	127.8

(b) Structure of labour resources (Figure 3)

- Decrease in the total number of workers by 4.2%.
- Growth of the number of citizens who are not dependent on work for their income.

(c) Supply and demand of manpower in the labour market

- Total numbers in work at the end of 1992 was about 4,050,000 people (79.4% of the total available resources).
- Total demand was 4,905,000 at the end of the year.
- Difference (total supply-total demand) was 135,000 people (that is the number of applicants in the job centers up to the last day in 1992 in the Czech Republic).

(d) Structure of employment

- The number of state owned companies has declined in favour of private ownership (Figure 4).
- Large companies (over 25 workers) reported falling employment (a reduction of about 11%) in favour of small companies (increasing by 91.2%).

These facts indicate trends in the development of employment in 1992 and looked set to continue in 1993 which was considered a decisive period for large privatization and was expected to bring fundamental structural changes. More dynamic changes in the structure of employment were expected. However the forecast rate of unemployment did not exceed 6.5% provided that improvements were implemented in finding new jobs and in advice and information activities; and perhaps in pursuing an active policy[1] of employment. The unemployment rate was 3.17% at the end of August 1993.

FIGURE 3. Labour Resources (distribution)–in thousands.

	1991	1992	Difference abs.	%
Total resources from:	6,420	6,348	−72	98.9
Working (main job)	4,976	4,766	−210	95.8
Women on the maternity leave	286	290	+4	101.4
Preparation for the profession	599	604	+5	100.8
Unable to work of productive age	174	175	+1	100.6
Other citizens of productive age	385	513	+128	133.2

FIGURE 4. Structure of Unemployment.

Type of Ownership

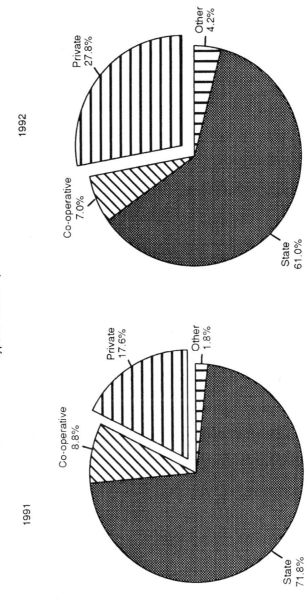

1992

Private
27.8%

Other
4.2%

Co-operative
7.0%

State
61.0%

1991

Private
17.6%

Co-operative
8.8%

Other
1.8%

State
71.8%

CONTEMPORARY PROBLEMS CONNECTED WITH UNEMPLOYMENT IN THE CZECH REPUBLIC

The previous section characterised the main trends in the development of unemployment in 1992. Now I will set out the fundamental changes in the field of unemployment. Along with the transition to a new tax system and the implementation of a fund economy,[2] there are increasing problems of finding optimal alternatives for organizational structure of employment services, including a way of financing employment policies.

Starting in January 1993 we have a new contribution system for paying for active and passive employment policies, with contributions included in the state budget. Payments for employment policies are provided by the state budget as well, in accord with regulations for job centers, together with the running costs of the job centers. In connection with finding optimal alternative organizational structures of services of employment, there are three basic possibilities (including ways of financing):

a. *Insurance company*–for example unemployment as an independent financial institution, ensuring choice and management of funds for employment and based on insurance principles. Next to this insurance institution would be the employment services system that would be engaged in looking for jobs, in ensuring retraining courses, and providing advice. One way to finance employment policies would be to carry out a form of payment by job centers, or a direct payment allowance to citizens. Another possibility admits to payment only of the allowance, and active employment policies would be stimulated from the state budget by job centers.

b. *An employment fund as a state fund or private non-profit institution* controlling funds for employment at the top level. Again, parallel functions of employment services are assumed as before.

c. *Employment services as an independent institution removed from the Ministry of Labour or a private institution.* Employment services management would manage job centers and take care of funds for employment and manage them with consideration for the labour market. These funds would be a component of the state budget or would be taken from the state budget in the case of a private institution.

The best contemporary alternative is considered to be the establishment of management employment services as an independent budgeted institution accountable to the Ministry of Labour. It would manage job centers and implement employment policies in accordance with legal regulations. This employment fund should be removed from the state budget and a state employment fund established. This solution will provide a basis for the future transition of additional independent institutions, and will bring employment services under general judicial principles.

A suggested alternative to re-organization of the structure of employment services and perhaps a way to finance employment policies would be to influence decision making in job centers, including through implementation of new information technology.

CHARACTERISTICS OF DECISION PROCESSES LEADING TO EMPLOYMENT IN JOB CENTERS IN NORTH MORAVIA

The job center officials in the North Moravia region requested cooperation from the Faculty of Economics in the Technical University in Ostrava. The main problem was "improving the process for finding suitable jobs" as a broad concept, starting with the initial registration through to finding a suitable job. The solution to this problem assumes great structural changes in this region expected during 1993 and 1994, and tries to prepare for re-structuring and to influence the supply side of the labour market.

The discussions with the job center officials showed the necessity of elaborating high quality information in the short term and creating organizational, technical and methodological assumptions for the efficient use of information systems. As new information technologies are developed and implemented along with computer networks in job centers in the North Moravia region, contemporary knowledge from the sphere of the artificial intelligence will be important. Most applications in this sphere are in expert systems.

On the basis of the above considerations, the following working hypothesis was formulated:–"*Implementation of information technology during the search process can improve the decision-making processes.*" The basic steps verifying this working hypothesis were:

- The description of contemporary situations during the job search process.
- The development of the prototype expert system for determining decision outcomes.

The results of the description of the decision processes during the job search was the formulation of the basic components and their interactive relations (Figure 5).

Knowledge was obtained on the basis of analysis of existing manual

FIGURE 5. The Basic Scheme of Process of Finding a Job (as a broad concept).

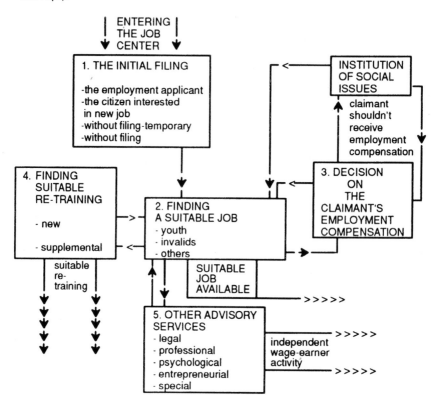

methods, firstly based on interviews with and observation of experienced job center workers, and secondly analysis of knowledge of the required documentation. The whole process of finding work starts with the initial registration by the applicant for a suitable job. On the basis of presented documents and through dialogue, the final decision may be arranged in the following categories:

- employment applicant
- citizens interested in a new job
- without temporary registration
- without registration.

The counsellor refers the registration card to the section mediating the job. The main assignment of this section is finding a suitable job for the applicant as soon as possible or a suitable re-qualification (mediating the job in the narrow sense). On the basis of experience and development of the structure of suitable jobs, it is possible to deduce that some groups of applicants have a very low probability of quickly finding a suitable new job. It is then necessary to complete the required information for this section. For obtaining employment compensation, the claimant must meet a series of conditions and legislative regulations. If there is no individual decision concerning the claimant's employment compensation and the job center is not able to find a suitable job or re-training, the counsellor sends the materials about the applicant to the decision section which considers and issues a decision on:

- awarding employment compensation
- refusal of claimant's unemployment compensation
- removing the applicant from registration
- discontinuing the claimant's employment compensation,
- in case of the award, subsequently stopping employment compensation.

In cases where it is impossible to find a suitable job, it is possible to classify the applicant to re-training courses, which are organized by the state, or at a region or company level. In cases of extended unemployment it is possible to use other advisory services such as private enterprise; professional; legal; youth services; new graduates; pregnant women or applicants older than 50.

On the basis of this broad knowledge about how to provide a job, there are stages of:

- providing a suitable job (in a narrow sense)
- the decision about the claimant's unemployment compensation
- providing suitable re-training
- providing special services and advisory sections in job centers.

The main position of the decision of the claimant's unemployment compensation during unemployment, from the financial point of view, was to pay attention to the implementation of the prototype expert system. Another part of the research work concentrated on the detailed description of the decision of the claimant's unemployment compensation. This is briefly summarized in Figure 6.

266

FIGURE 6. The Basic Scheme of the Decision of the Claimants Unemployment Compensation (CUC).

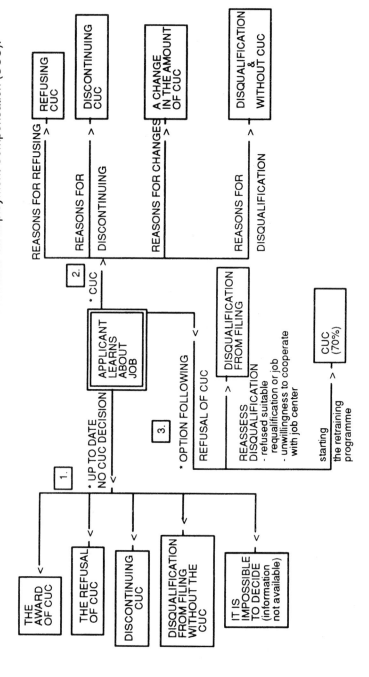

THE CONTEMPORARY STATE OF INFORMATION FOR THE DECISION MAKING PROCESS OF CLAIMANTS OF UNEMPLOYMENT COMPENSATION

Inquiry ensuring the decision making process in assessment of claimants for unemployment compensation is very different in individual job centers in the North Moravia region. Job centers do not have uniform organizational structures and technical equipment. Further it is necessary to say that officials in decision making sections and assessment of claimants for unemployment compensation do not use the same computer-based information system decision support. Most job centers use software called *"Mediating a new Job"* from KOŠICE in the Slovak Republic. It solves the problems of registering new applicants or people interested in suitable new employment. It is set up in the CLIPPER environment and the latest version provides:

- data registration about citizens (including current changes)
- searching for available working opportunities
- printing recommendations for jobs
- recording information from the contact at the job center.

When the Czech and Slovak Republics separated, development of this software package stopped. The Ministry of Labour arranged new software packages for job centers in the Czech Republic, but the organizational arrangements of employment services and ways of financing employment provision policies is not clear. Because of this difficult situation, job centers are building their own software support. Creation of these programmes is not coordinated among job centers in the North Moravia region and this contributes to their development time and duplication of solutions. On the basis of analysis of the decision making processes and information flows, we will approach the development of the prototype expert system for decision making support of claimants for unemployment compensation in the North Moravia region.

DEVELOPMENT OF A PROTOTYPE EXPERT SYSTEM TO SUPPORT DECISION MAKING AND PROVIDE ASSESSMENTS

One of the quickest ways to develop an expert system application is filling the knowledge base of a suitable shell expert system. This selection process is dependent on:

- financial restrictions
- the structure of the problem to be solved
- technical considerations
- available qualified specialists
- how knowledge is represented.

These factors were defined by the job center in Opava and by research at our Faculty of Economics. Analysis of the characteristics of the problem solving involved showed that the decision making process in assessment of claimants for unemployment assistance in the North Moravia region is a suitable, semi-structural problem for an expert system application from the following perspectives:

- An expert's judgement of real cases of applicants becomes an integral part of every day decision making in job centers.
- The decision for assessment of claimants with unemployment compensation assumes inference on the basis of actual law and regulation and real knowledge about the applicant.
- The decision should be completed in a given time, but based on a maximum understanding of the actual case.
- Expertise is one component of the decision process and should be used in other job centers in the North Moravia region to make available important new information from expertise in the individual job centers.
- The decision process results have great influence on actual social employment policies.
- The results of the decision should be legal, and the responsibility of officers in job centers for giving quality services to citizens.

In almost all job centers in the North Moravia region, insufficient modern finance software and hardware support is available. Job centers try to develop information systems without the support of necessary software and hardware. We also do not have knowledge of artificial intelligence implementation in practice. Since 1989, research institutes, universities and specialist software companies have begun building expert systems and are trying to fill a shell expert system. Our region has a shortage of knowledge engineers and experts for the employment fields.

During the selection of a suitable shell, various objectives were evaluated. However the dominant lack of funds forced a decision to use a demo-development version of the shell expert system EXSYS Professional, a product EXSYS Inc. from the USA. This shell expert system has many successful applications and has been positively evaluated in international publications. EXSYS Professional has rule-based representation of knowledge, five possibilities for confidence systems and forward and backward chaining in inference techniques.

On this basis, selection of the shell expert system and specification of the decision making situation led to the formulation of the basic exercises and main segments of the knowledge base, their structure of organization and the process of inference of the value of the new knowledge, including the goal recommendations of the expert system. A brief structure of the dependencies of knowledge segments and rules network is shown in Figure 7.

Expert system recommendations of the claimant's unemployment compensation follow three critical factors:

- the need of claimants for unemployment compensation
- restrictions set by legal regulations
- availability of other allowances.

The requirements show the need of the applicant for an allowance (type of applicant, re-training course decision making). Restrictions on unemployment compensation may be connected with legal conditions, the means available to the claimant and other conditions related to:

- previous employment
- period and place of insurance
- finding suitable retraining
- looking for a suitable job.

The final version of the prototype expert system included sixty-five rules with the structure IF-THEN-ELSE, which were framed by thirty-eight qualifiers. The prototype chose recommendations on the basis of seventeen final specifications of the claimant's unemployment compensation. Testing the knowledge base was completed in the Job Center in Opava, using a test database composed of real applicant cases. Testing the prototype confirmed the right formulation of the hypothesis.

THE BENEFITS OF THE PROTOTYPE EXPERT SYSTEM

Results of this research can be appreciated from two points of view—theoretical and practical benefits. The theoretical benefits consist in expansion of fundamentals of development of expert systems in the North Moravia region (an educational benefit). Benefits in practice can be formulated as:

FIGURE 7. Abstract of the Knowledge Segments and Rules Network.

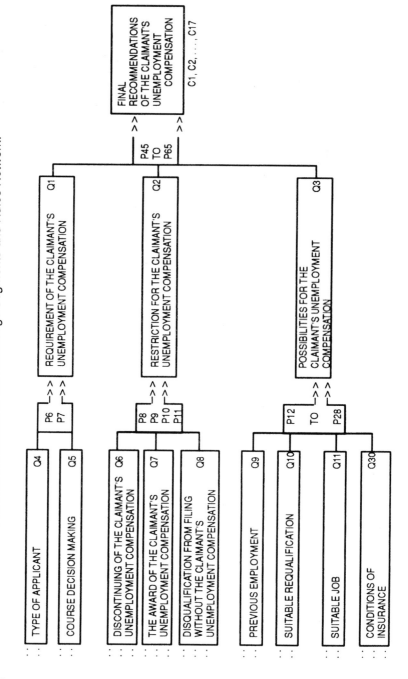

270

- Providing decisions leading to suitable new employment or retraining
- Filling the knowledge base on the actual demand in Opava
- Increased quality of employment services and less delay
- The prototype pays attention to all details and does not overlook relevant information.

In developing a prototype expert system, the main direction for improvement and expansion in the future are suggested as:

- To obtain the run-time/development version of a shell expert system with a rules network for knowledge representation
- Implementation of the expert system in the Czech environment (respect for Czech language and grammar)
- Extension of the prototype expert system to other job centers
- Inclusion of hypertext and a help system (for example hypertext with real law regulations)
- printing final administrative documents for applicants for new jobs
- to establish an adequate intellectual base for development of expert systems in the Moravia region and co-ordinate their research
- To pay attention to obtaining new financial resources for research in economics.

NOTES

1. Active employment policy represents the costs for active arrangement for employment support such as re-qualification, creation of new work opportunities-working places for public purpose.
2. A fund economy means the creation of relevant special purpose funds composed of employees' and employers' payments such as employment management, social and medical insurances.

REFERENCES

Carsky J.(1993). "The analysis of the development of employment in 1992," *Social Policy, Num. 5, Economia*, Prague.
Hanclova J.(1991). *"Computer Systems for Supporting Decision-Making,"* Technical University, Ostrava.
Parizkova, J. (1993). "Searching for optimal alternatives," *Social policy, Num. 5, Economia*, Prague.
Turban, E. (1990). *"Decision Support and Expert Systems,"* Macmillan Publishing Company, New York.

The Development of a Computerized Information System for Integrated Home Care in The Netherlands

Eric Verkaar

SUMMARY. In September 1992, The Netherlands Institute of Care and Welfare (NIZW) started development of GIRST, a computerized information system for the new integrated home care services in The Netherlands. These services integrated home nursing and family care services, with many institutions merging to facilitate the process. Integration of services required reorganization of all of the information processes and new technology provided the opportunity for improvement in their quality. These factors of reorganisation and of new technology opportunities stimulated NIZW to develop GIRST, which is designed as a tool to facilitate provision of care. It is not focused on managerial issues but on the information needs and concerns of those who actually provide care. The process of providing home care can be divided into four stages which correspond with the four modules of GIRST: care coordination–care allocation–care in practice–care evaluation.

Eric Verkaar studied sociology at Tilburg University in The Netherlands where he was also a researcher in the department for Policy and Management Science from 1985-1986. He then completed a doctorate at Erasmus University in Rotterdam on strategic management of patient organizations in Dutch health care. Since 1991 he has worked at the Home Care and Prevention section of The Netherlands Institute of Care and Welfare in Utrecht. Eric Verkaar's work focuses on managerial issues concerning integration of home nursing and family care and he is the manager of the GIRST project described in this chapter.

Address correspondence to: Eric Verkaar, Netherlands Institute of Care and Welfare, Catharijnesingel 47, PO Box 19152, 3501 DD Utrecht, The Netherlands.

[Haworth co-indexing entry note]: "The Development of a Computerized Information System for Integrated Home Care in The Netherlands." Verkaar, Eric. Co-published simultaneously in *Computers in Human Services* (The Haworth Press, Inc.) Vol. 12, No. 3/4, 1995, pp. 273-287; and: *Human Services in the Information Age* (ed: Jackie Rafferty, Jan Steyaert, and David Colombi) The Haworth Press, Inc., 1995, pp. 273-287. Single or multiple copies of this article are available from The Haworth Document Delivery Service [1-800-342-9678, 9:00 a.m. - 5:00 p.m. (EST)].

273

GIRST is being developed by a noncommercial institute for developing care and welfare in The Netherlands in cooperation with a few small specialized firms, not by a large commercial software firm. In developing GIRST particular ways of prototyping were chosen to formulate functional and technical descriptions. The choices of the developer and of the methodology are both unconventional but they enable development of a flexible and highly practical information system for home care services. *[Article copies available from The Haworth Document Delivery Service: 1-800-342-9678.]*

INTRODUCTION

In The Netherlands a new computerized information system for the recently integrated home care services is being developed by The Netherlands Institute of Care and Welfare (NIZW). This information system is abbreviated in Dutch as GIRST and in this paper I intend to characterize its aims and functionality. GIRST as a computerized information system consists of four modules which are described separately and in their mutual relationships and inter-connections. A short analysis of the preferred hardware platforms is also provided. Developing an information system like GIRST is a complex task and a non-traditional way of developing the software was chosen. This paper describes and explains the process of developing GIRST and discusses the role of different organizations involved in the process. Before outlining the functionality of GIRST, the reasons for developing a new information system for the home care services in The Netherlands are explained.

WHY DEVELOP A NEW INFORMATION SYSTEM?

The Dutch government report *Van samenwerken naar samengaan* ("From cooperation to consolidation," Ministry of Welfare, Health and Cultural Affairs, The Netherlands) inspired a wave of integration processes in many organizations for home nursing and family care throughout The Netherlands. Home care organizations offer a broad package of care services, the most important of which are district nursing, care for the elderly and child and maternity care. So far, integration has mainly affected district services but in the future will affect all services. Several organizations have already taken the first steps towards a completely integrated system of home care.

Integration involves more than a simple merger of two existing types of organizations; it creates a totally new organization with a completely new process of care provision. The integration of home nursing and family care was planned to improve both efficiency and quality. It enables a single organization (with one referral point) to offer better care by coordinating the expertise of the different care providers to meet needs more efficiently. The single referral point enables central assessment, provides sharing opportunities and encourages conditions that facilitate efficient coordination of care. These features of an integrated home care organization are developments that the government favours, as described in the policy document *Home care in the nineties* (Ministry of Welfare, Health and Cultural Affairs, 1992). Improvements in care provision can only be made if integrated home care organizations substantially reorganize their whole process of care provision. In particular, the greater variety of client problems and of care requests, together with greater diversity of expertise within the new organization, *necessitate* substantial changes.

CHANGED INFORMATION PROCESSES AND TECHNOLOGY

The task of establishing a new information and registration system goes hand in hand with that of developing a new integrated care process. Each care provision process involves exchanging and recording information. The goal of improving the quality and effectiveness of care requires a new process of information exchange. Information must be collected, recorded and passed on to support the provision of care and is central to decision-making for all aspects of care provision. The information, registration and communication processes in a new, integrated service differ from those needed for separate organizations for home nursing and family care.

The organization of care provision and the information procedures are not the only aspects which involve change: the technology and tools with which information is collected, stored and passed on will also differ. The first personal computers, hand-held and portable computers (notebooks) are being used in home care (Van Thiel, 1991) in addition to the mainframe and mini-computers which have been used for some time for administrative processes. These new tools and this technology enable us to collect, record and pass on far more information. Of course, the use of this technology costs a great deal of time and money, but that applies to established communication systems such as mail and telephone networks. Moreover relevant information is not stored and kept (except in the memory of the person involved) because it takes too much time to use older tools and systems such as archives. Current methods of keeping records are inefficient as the same information may be recorded several times and in several places. Use of modern information technology can improve this situation.

SUPPORTING THE PROVISION
OF CARE THROUGH INFORMATION

The main issue for this project is how new information technology and tools can be used to establish effective information and communication processes within the new integrated home care organizations. These processes, which aim to facilitate high-quality care, will ultimately be "translated" into a computerized information and registration system. NIZW started designing this system (GIRST) in order to establish the information, registration and communication processes needed. This system does not–due to the nature of NIZW's professional development goals–include all the communication processes within an integrated home care organization, but is restricted to processes which are directly relevant to the actual provision of care. Support of the primary activity, the direct provision of care, is the focus of concern.

The NIZW publication *"Van samengaan naar samenwerken"* (Verkaar, Slingerland and Van Amelsvoort, 1992) describes the future care provision process within an integrated home care organization. Broadly speaking, the home care process consists of four phases:

- *Care coordination* (formerly known as "intake" or "assessment"). This comprises processes such as assessment of needs, defining aims and determining the kind of care needed.
- *Care allocation.* Care is allocated on the basis of recommendations made throughout these processes. The expertise of various care professionals and the capacity present within an organization play an important role in allocation. Care must therefore be allocated on the basis of certain decision procedures which use information from the process of care coordination.
- *Care in practice.* The actual process of care starts after care has been allocated to a client and is provided by different care providers.
- *Evaluation.* When a client no longer needs care, the process is evaluated from the client's perspective and that of the care provider(s). Long-term care can involve periodic evaluations rather than just at the end.

MODULES AND SYSTEMS

Four registration, information and communication processes can be designed for the four care provision stages identified above. These processes can be "translated" into four modules or components of the GIRST information system. The modules can be considered as instruments which make the different processes possible. GIRST integrates the four components into a single whole and shows the links between them. In addition, GIRST allows links to existing computerized solutions in different fields of home care (such as client administration, salary administration or the purchasing system). In the future it will also be possible to link up to information systems of other care providers, such as general practitioners and hospitals.

In the next section the realization of the four modules of GIRST is discussed in greater detail. Figure 1 gives a schematic representation of the process of home care and of the GIRST modules.

FIGURE 1. Process of home care and GIRST.

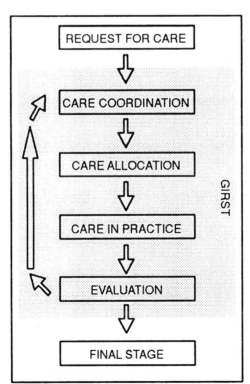

THE WORKING OF GIRST

This section discusses the aims of this project. It explains how GIRST will work, who it is intended for, the kind of information it will supply and to whom. NIZW has come up with an organizational design for the new home care service which focuses on team work. It is of course possible to design several different organizational structures for integrated home care, which would define professional units differently. An example is the present division between district nursing teams and family care teams. This distinction could either be maintained, or replaced by a new organization of the professional carers in which an integrated (multi-disciplinary) team would play an important part.

An integrated multi-disciplinary team unites all of the disciplines that are a part of home care: district nursing, district medical care, specialized family care and unlicensed carers. This approach enables the best possible coordination of care. An integrated team also best satisfies the quality requirements which are the basis for integration of services. There could still be tasks for single-disciplinary teams, such as straightforward "one-off" requests for domestic or health care.

The explanation of how GIRST works is based on the assumption that integrated teams will be providing the care. The system works in a similar way for non-integrated teams, but a simpler information procedure may suffice for less joint care. A team is made up of an operational manager and several care providers. A client's first contact with the team is normally with a care supervisor appointed to him or her. The care supervisor is responsible for all care given to the client by the home care organization, whilst the care is provided by an integrated team. In addition the care is coordinated by separate care coordinators. The final care evaluation is not performed by officials directly involved in delivery of care, but by a separate care evaluator or by the care coordinator. There is also an administrative official for home care in every working area. A home care office is used as headquarters by the officials and non-administrative personnel in a given working area. A more detailed description of those organizational concepts can be found in a recent publication: *Van samengaan naar samenwerken; modellen voor een geïntegreerde thuiszorg* ("From consolidation to cooperation; models for integrated home care," Verkaar, Slingerland and Van Amelsfoort, 1992).

Variations in Forms of Organization

Throughout this paper we have assumed for convenience that there is one way in which integrated home care takes place. There are other models which are not discussed here. However we have considered a variety of organizational structures in designing the information system–for instance differing relations of care coordination to care allocation. The pilot institutions vary in their structure and the information system must be applicable to as many variations as possible. In this way the care coordination module is not just for use by a specialist "registration official" but can also be used by the head of a team who is responsible for the "registration" or even by a care professional. GIRST is therefore designed to be used in as many forms of organization as possible.

Separate Use by Home Nursing and Family Care

Although GIRST is intended for integrated home care organizations, it is in principle applicable, at least in part, to home nursing institutions and to family care organizations. When these agencies share clients on whom they want to exchange information, it is necessary to make clear arrangements about management and exchange of this information. Arrangements must cover who is allowed to change what in a care plan, or in the care coordination data at each stage. In testing the system, experiments are carried out in this area to make the final system work in agencies which are not yet integrated. It is clear that, from an organizational perspective, this is more complex and that not all system options will be applicable.

NIZW's ideal concept of an integrated home care organization is used here to describe how the different modules of the information system are to operate. We must reiterate that the system is applicable to several organizational variants, not all of which are dealt with here.

THE CARE COORDINATION MODULE

A care coordinator can, as it were, "take immediate action" to find out what kind of care the client needs and what kind of support the institution (or other agencies) should provide. In order to obtain a complete picture of the care needs, a care coordinator has an assessment interview at the client's home and carries a notebook computer for this purpose. This has the GIRST care coordination module on it which replaces the old assessment forms. During the interview with a potential client all data relevant to care provision and of possible future importance is recorded. The care coordination module consists of a method of determining the care needs which results in a "home care diagnosis." This diagnosis includes goals which help determine the kind of care needed.

THE CARE ALLOCATION MODULE

The care coordinator returns from the home interview and transfers the data from the notebook computer to the office personal computer. The data from the home interview is used by the care coordinator to propose the combination of tasks to be carried out for the client. This proposal indicates from which discipline(s) care providers are needed and how long care provision will take. The first part of the care allocation module (care recommendation) is used for this stage and it also proposes a particular team, if there is a choice.

The care recommendations are passed on electronically to the operational manager (the supervisor) of the relevant team. The operational manager has an office at the home base of the teams and therefore uses the same computer (or network). The operational manager uses the second part of the module to organize the allocation of care which takes into account the availability of staff in the areas in which the client requires assistance. If, for instance, a district medical attendant in that discipline is not available, either a district nurse or a family care provider will be temporarily allocated to the client. Allocation depends on the complexity of care needed and on experience and expertise of the available care providers. The care allocation data must therefore include all client data which is relevant to needs, accompanied by an allocation of care for the tasks to be carried out and the time to be spent on these tasks.

THE MODULE FOR CARE IN PRACTICE

The care supervisors receive the care allocation data from their operational manager. The care supervisor then passes on this data and develops the care plan on the basis of this information using the computer at the home care office. Of course this is done after consultation with the client. The development of the care plan is the first element of the computerized GIRST module for care in practice. The module provides detailed lists of the kind of care needed, the actual care needs and of the care providers who will contribute (both from within and outside the home care organization). The care plan is in fact a complete inventory of the "whos," "whats," "wheres," "whens" and "whys."

All internal care providers working on the client's case receive a paper copy of the care plan and pass on proposals for changes during the care process to the care supervisor. Thus, the care plan is continually updated. The care plan focuses in particular on the goals and actions to be taken from the perspective of the client's needs. The plan made by the care supervisor is passed on to each care provider either on paper on a standard form or electronically. We will describe these variants briefly and examine their usefulness in the project. The second variant involves hand-held computers which can only hold a limited amount of data.

The first variant leads to a situation in which a care provider has been given a care plan on paper by the supervisor which is given to the client. Suggestions for changes are made orally or in writing to the care supervisor who decides whether to adopt them and passes on printed copies of the new care plan to all the care providers involved. The information on the care situation of the client is recorded in a logbook. In both variants, this logbook is a written record which remains with the client. The different care providers record relevant information in this logbook such as changes in the illness or the tasks which were carried out each day or week. The client also comments on his or her own situation in the logbook. It is helpful for this logbook to also be used by other care providers from outside the main agency.

In the second variant, the care provider enters the care plan which was developed by the care supervisor in a Personal Digital Assistant (PDA). This ensures that the information is always on hand and readily accessible during actual care provision. It also makes it possible to enter suggestions for changes in the care plan at the client's home. The PDA may also hold information files for the care provider, containing for instance useful addresses for the client or tools the client might be able to use. In the future it may be possible to create a practical support programme for care providers for instance as regards dressing wounds. In this way the quality of the care provided can be improved considerably. Less readily available knowledge may be stored in such a system and accessed when needed.

In the project, both variants (and possible combinations) are examined on their usefulness. In any case the information system will be constructed in such a way that both variants can be implemented by an agency as needed. The costs of investing in the equipment to be used by the care providers will determine, more than any other factor, which variant is chosen.

The information recorded by the care providers and stored in the system, can be retrieved by the team's operational manager. The report part of the module for care practice can be used to analyze the care provided, for instance, as compared to the care recommended. Moreover the progress of the care provision processes can be shown with the help of information from the care plans (and possibly from the logbooks). Based on these management reports an operational manager can draw up periodic plans.

Of course it is advisable to incorporate these reports at a later stage in the central management information system of the integrated home care organization.

THE CARE EVALUATION MODULE

An interim care evaluation will take place as specified in the care plan. This is carried out by the care supervisor and may lead to an adjustment of the care plan or even renewed care coordination. The interim care evaluation is the first element of this module. When a client no longer needs care, the provision is terminated. The final stage of care provision consists of an interview between the client and the care evaluator. In this interview the client may describe his or her experiences with the home care organization in general and with the particular care providers. The care evaluator uses a fairly standard formula for this interview with relevant information stored on a notebook computer and the data later transferred to the computer system in the home care office. The data gathered during the evaluation is of obvious importance to the operational manager of the team in charge of the care, as well as to the management of the entire organization or of a certain region. For this reason they issue a periodic report. Furthermore some of the data from the evaluation and the final stage of care should be linked to other information systems within the home care organization, such as the client registration or costs declaration systems (with care insurers).

THE HARDWARE PLATFORMS INVOLVED

The hardware chosen is an important factor in determining the performance, functionality and costs of developing the software, which is the central element of the system. Four different types of computers were mentioned above:

The central computer. The institutions already have central computers: mainframes or minis. However, these computers will be used as little as possible in processing the GIRST data. It will be necessary from time to time to link these computers to the equipment used for the GIRST. This link however falls outside of the scope of this project, since it depends on different systems.

The PCs or desk-top computers. Each home care office will be equipped with a PC or similar computer, with a printer, for use by the home care manager and the care providers for some tasks. This small network serves as a storage place for the data gathered by the team. In the light of our concern for a user-friendly approach in this project we chose to use software with a graphics interface. For the development period of GIRST, Apple Macintosh computers were chosen because of their excellent graphical user interface and development costs are relatively low.

This software can be adapted later for use on Microsoft Windows at a small additional cost (approx. 15%). We did not choose the Windows system initially because of its low speed, its high requirements in terms of equipment and its still imperfect reliability. The Apple Macintosh computers also have greater built-in connectivity which simplifies, and therefore cuts the costs of, writing communication software for instance for communicating with the central computer. The definitive GIRST will be available for computers using Windows.

The notebook (or powerbook) computer. The care coordinators and evaluators have to collect important data for GIRST from the client at home. For this they need a portable computer with a large screen with user friendly software to maintain productivity. For now we have opted for Apple Powerbooks but a later "translation" to Windows may be performed if the market so desires.

PDAs. Careproviders will also use small computers for recording data on a daily basis. GIRST will use pen-oriented hand-held PDA (Personal Digital Assistant) computers which are developed by Apple and other firms. The data contained in these hand-held computers will be transferred to the computer in the home care office.

THE PROCESS OF DEVELOPING GIRST

This section describes how the process of developing GIRST is being realized. We first explain the structure of the project–its different phases. The realization process of developing an integrated information and registration system for home care can be broken down into several phases. Hartman and Roos's system (1989) identified four phases: functional design–technical design–building–implementation. These phases reflect the traditional process of designing an information system, which consists of a linear development from design to operational system. The disadvantage of this process is that interim changes in the functional design cannot be incorporated as changes or improvements in the final system without a great deal of trouble (and expense). This is a much greater potential problem if the requirements a system will eventually have to meet are still unknown at the onset of its development.

The introduction of more advanced programming languages and tools has made it easier to build prototypes of parts of the information system at an early stage. Prototypes are working models of (parts of) an information system which have not yet been completed, but which operate and can be adjusted to meet the clients' wishes (cf. Bots, Van Hek and Van Swede, 1990, p. 843). Prototypes activate a cyclical or iterative process, which continually adjusts the functional design because the users can indicate their experiences when using the prototype. These wishes serve to determine both the functional design and the technical design in increasing detail. Ultimately, a completely tested prototype results in a well-balanced functional and technical design which is expanded to a final, definitive information system.

Functional Design

A number of activities take place in the functional design phase, which started in September 1992. It is essential that the foundations for the eventual system are laid during this phase. Actually this phase determines the nature of the future operation of the system. Designs are developed for the information exchange involved in the provision of care, based on problems NIZW anticipated in information processes in integrated home care, and on the diagnosis of future home care organizations. The module divisions already made and the related procedures are developed in great detail during this phase. In addition, the basic principles and criteria which the GIRST system must meet (connectivity, user-friendliness, etc.) are elaborated.

All the modules are completed and designed for the collection and processing of information, based on two NIZW trial projects. A description of the care coordination tool, which forms the basis for the care coordination module, is given in the publication *Thuiszorg bemiddeld* ("Coordinated home care," Slingerland and Van Amelsvoort, 1993). The care allocation tool, which forms the basis for the functional design of the care allocation module, is described separately in the publication *Op kwaliteit aangesproken* ("An appeal on quality," Van Amelsvoort, Slingerland and Verkaar, 1993). The functional concepts of the other two modules have not yet been published in detail.

The process of functional design is not linear before prototyping and technical design. Prototyping and functional design are phases which are circular, but which start with first description of desired functionality on the basis of an information analysis. After that prototypes are programmed and tested, leading to new information and alterations of the original functional designs.

Prototypes and Technical Design

The technical design phase involves specifications of the equipment and programs to be used. The system designs manual procedures, and develops data structures and processing rules. As our approach includes building prototypes, these already contain part of the technical design. Both the functional and the technical design are adjusted continually on the basis of the response and experiences of users of these prototypes. When prototype testing has concluded, a final functional and technical design is made. Testing the prototypes is in cooperation with workers from four home care institutions although several teams are interviewed for and shown the prototypes. They are built for use in practice by these different teams from different institutions.

Prototypes are not built by the NIZW, but through its contract with a specialized small programming firm. A very tight form of cooperation is necessary to make such a construction work. A programming firm tends to work in a solistic way and guided only by its own ideas. Very regular collaboration is necessary to guide the programmer in the direction desired by the contractor. Part of a functional design is also a complete description of the database structure which requires specialized technical knowledge. In this developing process the database structure is based on the prototypes by a specialized firm, which had already made database descriptions for information systems in the home care services. The phases of functional design, prototyping and technical design were completed at the end of 1993.

Building the System

To build a solid and professional information system for a critical market like institutions for home care services, a very professional, solid and experienced firm is required. In this developing process, flexibility and specialized knowledge is acquired by contracting specialized small firms. However these small firms cannot build a very complex information system like GIRST, so by means of a public tender a suitable firm will be selected to build the definitive system. This will only be the very complex programming work, because the functional and technical design is complete. The selection of the final builder was held at the end of 1993, for the definitive information system to be completed at the end of 1994.

Implementation: The Market of Home-Care Institutions

When GIRST is completed as a computerized information system at the end of 1994, it has to be implemented: people will need to work with it but will it have a role? The Netherlands Institute for Care and Welfare (NIZW) is an independent development foundation, subsidized by the Dutch Government, which has no power to force institutions to use GIRST or any other products. Home care services will have to be convinced by the qualities and value of GIRST in order to start buying it. So in essence GIRST is a commercial product which is developed through governmental finances. This governmental investment will reduce the price of this system but will not lead to public domain software!

In order to be sure of good maintenance and support of this information system, a commercial formula is used. An institution buys GIRST as an information system (mainly software) and can choose from several packages of support. By buying it, an institution identifies the product as worthwhile and pays for maintenance and continuity. The supplier will be a commercial software builder and distributor who will be responsible for selling, maintaining and supporting GIRST. Whether GIRST will be bought or not by home care institutions will depend on GIRST communicating with administrative information systems which are already operating (or will operate in the near future). To guarantee this, the database structure is designed so that import and export of significant data is possible with the few leading applications in the market for home-care information systems in The Netherlands.

CONCLUSION

In this paper I have pictured the process of developing GIRST, a new computerized information system for the home care services in The Netherlands. This system is not developed by a commercial software producer, but by an independent non-commercial developing institute for health care services, in cooperation with small specialized firms and in the end with a large commercial software producer and retailer. In this way every party can contribute its own strengths and flexibilities to this development process. It is essential that GIRST as an information system is designed and developed by people who are not software producers, but by developers in health care.

While developing GIRST, we have chosen prototyping as an essential part of our designing process. This seems to have been a successful approach. However prototypes are not complete full-grown pieces of software and workers in health care sometimes cannot wait to have their new instruments ready. So disappointment occurs when people think that their new prototype is already what they want it ultimately to be. Expectations of prototypes are sometimes too high and one can never be careful enough to explain elaborately the exact function of prototypes at the beginning of a developing process!

A strength is almost certainly also a weakness. The process of developing GIRST as described in this paper contains a lot of actors. This means mutual adjustment and potential conflict. A huge amount of work has been done and has to be done in the field of negotiating. The result will hopefully be a very useful and flexible information system for the home care services in The Netherlands. The price to be paid is a lot of work and risks and uncertainty during the developing process. Only time will tell whether or not this has been a successful approach. So far we can only be hopeful, but there are still a lot of problems to be solved to be successful in the end.

REFERENCES

Amelsvoort F. van, Slingerland P. and Verkaar E. (1991) *Criteria inzet menskracht geïntegreerde thuiszorg; basismodel voor de vaststelling van de inzet van menskracht*, Rapport NIZW, Utrecht, Juni 1991.
Amelsvoort F. van, Slingerland P. and Verkaar E. (1993) *Op kwaliteit aangesproken*, NIZW/Haeghepoorte, Utrecht/Den Haag.
Bots, J.M., van Heck E. and Swede V. van (1990) *Bestuurlijke informatiekunde*, Cap Gemini Publishing, Rijswijk.
Cayne D. (1990) *The personal computing scenario*, Gartner Group, Stamford USA.
Davies G.B. and Olson M.H. (1987) *Management informatiesystemen*, Academic Service, Schoonhoven.
Hartman, W. and Roos J.(1989) *Systeemontwikkeling*, Kluwer, Deventer.
Ministerie van WVC (1992) *Thuiszorg in de jaren '90*, DOP, SDU, 's-Gravenhage.
Ministerie van WVC (1990) *Van samenwerken naar samengaan; gezinsverzorging en kruiswerk naar een geïntegreerde thuiszorg*, DOP, SDU, 's-Gravenhage.
Slingerland, P. and Amelsvoort F. van (1991) *Thuiszorg bekeken, referentiekader voor te ontwikkelen instrumenten en protocollen voor het intakeproces binnen de Centra voor Thuiszorg te Den Haag*, NIZW, Utrecht, November 1991.
Slingerland, P. and Amelsvoort F. van (1993) *Thuiszorg bemiddeld*, NIZW/Haeghepoorte, Utrecht/Den Haag.
Stuurgroep Integratie Kruiswerk-Maatschappelijke Dienstverlening Midden en Noord Oost Twente (1991) *Modelstructuur Stichting Thuiszorg Centraal Twente*, Stichting Thuiszorg Centraal Twente, Hengelo.
Thiel E. van (1991) *In Rotterdam doen ze een deel van de WAS de deur uit*, MGZ, p. 10-14, April 1991.
Verkaar E., Slingerland P. and Amelsvoort F. van (1991) *Thuiszorg in Oost Gelderland; model voor een geïntegreerd hulpaanbod*, Rapport NIZW, Utrecht, December 1991.
Verkaar E., Slingerland P. and Amelsvoort F. van (1992) *Van samengaan naar samen werken; modellen voor een geïntegreerd zorgaanbod*, NIZW/Haeghepoorte, Utrecht/Den Haag.

INFORMATION SYSTEMS
FOR AGENCIES AND PRACTITIONERS

Introduction

Jan Steyaert

Without doubt the use of information systems for agencies and practitioners has been one of the most widely discussed applications of information technology in human services. Following the success of accounting systems and the hype of Management Information Systems (MIS) in the commercial sector, human services have looked for similar applications in their agencies. This has connected with the decade-old discussion on the use of client information systems and their alleged benefits/dangers. The papers in this section deal with the current state-of-the-art on these information systems. The first two discuss the major issues of organizational influences and integration, the following two relating to the important issue of reliability. The second of these introduces four perspectives on the introduction of a national uniform client registration system in the Netherlands, each discussing an aspect of this major development. The final

Jan Steyaert is Consultant at Causa, the innovation centre of the Institute of Higher Education, Faculty of Health Care and Social Work, Eindhoven, the Netherlands.

[Haworth co-indexing entry note]: "Introduction." Steyaert, Jan. Co-published simultaneously in *Computers in Human Services* (The Haworth Press, Inc.) Vol. 12, No. 3/4, 1995, pp. 289-293; and: *Human Services in the Information Age* (ed: Jackie Rafferty, Jan Steyaert, and David Colombi) The Haworth Press, Inc., 1995, pp. 289-293. Single or multiple copies of this article are available from The Haworth Document Delivery Service [1-800-342-9678, 9:00 a.m. - 5:00 p.m. (EST)].

289

contribution presents some challenging suggestions to take the issue of information systems beyond the existing thresholds.

The paper by Neugeboren gives an extensive overview of the literature on an important aspect of information systems in the human services. While others have focused on the technological innovations of new developments, Neugeboren raises the issue of organizational influences on management information systems. He notes that too often information systems have been developed whilst making false assumptions about the environment in which they function, thereby almost guaranteeing failure. The author describes some of the failures and successes of information systems in human services and the factors that were responsible. He then outlines the main barriers to the successful development and implementation of MIS. These include staff resistance and power structures, but also the focus on efficiency versus effectiveness and organizational change. Neugeboren concludes his paper by suggesting three key solutions that can be applied to overcome the described barriers. These are the structural location of MIS departments within the organization; the involvement of practitioners in the development and implementation of the information system; and using an organizational analysis as a prerequisite for a successful MIS. This paper gives an excellent overview of the different organizational issues involved in the development and implementation of information systems in human services, condensing decades of research and publications into a single text.

The next paper by Benbenishty and Oyserman introduces the concept of Integrated Information Systems (IIS). The IIS is in the first place a clinical information system, supporting the needs of professional practitioners. Without properly addressing these needs, Benbenishty and Oyserman argue that managerial and policy information systems are very costly and provide inaccurate data. The three main information needs of practitioners distinguished are monitoring, communication and learning from experience. In developing and implementing a computerized integrated information system that provides a tool for these needs, specific attention has been given to information gathering, information storage, data retrieval, information processing and reporting. This approach was used by the authors in different areas such as foster care agencies in Israel, child residential care and lately, foster care agencies in Michigan. The authors describe the way this approach was implemented in these settings and conclude their paper with an overview of the multiple benefits of integrated information systems.

While previous papers focused on the issue of organizational effect on information systems and the organizational encapsulation of information systems, the paper by Auslander and Cohen is concerned with the issue of data reliability and is based on their experiences in developing and implementing an information system for hospital social work in Israel. As shown elsewhere during the HUSITA 3 conference (Barnes, 1993), accuracy proves to be a major issue. Computers may induce a feeling of accuracy, but when one compares the computer data with the data in the paper files (not even with the "real life" data), one finds an average error rate of 24%. Auslander and Cohen describe two major causes for reliability problem, being problems inherent in the data (be it phenomenological or operational problems) and problems stemming from the staff. These staff have to fulfill three concurrent roles in the data collection process, each requiring special attention regarding reliability. In order to improve reliability in the information system of the Israeli hospital social work system, the authors used a three stage approach. At first, taxonomies for the different key variables were developed, during which preference was given to gross categories. While this was assumed to improve accuracy of the data, it also reduced the clinical relevance. This was however acceptable for a temporary solution. Secondly, the relevant reliability issues were identified for three situations, being accuracy in reporting on clients, variables with high face validity and those with low face validity. Thirdly, for each of these situations, detailed guidelines and definitions were developed. The reliability of the information system was tested after measures were taken by presenting case vignettes to social workers and comparing their results with the "correct" answers. Results on client reporting, high face validity and low face validity variables are given. This paper clearly describes the importance of the reliability of data in information systems and outlines some possible measures to make improvements. It also clearly demonstrates that the solution of the reliability problem is not a product (such as a good manual, or a help function in the software) but a process of learning, both for the organization and the staff.

The next paper continues issues raised in the previous two, but also opens a series of four contributions from the Netherlands with a common background. Van der Laan agrees with Neugeboren in that the rapid technological developments have not had a substantial impact on the content and quality of service provision. These are caught in slow processes that do not match the rapid processes of technological change. This paper disagrees with Auslander and Cohen's view of the use of gross categories in order to improve reliability, which for van der Laan is precisely the reason why information systems have such a low impact. The author refers to those broad categories as "garbage cans." The common background to this and the next three contributions are some major developments in the

Dutch social welfare system. With the new law on social welfare in 1988, the responsibility and funding of a whole range of social services was decentralised to the level of the local authorities. In order to improve accountability and to avoid disparity among social services, substantial efforts were made to develop and implement uniform data and information structures for all agencies. This resulted in a number of sectorial "GFOs" (Gemeenschappelijke Functionele Ontwerpen = Common Functional Designs) for different areas such as general social work and social service departments. By elaborating two examples on addicts and financial problems, van der Laan illustrates that the use of broad categories in collecting information generates useless information, that in no way relates to the costs of obtaining it. The author therefore strongly proposes the use of separate collection of the data at the source, rather then the use of "garbage cans." Data can always be aggregated when needed, but not disaggregated below the level used during the phase of data gathering. The author ends his contribution by linking this discussion on information quality with Habermas' work and the importance of the quality of communication.

While the previous paper described some of the issues that remained problematic in the new Dutch information system for general social work, Potting describes the history of this system and the advantages of having a database with information on all clients and agencies of general social work in the Netherlands. The author describes the three decades of gathering, processing and using the client information. Three major innovations can be followed through this historical account. The first is the increasing number of organisations that took part in a "uniform" national system. While these organisations were few at the beginning, they now form the overwhelming majority, with others likely to follow soon. The second development runs parallel with the first one and concerns the introduction of a national uniform way of dealing with client information. While there were three or four different, conflicting systems at the start of this process, each of them claiming to be the best, the introduction of the new law on social welfare provided the necessary incentive to integrate the different systems into one. The third main development throughout these three decades is the establishment of a national client databank where all client data are (anonymously) centralised and processed. The rich opportunities of such a database on a national level are described.

Although in a different area of human services (youth assistance), the paper by Smorenburg and Prickarts relates to the previous ones in that it describes concurrent developments of decentralising, regulatory and funding responsibilities (to the provincial level) while at the same time establishing a national uniform information policy. They start with describing some of the history of youth assistance in the Netherlands and the present day challenges of combining restricted funding and increase in demands. Within this history, the place and importance of a national centre for registration is situated. The authors outline some of the earlier attempts to create a national information policy for youth assistance agencies and the reasons of their failures. They continue to describe the options chosen at the time of the creation of the national centre, and how these were replaced with a more managerial focus and decentralised data-entry and processing. This situation created a local market for small-scale client information software, similar to, and overlapping with, the market for general social work mentioned in Potting's contribution. The paper concludes with developments likely to take place in the near future, with the establishment of regional registration points as an organisational change and the introduction of results flow charts as a methodological innovation. These charts will enable managers and policy makers to follow flows of youth between service organisations, without endangering clients' privacy.

This section concludes with a paper addressing a general approach regarding information systems for agencies and practitioners. Roosenboom, reacts against the widespread view that social work is slow in using information technology due to computer fear or anxiety for bureaucratisation. In order to put a new focus in the discussion, he elaborates on the difference between automation and informatisation. The first concept refers to the use of certain kinds of technology (automats) to make existing patterns of data and information more efficient. The second concept refers to the creation of new data and information flows, regardless of whether they are established with new technology or not. Roosenboom argues that social work is not lagging behind in automation processes, as accounting and word-processing are commonly done by using computers. Social work is behind other areas because it is faced with informatisation, rather than automation processes. In order to successfully carry out this necessary informatisation process, two different implementation efforts are needed, a technical one and a social one. The author concludes by proposing two levels at which solutions can be found, the level of implemented information and the level of technical progress.

Organizational Influences
on Management Information Systems
in the Human Services

Bernard Neugeboren

SUMMARY. Successful development and implementation of MIS requires an understanding of how organization goals and structures constrain and/or facilitate MIS. Some organizational factors influencing MIS are: ideology, staff resistance, power structure, efficiency vs. effectiveness; agency stability, leadership, organizational change and politics and self-interest. Strategies to overcome these barriers are: structural location of MIS; user involvement in MIS design and implementation; and organizational analysis as perquisites for MIS. *[Article copies available from The Haworth Document Delivery Service: 1-800-342-9678.]*

INTRODUCTION

Implementation of information systems in the human services depends not only on technical knowledge needed in the design of these systems, but also on the ability to overcome organizational barriers that impede the successful use of information in decision making for practice. The focus of this paper is on the effect that the organizational context has on the success or failure of Management Information Systems, MIS. Particular attention

Bernard Neugeboren is Full Professor at the Rutgers School of Social Work, Rutgers University, NJ USA.

[Haworth co-indexing entry note]: "Organizational Influences on Management Information Systems in the Human Services." Neugeboren, Bernard. Co-published simultaneously in *Computers in Human Services* (The Haworth Press, Inc.) Vol. 12, No. 3/4, 1995, pp. 295-310; and: *Human Services in the Information Age* (ed: Jackie Rafferty, Jan Steyaert, and David Colombi) The Haworth Press, Inc., 1995, pp. 295-310. Single or multiple copies of this article are available from The Haworth Document Delivery Service [1-800-342-9678, 9:00 a.m. - 5:00 p.m. (EST)].

is given to how organizational structures constrain and/or facilitate the establishment and implementation of MIS systems.

With the overcoming of the technological problems with MIS, there has been a shift in focus to the organizational and behavioral influences on the success of MIS (Lilly, 1986; Lucas, 1985; Schoech, 1982). Thus, there is recognition that the new information technology will have a major impact on the operation of human service agencies. Leavit and Whisler (1958) predict that computerized information systems will result in organizations becoming more centralized, with top executives less dependent on middle managers as computers take over their routine decision making tasks.

However, less recognized has been the influence that organizations have on MIS–how agency structures and processes constrain and/or facilitate the development and implementation of information systems. The effects of politics and power on MIS outcomes has not received adequate recognition as an explanatory factor in implementation of these systems (Lucas, 1975). The unanticipated consequences of information technology has not been taken into account (Ellul, 1964; LaMendola et al., 1989). The success or failure of MIS depends not only on rational technical considerations (McIntyre, Atkinson & Keller, 1977) but also on the organizational and political influences (Murphy & Pardeck, 1988). We need to understand how broader system management issues influence the development of effective decision support systems (Fuchs, 1989; Phillips, 1990).

Some examples of how MIS have not fulfilled expectations are: (1) the data collected is to meet needs of funding authorities or are used primarily to monitor services (Geiss & Viswanathan, 1986), with less utility to the service providers (Caputo, 1988; Macarov, 1990); (2) information and referral projects fail because of lack of cooperation between agencies; (3) MIS is favored by one administration which had a policy of service integration but was discontinued when another administration changed this policy (Geiss & Viswanathan, 1986).

Weissman (1987) cogently illustrates the effect of organizational context on an agency's ability to use information on client feedback to further service effectiveness. His scepticism of the value of client feedback is based on what he believes are unwarranted organizational assumptions. These assumptions include: agency agreement on goals and priorities; rationality rather than status and power as the most influential factors determining organizational decisions; organizations can transcend negative feedback; agencies are willing to change; and organizations are willing to accept limitations on their autonomy that feedback can impose. Thus, the organizational context in which MIS occurs needs to be considered in order to overcome the barriers for the successful planning for and implementation of these systems.

This paper will first review the factors associated with the success and failure of MIS. This is followed by an analysis of some of the organizational barriers to the development and implementation of MIS and strategies for overcoming them.

SUCCESS AND FAILURE OF MIS

Failure

Failure of MIS has been attributed to the tendency to concentrate on the technical aspects of systems overlooking organizational behavior problems (Lucas, 1975). An indicator of the lack of success of MIS is the low rate of utilization of information collected (Murphy & Pardeck, 1988; Nurius et al., 1988; Schervish, 1991). Utilization varies with staff level: executives are high users compared to middle managers (low users) and direct service staff are minimal users (Butterfield, 1988). Executive information use is primarily in the fiscal area (Caputo, 1988). Thus 78% of agencies use computers for financial operations in contrast to 28% used for direct service (Garrett, 1986). A review of nine social work journals in the 1970's found that computers were primarily used for clerical work and accounting (Boyd, Hylton & Price, 1976). There are no differences between professions (MBA vs MSW vs. MD vs Psych) in data use (Schervish, 1991). Lack of information usage may be associated with the de-emphasis in professional education on use of data in practice (Smith & Bolitho, 1990). However, an unanticipated consequence of MIS is that centrally stored data can be used for research purposes. For example, this author did a study of 250 psychiatric clinics using available data stored in a federally mandated state MIS (Neugeboren, 1970).

The lack of utilization resides in a more fundamental problem: human service agencies seldom determine the information needed to support the different kinds of decisions made by managers and practitioners (Schoech, 1990). This is in part influenced by the basic incompatibility of the political and value-laden nature of decision making processes (Neugeboren, 1991) with the rationally designed MIS (Caputo, 1988). An understanding of decision making processes should be a prelude to the introduction of computer support systems (Schoech, 1990; Vogel, 1985).

Failure has been associated with lack of administrative support (Briggs, 1991; Lynett, 1986; Tighe, 1991) and organizational uncertainty (Matheson, 1991). Pruger reports on a program that was not continued because of lack of administrative and political support in spite of its success in its achieving its objectives and its acceptance by operating staff. The failure in continuing the program may have been related to a "bottom up" implementation strategy which, although successfully involving the line staff, failed in having adequate participation of the top level. This suggests that the design of MIS should involve lower level staff in the establishment of the program in contrast to institutionalization of the program requiring executive participation.

LaMendola (1986) cites other examples of a failure of MIS due to organizational and political factors. Included were: power struggles over control of information; conflicting data demands of funding authorities; and fear of loss of jobs. A general criticism of MIS is that the data available was not found to be useful (Nurius & Anderson, 1988; Poertner & Rapp, 1984). Problems in information usage by managers include: reports are not understood; more information reported than needed; reports not received on timely basis; information not relevant for decision making needs; and the presence of staff informational freelancing where they develop their own information systems (Palmer et al., 1991). Information overload in which large amounts of data is provided which cannot be digested by the decision maker is frequently reported (Lucas, 1975; Schoech, 1982). *"We are drowning in information but starved for knowledge"* (Naisbitt, 1982). *"Agencies are tremendous information generators, but inadequate information users"* (Schoech, 1992).

Success

Success in initiation and implementation of MIS has been associated with opposite conditions of failure, e.g., staff stability (Briggs, 1991); innovative individuals; goal clarity; resource availability; and commitment of senior managers (Matheson, 1991).

Pruger (1986) reported on the success of a decision support system in terms of worker acceptance after realizing that their worst fears (e.g., computer would replace them; clients would be dehumanized; worker discretion would be taken away) were unjustified. Success was also measured by a reduction in paperwork, less need for supervision and in a more equitable service system. Phillips (1990) reports success in the welfare rights arena in which clients using computers led to an increase in their claiming of benefits.

Velasquez (1992) reports on a successful MIS in a public welfare organization with an increase of over 30% worker productivity. The MIS development process included active management support as well as participation of line staff and a gradual introduction of the system into the work environment.

Stress reduction in clerks in a public child welfare agency was found to be associated with the use of microcomputers to reduce paperwork (Cahill & Feldman, 1989).

BARRIERS TO THE DEVELOPMENT
AND IMPLEMENTATION OF MIS

The barriers to the development and implementation of MIS has been associated with a variety of factors, including: staff resistance, power structure, agency stability; agency efficiency vs. effectiveness, leadership, organizational change, MIS design, politics and self-interests.

Ideological Barriers

Human service organizations tend to favor particular philosophies which shape specific goals and interventions (Neugeboren, 1991). When information systems based on rational assumptions such as a treatment modality that has been found to work conflicts with the prevailing agency philosophy which favors a different intervention modality, then the rational approach will be rejected. For example, a computer program for the training of therapists in the field of alcoholism provided information on the intervention that was most effective based on research. When these recommendations conflicted with the existing agency ideology regarding intervention, the therapist attempting to use this "deviant" intervention was constrained by the supervisor who indicated that *"we find this intervention unacceptable since the one we currently use has been found to be most effective"* (Carlson, 1991).

Staff Resistance

Fuchs (1989) found that attitudes towards computer technology varied with position–managers found MIS more useful. The majority of staff did not find the system useful, accurate or relevant. A survey of social workers in Minnesota found that 47% thought that information collected served no important purpose, 20% falsified data and one third ignored requests for data (O'Brien et al., 1992). In contrast to the prevailing belief regarding negative staff attitudes toward computers, other studies found that this was not the case (Cwikel & Monnickendam, 1991; Mutschler & Hoefer, 1990).

Fearfulness of staff to use the computer (computer phobia) is believed to be widely prevalent. This barrier was overcome in one instance by use of a strategy of instituting an electronic mail system which forced the staff to use computers (Carlson, 1991). In this instance a forced change in staff behavior reduced their negative attitudes.

Forrest and Williams (1987) suggests that human service staff resistance to information generated by computer systems may rest in their predilection to favor oral and personal information sources rather than that coming from more impersonal origins and therefore deemed "dehumanizing" (Schoech, 1982). Staff resistance has been also linked with power relationships with concern that computerization would increase top level power and control (Mandell, 1989).

In summary, staff resistance may be attributed to three sources: staff alienation to information usage, lack of utility of the information for practice decision making and power. If the lack of utility is the principal cause, then attributing resistance to the staff is in a sense "blaming the victim."

Power Structure

If "information is power," its control as an essential resource can influence agency power structure (Caputo, 1987; Davidson, 1989; Phillips, 1990). Computerizing of information systems can result in greater centralization of power with a reduction of discretion and autonomy on the lower levels (Bronson et al., 1988; Taylor, 1981). Power has been associated with reduction in organizational uncertainty. Computer departments increase their power by the dependence created when other departments rely on them for information to reduce uncertainty (Lucas, 1985). Information systems also have potential for stimulating conflict derived from inter-dependencies between user and information departments (Lucas, 1973).

Type of computer technology used can affect centralization/decentralization of power. For example, use of PCs in contrast to centralized computer networks resulted in the hoarding of information by individual practitioners (McTanney, 1991) with consequences of decentralization of power (Cowen, 1991; Montgomery et al., 1991). "The political implications of data control passing to multiple, decentralized data bases alters fundamental concepts of organizational control and social innovation" (LaMendola, 1986). In library information systems middle managers were able to control the information fed to the organization's higher management levels. In public libraries, the control of computers by municipal authorities reduced the control by the library managers (Homer, 1986). Interdepartmental competition and fragmentation can be accentuated when each department establishes separate data systems resulting in hoarding of information (Pardeck & Murphy, 1990).

As clerks increase their expertise in use of computers, their power and control may be enhanced in relationship to professional staff (Macarov, 1990). The opposite can also occur: as professionals gain computer expertise (e.g., word processing) their dependence on clerks is reduced (Weinbach, 1991), thus diminishing their power (Mechanic, 1962). Staff who have word processing skills can enhance their power in relation to their colleagues who lack these skills by their ability to reduce the turnaround time to produce reports and memos which places them in an advantageous position in their competition with these colleagues.

MIS organizational feasibility (the extent an organization is ready to accept and use a particular information system) is influenced by structural components. When an information system's focus is on operational needs of a department, data was collected relevant for structured decisions, neglecting the needs of upper level managers for information needed for non-structured decisions required for strategic planning (Homer, 1986).

Power struggles between staff on different organizational levels can be engendered by the introduction of MIS systems (Schoech, 1982). In one instance direct service level staff were empowered to provide information to upper level personnel and in the process bypassed the secretary and middle managers, generating jealousy and resentment (Briggs, 1991).

Source of funding can also be a factor that generates power struggles over control of data and equipment (LaMendola, 1986). In one situation a power struggle between federal, state and local agencies was solved under the principle of "he who pays the piper called the tune;" the state and federal source of funds determined ownership even though local level collected the data (Montgomery et al., 1991). The hierarchical structure can also be affected by the introduction of MIS systems. In one instance a decision support system reduced the need for a detailed hierarchical supervision (Pruger, 1986).

Agency Stability

High staff turnover and unanticipated organizational changes can affect the continuity and implementation of MIS (Caputo, 1987). Instability in one agency resulted in inability to meet deadlines; to complete data entry; eventual abandonment of the electronic system and return to a manual system (Tighe, 1991). Agency stability can be adversely affected by negative public reaction to media case sensationalization, resulting in constraints on the development of MIS and systematic planning (Fuchs, 1989).

Efficiency vs. Effectiveness

Evaluation of MIS has stressed efficiency (economic benefit) as a principal outcome. The lack of success of MIS may in part be due to the lack of attention to effectiveness outcomes (i.e., client benefit) (Caputo, 1991). Examples of client benefit outcomes are: a more equitable service system (Pruger, 1986) and increased client access to services (Phillips, 1990). Although efficiency is certainly important to administrators and funding authorities, the legitimation and professional acceptance of MIS may be more readily accomplished if more attention is given to effectiveness–client outcomes (Patti et al., 1987).

Evaluation of efficiency of the introduction of MIS needs to take into account different costs. Dukler (1989) highlights operating, opportunity and political costs. He includes (1) resources to explore the operating environment and its problems; (2) resource needs to involve various stakeholders (Briggs et al., 1991), interest groups and politicians to ensure that the changes are supported; (3) costs of maintaining two information systems while the new system is being tested and installed; and (4) costs associated with resistance to change. Schoech (1982) cites "hidden costs" such as disruption of agency; staff displacement; loss of work effort due to frustration and change.

The issue of costs highlights the unwarranted assumption that MIS will invariably lead to greater efficiency. Van Hove (1989) refers to the "myth of computer efficiency" in that computers are expected to bring order out of chaos, which is unrealistic.

Leadership

It has been suggested that good administration facilitates computerization and use of information technology (Lingham & Law 1990; Schoech, 1982). Executive commitment to computerization can foster automation by providing incentives and rewards (Bronson et al., 1988). As indicated previously, lack of managerial support can adversely affect MIS outcomes (LaMendola, 1986; Briggs, 1991; Pruger, 1986; Lynett, 1986). Leadership style also affects implementation of MIS (Briggs, 1991). A participatory management style would facilitate the involvement of lower level staff in the development and implementation of MIS (Tripp, 1991). However, as with any significant organizational change that affects agency power structure, leadership will probably need to consider also the use of a power strategy to effect the change (Neugeboren, 1991).

MIS Design

Information systems designers are like architects; they should work with users to identify goals and shape of the new system (Lucas, 1985). It requires technical as well as behavioral knowledge and skill. Design of MIS needs to take into account differences in influence of staff at different levels. Thus one justification for designing systems from the bottom up is that worker discretion is beyond the control of superiors and therefore the administration needs the voluntary cooperation of lower level staff for successful implementation of MIS (Calica, 1986). User involvement with MIS design improves MIS performance (Bozeman & Bretschneider, 1986).

Design of MIS needs to take into account the problems associated with the transition from manual to electronic systems (Briggs, 1991). Thus, time delays in the implementation of electronic system may foster staff resistance in giving up a functional manual system.

Organizational Change

Introduction of MIS should be viewed in the context of system change (Lucas, 1985) and therefore the change process should require as much or more attention as the technical details of system design. The dynamics of organizations require that we "develop models of organizational change and system development that are consonant with the values of our profession and that adequately account for the political problems that will arise" (Keen & Morton, 1978). The evolution in the initiation and development of MIS has been linked to the organizational life cycle involving the following stages: missionary, consolidation, institutionalization, and diffusion of innovation (Keen & Morton, 1978). Strategies for introduction of MIS needs to take into account these organizational stages since they will have varying effects.

For example, in an agency with which I consulted, the administrator first had to solve various organizational problems prior to considering the development of an MIS system. She had to move the agency from the missionary to the consolidation stage of development. It took her two years to make the following changes: centralizing the agency structure to better integrate the various programs in the agency; replacing staff, changing the service delivery and fiscal procedures and educating the Board as to the need for more efficient administrative structures. When the administrator took over, the agency was in disarray, so that effort had to focus on short term problems. Once these changes were made the administrator could devote time to long range planning which required a more comprehensive information system to accomplish such tasks of computerizing demographic information to do need assessments for use in grant applications.

Theories on organizational change (Hage & Aiken, 1970) which prescribe different strategies (e.g., consensus vs. power) for the initiation and
implementation of the change could be applied to MIS innovations.
Weinbach (1991) indicates that the requirements for change during computerization can cause organizational disruption, particularly in the informal
power and communication structures increasing the likelihood of resistance to change. Suggested management strategies to minimize this resistance include: reassurance of fair and equitable treatment; providing staff
assurances about continuity in daily operations; replacing lost face-to-face
communication and compensating for individual staff loss of status.
    Incremental change is the preferred strategy in contrast to major rapid
change (Weinbach, 1991). An evolutionary process based on a series of
compromises (Miller, 1991) requires a gradual introduction of change in
information systems.

Politics–Self-Interests

    The varying self-interests of the different actors in a system need to be
taken into account in the planning for and implementation of MIS. The
political process of information systems planning depends on organizational
and social relationships of three managerial "stakeholder" groups: top
management, user management and information system management (Ruohonen, 1991).
    The influence of politics and self-interests was evident in one instance
where legislators, government agency administrators, line workers and
university professors had different interests and motives for supporting or
resisting the use of technology (Calica, 1986). The integration of information systems among agencies on different levels of government can be
limited by competing political priorities (Fuchs, 1989).
    In another example, successful political action overcame state bureau-
cratic timidity in the establishing of MIS. This was accomplished by
organized pressure from county officials and threat of legislative action
(Pruger, 1986). However, MIS staff often lack the skills to respond to these
kinds of barriers. Also university staff had difficulty seeing their limitations in the political area (Pruger, 1986).

SOLUTIONS FOR OVERCOMING BARRIERS

Structural Location of MIS

    Location of MIS departments on the upper levels of hierarchy can help
deal with the problem of lack of administrative support (Caputo, 1988;

Schoech, 1982). However, distance from the operational level has the drawback of lack of familiarity with the information needed for decision making on that level.

Involvement of Practitioners in MIS

As indicated above, a prerequisite for the development and implementation of an effective MIS is sufficient understanding of the decision making processes involved in practice, whether it be on management or service delivery level. A strategy for accomplishing this would be the collaboration between information specialists and practitioners in the planning of MIS (Lucas, 1985; Pardeck & Murphy, 1990; Schoech, 1982). Lilly (1986) suggests involvement of administrators in the system's development, testing and implementation. Issues of power and control between these different staff levels would have to be taken into account for successful practitioner/administrator collaboration (Weinbach, 1991). An internal user survey mechanism can facilitate this collaboration (Palmer, 1991). The benefits of user involvement will be maximized if it is done with an understanding of the agency context which requires an organizational analysis.

Organizational Analysis As Prerequisite for MIS

Since the organizational context is a critical factor influencing the success or failure of MIS (Lucas, 1975; Rosenberg & Rehr, 1979), an analysis of agency policies including its goals, structure and processes should be a prerequisite for the development and implementation of MIS. An analysis of the organizational opportunities and constraints on MIS is required (Ruohonen, 1991). As indicated previously, one of the barriers to the institutionalization of MIS is the effect of changing policies. A strategy for insuring that the MIS will continue beyond the current administration is to link it with agency goals (Schoech, 1982) which are usually fairly stable. This will be possible if the MIS provides the data to determine organizational effectiveness (i.e., the accomplishment of organizational goals).

In addition to the assessment of organizational goals, the analysis should also assess the existing organizational structure (official and operative): communication, role, power, reward and inter-organizational structures (Neugeboren, 1991) to determine how the structure constrains or facilitates the MIS system. It is also important to determine the reverse: how the MIS may affect organizational structure to become aware of potential sources of resistance to the MIS.

As indicated above, it is important to take into account an agency's POWER structure to insure that the support of the "stakeholders" in the MIS will be obtained. Analysis of the existing COMMUNICATION structure will be necessary to ensure integration of MIS into that structure. Study of the ROLE structure (i.e., staff job responsibilities) will be needed if the information system is to provide data on staff tasks and activities which is integrated with the existing role structure. Knowledge of the existing REWARD structure (criteria and procedures for staff rewards and sanctions) is needed if the goal of the information system is to provide objective information to implement a more equitable reward system. Information on the INTER-ORGANIZATIONAL structure is relevant if the agency is involved in inter-agency collaborative agreements requiring procedure for monitoring these inter-organizational arrangements.

A thorough organizational analysis may provide information on the feasibility of an MIS in a particular agency. This analysis could provide suggestions on the organizational steps needed to prepare the organization for the introduction of an MIS system (Weinbach, 1991). A delay or postponement of the establishment of an MIS may be indicated if the analysis determines that the organizational barriers are too formidable.

CONCLUSIONS

The organizational influences on the development and implementation of MIS has been the focus of this paper. Given the organizational constraints on the successful development and implementation of MIS, and the considerable resources required, information specialists need to collaborate with those who are in a position to inform them of potential organizational opportunities and constraints on the establishment and implementation of management information systems.

REFERENCES

Bozeman, B. & S. Bretschneider. (1986). Public management information systems: Theory and Prescription. *Public Administration Review.* 46 (Special Issue): 475-487.

Boyd, L.H., J.H. Hylton & S.V. Price. (1978). Computer in social work practice : A review. *Social Work*, 23 (368-371).

Briggs, P.P. Kindler & N. Smith. (1991). Bridging the gap between information technology and human services. Paper presented at HUSITA-2 International Conference. New Brunswick, New Jersey.

Bronson, D.E., D.C. Pelz & E. Trzcinsk. (1988). *Computerizing Your Agency's Information System*. Newbury Park, Ca: Sage.

Butterfield, W.H. (1988). Artificial intelligence: An introduction. *Computers in Human Services*. 3(1/2): 23-36.

Cahill, J. & L. Feldman. (1989). Computers and stress reduction in a child protection agency. Paper presented at, Boston, Mass. Nov. 1989. American Public Health Association Meeting.

Calica, R.H. (1986). Discussion of information technology in support of service delivery decisions. In the Human edge: Information technology and helping people. G.R. Geiss & N. Viswanathan, Eds. New York: Haworth.

Caputo, R.K. (1988). Management and information systems in human services: Implications for the distribution of authority and decision making. New York: Haworth.

Caputo, R. (1991). Managing information systems: An ethical framework and information needs matrix. *Administration In Social Work*. 15(4): 53-64.

Carlson, R. (1991). Capturing Expertise to Support Human Services Decision Making. Paper presented at HUSITA-2 International Conference. New Brunswick, N.J.

Cowen, L. (1991). Reorganizing organization and information: How knowledge technologies squash hierarchy and alter the role of information. *Documentation Image Information*. 11(5): 288-294.

Davidson, M.E. (1989). Enhancing equity in service delivery in minority populations. *Computers in Human Services*. 4(1/2): 55-64.

Dukler, M.A. (1989). Improving the quality and reducing the cost of human services through on-line transaction processing. *Computers in Human Services*. 4(3/4): 205-216.

Ellul, J. (1964). *The Technological Society*. New York: Random House.

Forrest, J. & S. Williams (1987). *New technology and information exchange in social services*. London: Policy Studies Institute, pp. 3-10.

Fuchs, D.M. (1989). Integrated information system for child welfare agency: Evolution in two Canadian case studies. *Computers in Human Services*. 4(3/4): 191-204.

Garrett, W.J. (1986). Information technology in direct service to clients. In *The human edge: Information technology and helping people*. Geiss, G.R. & N. Viswanathan, Eds. New York: Haworth.

Geiss G.R. & N. Viswanathan, Eds (1986). *The human edge: Information technology and helping people*. New York: Haworth.

Hage, J. & M. Aiken. (1970). *Social Change In Complex Organizations*. New York: Random House.

Homer, G. (1986). Management information systems can help senior library managers. *Canadian Library Journal*. 43(3): 141-145.

Keen, P.G.W. & Scott Morton, M.S. (1978). *Decision support systems: An organizational perspective*. Reading, Mass.: Addison Wesley.

LaMendola, W. (1986). Discussion of information technology applied to facilitating practice. In *The human edge: Information technology and helping people.* G.R. Geiss & N. Viswanathan (Eds.) New York: Haworth.

LaMendola, W., B. Glastonbury & S. Toole, Eds. A casebook of computer applications in the social and human services: Part I. *Computers in Human Services.* 4(1/2): 10.

Leavit, H.J. & T.L. Whisler. (1958). Management in the 1980's. *Harvard Business Review.* 36: 41-44.

Lilly, E.R. (1986). *Implementation of computer based management Information systems: A Behavioral perspective.* Education Resources Information Center.

Lingham, R. & M. Law. (1990). Using computers for better administration of social service departments. *Computers in Human Services.* 5(1/2): 117-132.

Lucas, Jr., H.C. (1973). Problems of politics of change: Power, conflict and information services subunit. In F. Gruenberger (ed.). *Effective Vs. Efficient Computing.* Englewood Cliffs, N.J.: Prentice Hall.

Lucas, Jr., H.C. (1975). *Why Information Systems Fail.* New York: Columbia.

Lucas, Jr., H.C. (1985). *The Analysis, Design, And Implementation of Information Systems.* New York: McGraw Hill.

Lynett, P. (1986). Information technology in professional preparation and delivery of services. In *The human edge: Information technology and helping people.* G.R. Geiss & N. Viswanathan, (Eds.). New York: Haworth.

Macarov, D. (1990). Computer in the Social Services. *International Journal of Sociology and Social Policy.* 10, Nos. 4/5/6.

Mandell, S.F. (1989). Resistance and power: The perceived effect that computerization has on a social agency's power relationship. *Computers in Human Services.* 4(1/2): 29-40.

Matheson, A.D. (1991). Innovative use of computers for planning in human service organizations. Paper presented at HUSITA-2 International Conference. New Brunswick, N.J.

McIntyre, M.H., Atkinson, C.C. & Keller, T.W. (1977). Components of program evaluation capability in community mental centers. In W.A. Hargraves, C.C. Atkinson & J.E. Sorenson (eds.) *Resource materials for community mental health program evaluation.* (pp. 4-15). Washington, D.C.: DHEW.

McTanney, (1991). Paper presented at HUSITA-2 International Conference. New Brunswick, N.J.

Mechanic, D. D. (1962). Sources of power of lower participants in complex organizations. *Administrative Science Quarterly.* 7(3): 349-364.

Miller, H.W. (1991). Information technology creation or evolution. *Journal of Systems Management.* 42(4): 23-27.

Montgomery R., J. Kennedy & K. House. (1991). Whose data is it: Exploring tension between local, state and federal information needs. Paper presented at HUSITA-2 International Conference, New Brunswick, N.J.

Monnickendam, M. & A.S. Eaglstein (1991). Social Workers Resistance to Computer Implementation: A Second Look. Paper presented at HUSITA-2 International Conference. New Brunswick, New Jersey.

Murphy & Pardeck. (1988). *Computers in Human Services.* 3 (1/2): 1-8.

Mutschler, E. & R. Hoefer. (1990). Factors affecting the use of computer technology in human service organizations. *Administration In Social Work.* 14(1): 87-101.

Naisbitt, J. (1982). *Megatrends: Ten directions transforming our lives.* New York: Warner Books.

Neugeboren, B. (1970). *Psychiatric Clinics: A Typology of Service Patterns.* Metuchen, N.J.: Scarecrow Press.

Neugeboren, B. (1991). Organization, Policy and Practice. In *The Human Services.* Binghamton, N.Y. Haworth.

Nurius, P.S. & W. Hudson. (1988a). Computer based practice: Future dream or current technology. *Social Work.* 33(4): 357-362.

Nurius, P., A. Hooyman & A. Nichol (1988b). The changing Face of computer utilization in social work settings. *Journal of Social Work Education.* 24, 2, 186-197.

O'Brien, N. McCllan & D. Alfs. (1992). Data collection: Are social workers reliable? *Administration In Social Work.* 16(2): 89-99.

Palmer, R.J., M. Tucker & J.B. King II. (1991). A diagnostic approach to information management problems in the organization. *Journal of Systems Management.* 42(6): 13-16.

Pardeck, J.T. & J.W. Murphy. (1990). *Computers In Human Services.* New York: Harwood.

Patti, R., J. Poertner & C.A. Rapp. (1987). Management For Service Effectiveness in Social Welfare Organizations. *Administration In Social Work.* 11(3/4).

Phillips, D. (1990). The underdevelopment of computing in social work practice. Computers in the Social Services: Papers from a consultation. D. Macarov (Ed.) *International Journal of Sociology and Social Policy.* 10(4,5,6): 9-29.

Poertner, J. & C. Rapp. (1980). Information system design in foster care. *Social Work.* 25(114-119).

Pruger, R. (1986). Information technology in support of service-delivery decisions. In *The human edge: Information technology and helping people.* Eds. G.R. Geiss & N. Viswanathan. New York: Haworth.

Rosenberg, G. Rehr, H. (1970). Quality assurance and structural standards. In *Professional accountability for social work practice.* New York: Rehr, Prodist.

Ruohonen, M. (1991). Stakeholders of strategic information systems planning: theoretical concepts and empirical examples. *Journal of Strategic Information Systems.* 1(1): 15-28.

Schervish, P.H. (1991). Patterns of information use by levels in human service organizations. Paper presented at HUSITA-2 International Conference. New Brunswick, New Jersey.

Schoech, D. (1982). *Computer use in human services: A guide to information management.* New York: Human Sciences Press.

Schoech, D. (1990). *Human service computing: Concepts & applications.* Binghamton, N.Y. Haworth.

Smith, N.J. & F.H. Bolitho (1989). Information: The hydra headed concept in the human services. *Computers in Human Services.* 5(3/4): 83-98.

Taylor, J.B. (1981). *Using Computers In Social Agencies.* Sage Human Service Guide #19. Beverly Hills, CA. Sage.

Tighe, R. (1991). Organizational development and information systems: A case study. Paper presented at HUSITA-2 International Conference. New Brunswick, New Jersey.

Tripp, R.S. (1991). Managing the political and cultural aspects of large scale MIS projects: A case study of participative systems development. *Information Resource Management Journal.* 4(4): 2-13.

Van Hove, E. (1989). Three lessons from automating social services in Belgium. *New Technology in the Human Services.* (2): 10-14.

Velasquez, Joan. (1992). GAIN: A locally based computer system which successfully supports line staff. *Administration In Social Work.* 16(1): 41-54.

Vogel, L.H. (1985). Decision support systems in the human services: Discovering limits to a promising technology. *Computers in Human Services.* 1(1): 67-80.

Weinbach, R.W. (1991). Proactive management to minimize the cost of computerization. *Computer Use in Social Services Network.* 11(4): 24-27.

Weissman, H. (1987). Planning for client feedback: Content and context. *Administration In Social Work.* 11(3/4): 205-220.

Integrated Information Systems
for Human Services:
A Conceptual Framework, Methodology
and Technology

Rami Benbenishty
Daphna Oyserman

SUMMARY. A conceptual framework and methodology to design and implement clinical information systems to support direct practice is described. This article presents an analysis of the information needs of clinicians in human service organizations. Three main uses of information are identified: monitoring/tracking, communicating/reporting and learning from experience. In order to meet these needs, practitioners have to gather information, store it and process it. The article demonstrates the methodology and conceptual framework with a series of examples of applications. *[Article copies available from The Haworth Document Delivery Service: 1-800-342-9678.]*

In recent years there has been a growing emphasis on accountability in the human services. Concerns about accountability have permeated at-

---

Rami Benbenishty is Professor at the Paul Baerwald School of Social Work, Hebrew University, Jerusalem, Israel, currently on sabbatical at the Merril Palmer Institute, Wayne State University, Detroit, MI.

Daphna Oyserman is Associate Researcher at Merril Palmer Institute, Wayne State University, Detroit, MI.

[Haworth co-indexing entry note]: "Integrated Information Systems for Human Services: A Conceptual Framework, Methodology and Technology." Benbenishty, Rami, and Daphna Oyserman. Co-published simultaneously in *Computers in Human Services* (The Haworth Press, Inc.) Vol. 12, No. 3/4, 1995, pp. 311-325; and: *Human Services in the Information Age* (ed: Jackie Rafferty, Jan Steyaert, and David Colombi) The Haworth Press, Inc., 1995, pp. 311-325. Single or multiple copies of this article are available from The Haworth Document Delivery Service [1-800-342-9678, 9:00 a.m. - 5:00 p.m. (EST)].

311

tempts to improve effectiveness and efficiency of practice through methods such as single case design, evaluation research, effectiveness research, management information systems, clinical information systems, integration of research and practice, decision support and expert systems (Bloom, Fischer and Orne, 1993; Blythe, 1992; Fischer, 1981; Gingerich 1990; Grasso & Epstein, 1989, 1992; Hudson & Nurius, 1993; Jayaratne & Levi, 1979; Kratochwill, 1978; Poertner, 1987; Wick & Schoech, 1988).

Much progress has been made in raising awareness to issues of accountability and the importance of basing practice on empirical evidence of effectiveness. However, less progress has been made in implementing and disseminating effective and accountable practice methods. Practice in human service organizations thus continues to be characterized by the same problems that led to calls for increased accountability and empirically based practice.

The challenge, therefore, is to collect clinically relevant data systematically, process and analyze it in ways that will inform practice, and to fold these insights back into daily practice. Efforts to collect and effectively use information underlie single subject design, program evaluation and management information systems. Building on these previous efforts, we have been working for a number of years on a conceptual framework and methodology to address the various aspects of this central concern for human service organizations (Benbenishty, 1989; Oyserman & Benbenishty, 1993).

In this paper we present a conceptual framework and methodology for the design of Integrated Information Systems (IIS) that aims at providing a more comprehensive response to the information needs of human service organizations than previous efforts described in the literature (Mutschler & Hasenfeld, 1986). We will then describe the elements of the IIS, and briefly review their powerful impact on practice, management and policy making.

Front line clinicians and clients are the most directly involved in information collection and documentation. It is on the basis of this information that each of the other partners receives information necessary to carry out their tasks. Therefore, direct line workers, clients and client groups should have a major role in determining what information should be collected, processed and disseminated to others. Involvement of these parties and careful consideration of their needs will ensure that clinicians and clients will have a stake at providing timely and accurate information. Hence, some of the thorniest problems of information systems today, namely inaccurate and dated reporting, can be reduced dramatically.

INFORMATION NEEDS

Of the numerous information needs of human service agencies we are focusing on three categories of needs.

Monitoring

This refers to the need to have a "finger on the pulse," to know what is currently happening in the agency. Monitoring addresses the client population, services and interventions provided, and the outcomes of these services (Benbenishty, 1989a, 1989b; Benbenishty & Oyserman, 1991; Oyserman & Benbenishty, 1993). In the present context it is important to point out that direct service staff, supervisors, administrators and policy makers need to use information to monitor issues of relevance to them. Direct service staff need to monitor their clients, supervisors need to know about specific clients and have a picture of whole case loads, administrators need to monitor clients and interventions, and policy makers need to monitor key characteristics of the population and of services provided. Throughout the service delivery process, program compliance, process and outcome quality should be continuously monitored by staff at all levels.

Communication

This refers to the need to share information both within the human service organization and between related service providers. Human service organizations depend on the cooperation and joint efforts of many individuals, programs and departments. To provide quality care, direct service staff are dependent on colleagues who provide related services, on administrators, on managers, and on funding agencies. Similarly, supervisors, managers and policy makers need to receive accurate and timely information from service staff, as well as disseminate information such as agency directives and policy guidelines back to practitioners.

Due to the complex interdependency between various human service organizations, there is always the need to share information with appropriate and relevant agencies (provided that confidentiality and client rights are protected). Thus, for example, most foster care agencies deal with clients who have been referred via Protective Services. The information which led to this referral should be communicated to the foster care agency. Children exiting foster care are likely to be referred to residential care and adoption services, as well as to a range of community based programs given continued care responsibilities. In addition, clients are likely to receive services simultaneously from several agencies. Clearly, information gathered over the course of foster care should be communicated to these continued care agencies.

Furthermore, because human service organizations should be accountable to informal and formal social institutions, they need to provide comprehensive and accurate information. Thus, for instance, an adoption service should be communicating with the court with regard to the placement plan for a specific child and with state authorities with regard to the number of children waiting for placement more than six months. Foster care agencies need to be able to describe the services they provided to promote attainment of a treatment plan, as well as be accountable for the decisions leading up to development of these plans.

Learning from Experience

This refers to the need to use information effectively in order to learn lessons from accumulated experience and to generate knowledge to guide future actions. Human service organizations operate in environments that are characterized by change and high levels of uncertainty and ambiguity. The current level of knowledge in many areas limits to a great extent the ability to predict the possible impact of various lines of action. Furthermore, much of the operation of service agencies is context-specific and dependent on local conditions, limiting the ability to generalize from the experience of other agencies (Benbenishty, Ben-Zaken and Yekel, 1991). For instance, a New York City agency trying to assess the effectiveness of "meals-on-wheels" program for elderly, may be cautious in accepting conclusions drawn from a study of such a program in rural Idaho. Thus, it is clear that even when valid and generalizable knowledge does exist, human service organizations need to "learn" their environment in order to adapt and adjust to a fast changing milieu.

THE INTEGRATED INFORMATION SYSTEM APPROACH

In order to respond to this array of information needs we have developed a methodology appropriate and relevant to the needs of direct service staff, supervisors, administrators, policy makers, and public interest groups. The rationale and details of this methodology were described earlier (Benbenishty, 1989; Benbenishty & Oyserman, 1991; Oyserman & Benbenishty, 1993). The basic principle is that the information needs of the human service organization should be addressed on the agency level.

According to this approach, each client is monitored systematically and continuously, on aspects relevant to all partners in the agency, using language and structure shared across the agency. Information gathered is immediately processed, shared and stored, accumulating a dynamic data base that serves to inform all partners, enables learning and provides guidelines for future action.

The only feasible way to provide a comprehensive response to the broad and complex information needs discussed is a computerized Integrated Information System (IIS). The specifications, design and implementation of this system should follow very closely the rationale and methodology outlined above. In general, the impact of an integrated information system is achieved by improving the gathering, storage, retrieval, processing and the analysis of information (Oyserman and Benbenishty, 1993). The system serves as a mechanism to connect partners, facilitating communication and knowledge dissemination among all partners in the agency. In the following sections we will review the basic elements of the IIS.

Information Gathering

The information gathered by practitioners in service agencies is of crucial importance. This information serves as the basis for numerous judgments and decisions of front line workers, supervisors, administrators and policy makers.

Information gathering in human service organizations is an active, selective and informed process. In addition to receiving information from other sources, practitioners need to initiate information searches: ask questions, observe, and scan available documents. Given the enormous amount of potentially relevant information, information gathering should be selective and focused. Thus, important information should not be omitted and superfluous information should not be collected. This active and selective information gathering should be based on professional knowledge. To determine what information is relevant and when, may require high levels of skill and expertise. In fact, effective information gathering may be considered a hallmark of expertise.

Because the front line is where most information is being gathered, the Integrated Information System structures and supports this crucial task at the front line. In this way, the IIS moves expertise to the front line. The implication is that the data gathering component of the IIS should be designed by domain experts who have deep understanding of the needs and requirements of the clinical task at hand. Past efforts to develop information systems for clinical settings have often been crippled when systems analysts and programmers without human service expertise have attempted to define information gathering requirements (Kettelhut & Schkade, 1991).

Assurance of practice standards in information gathering is achieved in several ways. Integrated information systems implement tools, such as forms, screens and checklists, to structure the process and capture all information to meet practice needs, as well as reporting and licensing requirements. Forms, checklists and "help screens" are designed after a thorough analysis of the expertise elicited from practitioners, supervisors, administrators, policy makers, and, whenever relevant, from clients. Also, the professional literature, policy guidelines, service manuals, and other material are studied to identify relevant and necessary information.

In addition to providing guidance in information collection, the IIS reduces errors. This could be on a simple level of avoiding spelling errors and out-of-range values. Error reduction can address more complicated issues by examining whether information collected is contradictory, or is at odds with policy guidelines. For instance, in the State of Michigan, policy guidelines for foster care mandate that a child under age 14 should not have a treatment plan of permanent foster care unless this has been specifically cleared with the Department of Social Services. An integrated information system for foster care would provide feedback to workers that their treatment plan is age inappropriate, prompt for corrections, and suggest alternatives.

Information Storage

The IIS stores information gathered by members of the service agency so that it can be retrieved and processed. Modern computerized systems offer efficient information storage capabilities that facilitate retrieval and processing. Data are stored in relational databases that accumulate over time, and allow juxtaposing data from several sources. Integrated information systems should be designed around data bases that are both interrelated and independent. As to interrelatedness, most agencies recognize the need to link data bases and information systems so that they connect the various components of the agency, and the agency to other neighboring or superordinate agencies.

Yet, emphasis on interrelatedness overlooks the importance of independence of information systems. Focusing only on interrelatedness stifles attempts to create information systems which suit particular programs. Thus an agency or a State may mistakenly attempt to create one information system to meet the diverse information needs of distinct programs such as foster care, juvenile corrections, and adoptions. A balance between interrelatedness and independence can be achieved by designing a series of integrated information systems that share a common core. While each IIS is tailored to a specific program's needs, it contains the basic information structures necessary to coordinate the various information systems. This design creates a seamless integration of services, facilitating provision of proper care and efficient resource management.

IIS provides storage capacity for numeric as well as for text data. Since much of the data needed by front line practitioners cannot be classified and precoded into a limited number of numeric codes or fixed length data fields, IIS can store virtually unlimited free text data. This stored information can be later retrieved, incorporated into reports and used in qualitative data analysis. Furthermore, in certain contexts it may be useful to store pictorial information. For instance, an interdisciplinary team in the area of child abuse may need to store photos of bruises and burns allegedly related to physical abuse. These may help assessment and comparisons in the unfortunate event that another incidence occurs.

Data Retrieval

The IIS addresses both the content and the form of information retrieval. Since these systems are designed to accommodate many partners with different skills and information needs, data retrieval capabilities are versatile. Current information systems are designed mainly to respond to data retrieval needs of administrators, managers and policy makers. These include interfaces that allow access to individual files, as well as to lists of clients, services received, payments or other resources allocated.

In addition to responding to these data retrieval needs, integrated information systems provide clinicians with access to the information they need. The IIS provides clinicians with the capacity to browse through their client files as well as access to relevant information collected by other members of the agency. The IIS also provides "tickler systems" which organize and retrieve important dates and activities and present them to practitioners as "to do" or tracking lists (see Bhattacharyya, 1992 for an example). Sophisticated IIS interfaces can allow for natural language requests from the data base. Thus, clinicians can request retrieval of previous cases sharing characteristics with a current one. In addition, policy guidelines, service manuals, practice tips, abstracts of professional literature, and guides to services provided by other agencies, can all be accessed and retrieved from the IIS.

Given the emphasis on integration and on inclusion of as many partners as possible, issues of confidentiality and access are of prime importance. Much attention is given to the delicate balance between improved accessibility and retrieval of information, and protecting clients and workers from unacceptable intrusion of privacy. Involving as many partners as possible in the design process helps in fine tuning this vital balance.

Information Processing

Computers provide a powerful means of processing and analyzing large amounts of information quickly. The challenge is to use this power to maximize the goals of the IIS. The most common way to process information in information systems is to aggregate information across cases. Thus, information systems count cases which satisfy certain criteria, cross-tabulate them, and compute various statistics. For instance, Harrison and her associates (Harrison, Washington, Williams & Esterline, 1993) counted how many cases in a given period were under Protective Services investigation, and the distribution of the length of time needed to complete these investigations. To better satisfy the information needs of front line clinicians, Integrated Information Systems emphasize aggregating and processing information pertaining to individual clients. This includes the analysis of many separate information items relating to a specific client in order to reach an overall assessment (see Nurius, 1990 for a review of automated assessment). Thus, for instance, when a behavior checklist such as the Adaptive Behavior Scale (Hile, 1989) is used to gather data on a client, the IIS analyzes the client responses, provides a client profile, and indicates to what extent this client deviates from known norms. Similarly, IIS may process all the information regarding a client unit in order to assess risk, to ascertain eligibility or to recommend the appropriate basket of services. Furthermore, the IIS facilitates client tracking by processing information regarding the client unit, collected at several points in time.

It is useful to distinguish between information processing that is programmed in advance, performed routinely and automatically as part of everyday use of the system, and processing which is more long term and requires reflection. The more automatic processing can be used for tasks such as assessing risk levels of clients, computing program compliance and quality assurance statistics, management and administrative housekeeping statistics, etc.

Longer term, reflexive, and sequential analyses are also possible as data accumulate in the IIS data base. These data allow more in-depth analyses, enabling researchers and agency staff to explore issues involved in the process and outcomes of interventions. Sophisticated statistical analyses address issues such as clients' characteristics, services provided, performance and outcome assessments, client and service profile analysis, program retention and its predictors, and many more relevant analyses (Caputo, 1986). On the basis of these analyses, decision aids can be designed and incorporated into the IIS.

Sicoly (1990) describes the development of a decision aid based on a statistical model predicting important service events. This statistical model can then become part of the IIS and be used to predict this event in the future. Argles (1983, as cited in Sicoly, 1989, p. 48) used this approach to predict duration of child's stay in care, Stone and Stone (1983, as cited in Sicoly, 1989, p. 48) performed multivariate analyses to statistically model the likelihood of placement breakdown or success, and Johnson and L'Esperance (1984) attempted to predict recurrence of abuse. These type of analyses can be performed easily within an IIS environment as the Integrated Information System routinely collects the data needed for statistical modelling of relevant critical events.

Reporting

Reporting capabilities are a crucial element of the IIS. As information is gathered, stored, retrieved and analyzed, it should be communicated and reported in a timely and accurate manner. Integrated Information Systems provide a wide array of reporting mechanisms in order to address the needs of all partners. A series of preprogrammed, "canned reports," are readily available for routine use by administrators, managers, supervisors and direct line workers. A user friendly report generator should provide the ability to design "ad hoc" reports, and to allow users to tailor existing reports to suit their individual needs.

Further, to increase connectivity among various components of the agency, programs and services, and between the information systems of agencies and county- and State-level systems, reports can also be designed in the form of data files. These files can be transferred and shared by many relevant and appropriate users. Traditionally, reports reflect the emphasis on the aggregation of data across many cases. Thus, most reports consist of lists, and of numbers describing classes of clients and of services. For instance, a report generated by Texas Department of Protective & Regulatory Services (Harrison et al., 1993) describes for each stage of service what is the duration of that stage, and how this duration differs across programs and regions.

The IIS emphasis on the information needs of clinicians and on client-level processing, requires additional modes of reporting. To facilitate reporting on the client level, and to ease the heavy burden of reporting placed upon the individual clinician, a "client report" is generated. This is a text report that resembles current written reports and can replace the hand written or typed report. This type of report takes all the relevant information from the client's file and implants it in sentences and paragraphs that are a hybrid of computer generated segments and free text entered by the worker at the data collection phase.

Various client reports are designed to meet different reporting requirements. For example, using the same data file of a client in a drug treatment program, different client reports can be generated for the court, the health insurance company, the clinical supervisor, and for the administration of the clinic. Thus, whereas data are entered only once, the IIS stores the information, retrieves it and uses it for as many different reports as necessary.

IMPLEMENTATION

The conceptual framework outlined above and the methodology described here were the basis for a number of efforts to design effective methods to utilize information for practice. During the years we have designed systems to support family therapy, child residential care, and foster care (Benbenishty, 1991; Benbenishty & Ben-Zaken, 1988; Benbenishty & Oyserman, 1991). Presently we are implementing an Integrated Information System for Foster Care in Michigan (Benbenishty & Oyserman, 1993; Oyserman & Benbenishty, 1993).

We are implementing an IIS for Foster Care (IIS-FC) at a multi-site private nonprofit foster care agency, serving children in metropolitan Detroit area as well as throughout Eastern Michigan. The system we have designed is based on a review of the foster care literature, State-level policy guidelines and directives, review of existing case files, and extensive interaction with agency clinical and administrative staff. The IIS-FC uses a relational data base that consists of a series of interrelated data bases about each child's demographic and family information, psychosocial development, legal status, treatment plans and goals, and services received. The database structure makes it possible to monitor each child, sibship and family over time.

The system consists of two main modules, one focusing on children and their families and the other on foster families. These modules are interlinked so that intake workers can access foster families files and identify available and appropriate placements. Further, when children enter care and move through the system, information passes automatically to the foster family file, updating vacancy reports.

The IIS-FC uses an extensive array of screens to structure information gathering and data entry needed for monitoring children, families, and services. These screens address the process of care in its entirety, covering background, assessments, plans, goals, psychosocial interventions, services provided, and follow-up. Screens provide several means of data entry: single and multiple choice lists and text fields. Text fields allow for unlimited documentation, storage and retrieval.

All information entered in these information screens can be immediately translated into text reports that can be filed in child's case file as well as sent to the court and Department of Social Services. The system also provides numerous preprogrammed reports listing information such as children in care, dates due in court, and foster family vacancies. Reports are specifically designed to meet the needs of each partner in the agency. In addition, the ISS-FC includes a report generator that can be used by practitioners and administrators to create new reports as the need arises.

IIS IMPACT ON PRACTICE, MANAGEMENT AND POLICY MAKING

Implementing an IIS in an agency may have major impact on almost every aspect of the agency's functioning and on the relationship of the agency to other related organizations (Oyserman & Benbenishty, 1993). A complete review of the impact of an IIS is beyond the scope of this paper. The following sections will highlight areas in which IIS may have a major impact.

IIS Supports a Quality Process of Service Delivery

As the system structures data gathering, processing, communicating and reporting, it assures that all professional, legal and administrative directives are being followed. The expertise of the most knowledgeable people in the agency and in the professional literature is embedded in the system and guides practitioners, some of them novice and inexperienced.

IIS Improves Decision Making

IIS provides support for decision making on all levels in several ways. The system ensures that all data needed for decisions have been collected properly and communicated to the appropriate decision maker on a timely basis. Further, the IIS can provide an array of decision aids ranging from help screens, access to relevant literature reviews (Schoech, 1993), risk assessment scales, expert system modules (Schuerman, Mullen, Stagner & Johnson, 1989), predictive statistical models (Sicoly, 1989), and other aids relevant to a specific domain.

IIS Saves Time and Cuts Cost

Information systems eliminate redundancies in data collection and reporting. Information items are entered only once and then copied and moved as needed. The time consuming process of report preparation is streamlined and shortened. The need for support staff to type various reports, check for errors and retrieve information from files is reduced significantly.

IIS Improves Quality of Data

The information system provides means to ensure the quality and correctness of data at the point of entry. By providing lists, checklists and edit checks, the probability of omissions, contradictions, and typing errors is greatly reduced. Furthermore, because practitioners use the data daily and depend on these data for their work, they pay close attention to the completeness and accuracy of their documentation.

IIS Strengthens Reporting and Data Transfer

Data entered into the system are immediately available to all partners in the organization, cutting the time and effort involved in keeping each of the organization's departments and programs updated. A virtually unlimited number of reports designed to suit the agency needs combined with a flexible and user-friendly report generator, greatly enhance reporting capabilities. The system's ability to transfer data to other information systems is extensive. Data can be transferred electronically using various data formats to fit the characteristics of these related information systems.

IIS Enriches Program Monitoring and Research

The quality, extensiveness and immediate availability of data stored in the system make program monitoring and evaluation, quality assurance and research integral parts of practice and of policy making. In addition, the information system can serve as a platform for data collection efforts needed for research and other purposes such as program development or funding acquisition. For instance, a questionnaire may be added for a limited time to assess the need for a new service.

IIS IMPACT

Our work in this area so far has been well received. Line staff, supervisors, and administrators each emphasize different aspects of the impact and the promise of this approach to practice. In the near future, as more experience accumulates, the impact of integrated information systems for human services on accountability, quality of care, and the development of empirical practice should be studied and evaluated systematically.

REFERENCES

Benbenishty, R. (1988). Assessment of task-oriented family interventions with families in Israel. *Social Service Research*, 11(4), 19-43.

Benbenishty, R. (1989a). Combining the single-system and group approaches to evaluate treatment effectiveness on the agency level. *Journal of Social Service Research*, 12, 31-47.

Benbenishty, R. (1989b). Designing computerized clinical information systems to monitor interventions on the agency level. *Computers in Human Services*, 5, 69-88.

Benbenishty, R. (1991). Monitoring practice on the agency level:An application in a residential care facility. *Research on Social Work Practice*, 1, 371-386.

Benbenishty, R., & Ben-Zaken, A. (1988). Computer-aided process of monitoring task-centered family interventions. *Social Work Research and Abstracts*, 24(1), 7-9.

Benbenishty, R., Ben-Zaken, A., & Yekel, H. (1991). Monitoring interventions with young Israeli families. *British Journal of Social Work*, 21, 143-155.

Benbenishty, R., & Oyserman, D. (1991). A clinical information system for foster care in Israel. *Child Welfare*, 70(2), 229-242.

Benbenishty, R., & Oyserman, D. (1993). *The design and implementation of an integrated information system to support foster care.* Workshop presented at National Association for Welfare Research and Statistics. Scarsdale, Arizona.

Bhattacharyya, A. (1992). Tickler: An automated system to monitor assessment dates for psychiatric care. *Computers in Human Services*, 8, 87-119.

Bloom, M., Fischer, J., & Orme, J. G. (1993). *Evaluating practice: Guidelines for the accountable professional* (2nd ed.). Englewood Cliffs, NJ: Prentice-Hall.

Blythe, B. (1992). *Evolving and future development of clinical research utilization in agency settings.* In A. J. Grasso, & I. Epstein (eds), *Research utilization in the social services: Innovations for practice and administration*, (pp. 281-299). New York: The Haworth Press.

Blythe, B., & Briar, S. (1985). Developing empirically based models of practice. *Social Work*, 30, 483-488.

Caputo, R. K. (1986). The role of information systems in evaluation research. *Administration in Social Work*, 10, 67-77.

Fanshel, D., Marsters, P. A., Finch, S., & Grundy, J. F. (1992). *Strategies for the analysis of databases in social service systems.* In A. J. Grasso, & I. Epstein (eds.), *Research utilization in the social services: Innovations for practice and administration* (pp. 301-323). New York: The Haworth Press.

Fischer, J. (1981). The social work revolution. *Social Work*, 26, 199-206.

Fluke, J. &. O'Beirne, G. (1989). Artificial intelligence–An aid in child protective services caseload control systems. *Computers in Human Services,* 4, 101-109.

Gingerich, W. J. (1990). Expert systems and their potential uses in social work. *Families in Society,* 71, 220-228.

Gleeson, J. P. (1987). Implementing structured decision making procedures at child welfare intake. *Child Welfare,* 66, 101-112.

Grasso, A. J. (1992). *Conclusion-Information utilization: A decade of practice.* In A. J. Grasso, & E. Epstein (Eds), *Research utilization in the social services: Innovations for practice and administration,* (pp. 437-450). New York: The Haworth Press.

Grasso, A. J., & Epstein, I. (1989). The Boysville experience: Integrating Practice decision-making, program evaluation, and management information. *Computers in Human Services,* 4, 85-94.

Grasso, A. J., & Epstein, I. (Eds). (1992). *Research utilization in the social services: Innovations for practice and administration.* New York: The Haworth Press.

Harrison, J. G., Estrline, J., Washington, D., & Williams, D. (1993). *Five-Year history of stages of services in child protective services.* Scottsdale, Arizona: 33rd Annual Workshop of the National Association for Welfare Research and Statistics.

Hile, M. G. (1989). Two automated systems for behavioral assessment of clients with mental retardation or developmental disabilities. *Computers in Human Services,* 5, 183-191.

Jayaratne, S., & Levy, R. (1979). *Empirical clinical practice.* New York: Columbia University Press.

Johnson, W. & L'Esperance, J. (1984). Predicting the occurrence of child abuse. *Social Work Research and Abstracts,* 20,21-26.

Kettelhut, M. C., & Schkade, L. L. (1991). Programmers, analysts and human service workers: Cognitive styles and task implications for system design. *Computers in Human Services,* 8, 57-79.

Kratochwill, T. R. (ed.) (1978). *Single subject research: Strategies for evaluating change.* New York: Academic Press.

Mutschler, E., & Hasenfeld, Y. (1986). Integrated information systems for social work practice. *Social Work,* 31, 345-349.

Nurius P. S. (1990). A review of automated assessment. *Computers in Human Services,* 6, 265-281.

Nurius P. S., & Hudson, W. W. (1993). *Human services practice, evaluation, and computers.* Pacific Grove, Cal: Brooks/Cole.

Oyserman, D., & Benbenishty, R. (1993a). *A clinical information system to support direct practice.* Workshop presented at HUSITA-3. Maastricht, Netherlands.

Oyserman, D., & Benbenishty, R. (1993b). The impact of clinical information systems on human service organizations. *Computers in Human Services.* 9(3/4), pp. 425-438.

Poertner, J. &. Rapp C. (1987). Designing social work management information systems: The case for performance guidance system. *Administration in Social Work*, 11, 177-190.

Raider, M., & Moxley, D. (1990). A computer-integrated approach to program evaluation: A practical application within residential services. *Computers in Human Services*, 6, 133-148.

Schoech, D. (1993). *"Beyond Information Systems to Electronic Performance Support."* Presented at the Clinical Technologies Conference, Trieschman Center, Cambridge, Massachusetts.

Schuerman, J. R. (1987). Expert consulting systems in social welfare. *Social Work Research and Abstracts*, 23, 14-18.

Schuerman, J., Mullen, E., Stagner, M., & Johnson, P. (1989). *First generation expert systems in social welfare*. In W. LaMendola, B. Glastonbury, & S. Toole (Eds.), *A casebook of computer applications in the social and human services*, (pp. 111-122). New York: The Haworth Press.

Sicoly, F. (1989). Prediction and decision making in child welfare. *Computers in Human Services*, 5, 43-56.

Stone, N. & Stone S. (1983). The prediction of successful foster placement. *Social Casework*, 64, 11-17.

Wick, J., & Schoech, D. (1988). Computerizing protective services intake expertise: Preliminary research. *Children and Youth Services Review*, 10, 233-252.

Reliability Issues in the Development of Computerized Information Systems

Gail Auslander
Miriam Cohen

SUMARY. This paper examines issues of reliability in the development of computerized information systems and presents several strategies for dealing with them. It is based on our experience in developing a national hospital social work information system in Israel. Strategies included the careful and explicit definition of categories and the assessment of inter-rater reliability based on case records and on the systematic manipulation of key variables. Analysis of the data confirmed the reliability of most items of the system. It also pointed out a number of problem areas, and service as the basis for further refining variable categories and definitions to overcome difficulties revealed in the study. *[Article copies available from The Haworth Document Delivery Service: 1-800-342-9678.]*

INTRODUCTION

The reliability of measures is a major factor in the degree to which computerized information systems can provide usable information. This is

Gail Auslander is a member of the faculty of the Paul Baerwald School of Social Work, Hebrew University, Jerusalem, Israel. Miriam Cohen is a staff member, JDC-Brookdale Institute of Gerontology & Adult Human Development in Israel.

Address correspondence to: Gail Auslander, School of Social Work, Hebrew University of Jerusalem, Mt. Scopus, Jerusalem 91905, Israel.

[Haworth co-indexing entry note]: "Reliability Issues in the Development of Computerized Information Systems." Auslander, Gail, and Miriam Cohen. Co-published simultaneously in *Computers in Human Services* (The Haworth Press, Inc.) Vol. 12, No. 3/4, 1995, pp. 327-338; and: *Human Services in the Information Age* (ed: Jackie Rafferty, Jan Steyaert, and David Colombi) The Haworth Press, Inc., 1995, pp. 327-338. Single or multiple copies of this article are available from The Haworth Document Delivery Service [1-800-342-9678, 9:00 a.m. - 5:00 p.m. (EST)].

particularly true with regard to large systems which are used at multiple sites and by numerous workers in different positions. Yet it is frequently overlooked in system development, and when noted, it is usually about its absence. This paper examines the issue and presents several strategies for improving the reliability of measurement, based on our experience in developing a national hospital social work information system in Israel (INHSWIS).

Reliability refers to the degree to which information generated by the computerized information system is supported by judgments which are stable, reproducible and error free. In research methodology reliability is considered a necessary, although not sufficient, condition for the validity of findings (Cook & Campbell, 1979).

During the development stages of the INHSWIS, considerable time, thought and energy was invested in uncovering reliability problems. While many of them were in fact resolved, no solutions are 100% effective, nor can we be certain that no additional problems will arise. The purpose of this paper is to delineate some of the reasons why reliability is an issue of major importance, its various sources and some of the options available for dealing with it.

The Israel National Health Social Work Information System (INHSWIS) is a joint project involving Israel's major health care providers (the Sick Fund of the General Labor Federation, the Ministry of Health, and the Hadassah Medical Organization). These organizations provide health care for almost all of the country's patients, in 28 acute care facilities throughout the country, in addition to ambulatory and mental health services.

The INHSWIS collects and organizes data on individual clients and aims at providing information to direct service workers, supervisors and managers. It attempts to provide information on the scope of care, addressing the following questions:

1. Who are the clients served?
2. How do clients reach social workers?
3. What are the psychosocial problems dealt with?
4. What is the extent and nature of the care provided?
5. What is the status of clients at discharge or termination of treatment?
6. To which agencies are clients referred?
7. What are the extent and reasons for discharge delays?

IMPORTANCE OF RELIABILITY

There are several key reasons why the issue of reliability demands attention in the development and implementation of clinical information systems:

1. Product value. Computerization requires that social workers make changes in the way they think about cases, observe clients and record data, often employing new taxonomies and concepts (Gripton, Licker & de Grooty, 1988). Some claim that this alone is a major contribution of the process; others that it can distort reality (Murphy & Pardeck, 1992). In either case it is clear that if the data entered into the computer are unreliable, the system's reports and other products will be worthless (Benbenishty, 1993).

2. Trust and professional relationships. Problems of reliability can also damage the efforts of systems developers to establish effective working relationships and trust with the users of computer systems (Benbenishty, 1993; Williams & Forrest, 1988). Human service professionals are often skeptical about the contribution of such systems to their job performance and professional role (Bronson et al., 1988; Mutschler & Hoefer, 1990). If social workers are unsure about the reliability of the data they themselves gather, it is unlikely that they will trust the reports that are based on those data. And if they see no use in the output, it is difficult to imagine that they will be willing partners in the computerization effort. A recent survey illustrates the seriousness of the situation with 75% of workers questioning the accuracy of data recorded, 20% reporting they had falsified data and 30% ignoring requests for data (O'Brien, McClellan, & Alfs, 1992).

3. Networking. Reliability is especially important when a number of agencies want to network among themselves, sharing, comparing and compiling information on client populations or programs. Problems with using new concepts and taxonomies are magnified when users are located at different, often distant sites with no ongoing mechanism for face-to-face contact and mutual support.

4. Marketing. Prospective consumers of information systems are being urged to examine the reliability and testing procedures of the various programs available to them (Finnegan, Ivanoff & Smyth, 1991; Witkin, 1988). Yet a search of the human services-computer literature turned up a negligible number of references to reliability of specific systems, beyond theoretical pieces, which bemoaned the failure to relate to the reliability of measures. However, it seems reasonable to expect that, in the future, systems which provide evidence of the reliability of the measures employed will have a distinct marketing advantage over alternative systems.

THE NATURE OF THE PROBLEM

There are two main sources of reliability problems: the data themselves and the persons who work with them.

1. Problems inherent in the data. Problems stemming from the nature of the data themselves exist on both the phenomenological and operational levels. On the phenomenological side, social work has long been characterized by the use of vague terminology representing complex and amorphous situations and interpretations. Some writers have claimed that all data "are united inextricably with values, beliefs, and commitments" and that the attempt to quantify these phenomena objectively actually distorts their nature (Murphy & Pardeck, 1992, p. 64). Minimizing these distortions in a way that is acceptable to both practitioners and system designers requires a high level of mutual cooperation as well as skill. Clearly when categorization of such phenomena requires judgment or interpretation, then reliability problems are likely.

On the operational side, it is often difficult to arrive at a balanced taxonomy or category list. On the one hand categories should not be overly specific. The finer the distinguishing points between categories, the greater the knowledge required for consistent judgment and the greater the threat to reliability. Furthermore, if they are too specific the number of cases in each category will likely be too small for meaningful comparisons and decision-making. On the other hand, using categories which are broad or general can improve reliability, but they may lack sensitivity and risk being trivial and even meaningless (Selitz et al.,1959).

2. Problems stemming from personnel. The second source of problems of reliability is our reliance on the "two-legged meter," that is the persons who work with the data (Cohen, 1960). In our case, the problem is particularly acute because social workers play three concurrent roles in the data collection process–respondent, interviewer and coder. Each role engenders special challenges to reliability.

At the level of the respondent, one needs to be sure that requests for data and questions are phrased in a way that is both clear and relevant. The respondent must also be able to provide the data requested in sufficient detail to allow for accurate categorization. For example, social workers may not be the best source of data on clients' medical diagnoses.

At the level of the interviewer, reliability is particularly problematic among interviewers who code only the data they themselves collect (Selitz et al., 1959). In such situations interviewers tend to develop a frame of reference which is appropriate to their limited materials. For example, interviewers on one unit may see numerous problems of an emotional nature, and thus become more attuned to sub-categories of such problems. Interviewers on another unit may see more problems of physical function and thus become adept at distinguishing between sub-types of function while remaining relatively unskilled in areas which they see less often.

Third are problems which are common to coders, regardless of whether or not they are also interviewers. These stem primarily from variations in judgment and difficulties in understanding and differentiating clearly among a set of categories.

In most clinical information systems, the social workers play all three roles, responding and coding answers to questions relating to their own individual work. When this is multiplied by the number of workers involved in operating the system—in the INHSWIS case over 400 workers at 30 to 40 sites of varying sizes and functions—the magnitude of the threat to reliability is overwhelming.

IMPROVING RELIABILITY

What can be done in the face of reliability threats of such enormity? Some systems use standard instruments and multiple-item scales whose internal consistency can be measured (Nurius & Hudson, 1989; Raider & Moxley, 1990; Thomas, 1990).

However, these instruments are most appropriate for systems that interact with clients rather than with workers, or that have a major diagnostic element rather than a monitoring or quality assurance focus. They can be cumbersome and time-consuming for reporting on large caseloads with frequent turnover.

In the light of the lack of reported experience from the field, we attempted to develop our own strategy to maximize the reliability of the INHSWIS. It is largely based on accepted research methodology for dealing with categorical data, that is by trying to achieve maximum agreement among independent judges. This was done in several stages:

1. The issue was first addressed in the earliest stages of system design, in conceptualizing and delineating taxonomies of categories for key variables. When available, taxonomies which had already been tested and were in use locally were adapted for use in the INHSWIS (Soskolne, 1986). In other cases original taxonomies had to be developed. In both situations detailed category lists were collapsed, preference being given to relatively gross categories. As expected this led many social workers to question the relevance and sensitivity of the system. However, system development was seen as a multi-stage process; at a later stage it will be possible to further specify selected subcategories, both nationally and locally. To this end codes were created with an extra digit left free for further specification.

In the initial category list, efforts focused on insuring that categories were exhaustive and mutually exclusive, covering all eventualities. For instance, an issue of central importance in hospital social work is determining how potential clients reach the social services department. In the project's early stages six possibilities were specified: social work screening, patient/family, hospital staff, other medical personnel, non-medical personnel, and psychiatric referral sources. However, further examination showed that not all referrals come through one of these paths. For instance, in some units, e.g., dialysis and oncology, all patients are automatically seen by a social worker. Hence additional categories were added to cover this and other contingencies.

2. The next stage required identifying the different reliability issues faced by the system. Three clear classes of issues were determined:

a. Accuracy in identifying clients to be reported on. Hospital social workers interact with numerous patients during the course of their day-to-day activities. Not all of them are clients on whom full reporting is required.
b. Accuracy in reporting on variables with high face validity whose categorization requires little or no discretion or judgment. This includes variables such as sex, marital status, and so on, as well as a variety of significant dates in the patient's hospitalization experience.
c. Accuracy in reporting of variables whose categorization requires a moderate to high degree of discretion or judgment. This is particularly true for variables relating to the intervention process, for example, psychosocial problems for treatment, worker activities, problem status at discharge.

3. The third stage involved developing detailed guidelines and definitions of categories, with an eye to addressing the appropriate reliability issue. For instance, clear guidelines had to be spelled out for differentiating between persons who are to be considered social work clients and those who are not. Thus clients were defined as: "patients who are receiving care within the medical setting, are receiving social services to promote their emotional or physical health, and are personally known to the social worker."

For other variables, especially those demanding judgment or discretion on the part of the worker, detailed definitions of the categories were provided. Definitions could include up to three elements: a conceptual and operational definition, a list of examples of what was to be included, and a list of examples of what was to be excluded. For example the activity of providing information and advice was defined as "giving information or a professional opinion to the patient or family about the patient's condition, characteristics of medical care and services available to assist them. Cite this category only if the activity was actually intended to provide information and not if it occurs as a marginal element in a therapy session."

These guidelines, category lists and definitions were then put into use in the first pilot tests of the project. During this period, project staff met repeatedly with participating social workers, to discuss difficulties and further refine definitions and guidelines.

4. The fourth stage of the process was systematic testing of the reliability of the system components. The testing consisted of two main pieces–distinguishing between persons considered clients and those not considered clients, and the recording of standardized material on clients.

RELIABILITY TESTING METHODOLOGY

Testing was carried out among 53 workers at three sites. All participating workers had undergone training in using the data collection instruments, including their variables and categories and definitions. They had been using the instruments for at least six weeks prior to the testing. The test was administered at staff meetings at each site.

In order to test the reliability of the selection criteria for inclusion as clients, a series of eight short vignettes was developed in which the description of the relationship between worker and patient was systematically varied in line with the selection criteria. Each social worker was randomly given one vignette and asked whether he or she would consider this person a client to be reported on. Three of the vignettes represented situations which failed to meet the criteria for reporting on a case. The other five vignettes represented situations in which the case should have been reported.

The second part of the test was aimed at testing the reliability of categories, both those with high face validity and those requiring discretion or judgment on the part of the workers. To this end eight case examples were developed in which most of the key variables and categories appeared. Workers were asked to complete the reporting forms in use at that site on each of two case examples, distributed randomly among the workers.

"Correct" responses were predetermined for all variables, and worker responses compared to the standard. For the discretionary judgment categories, it was also planned to analyze statistically the level of agreement between workers, in order to determine common areas of misunderstanding and lack of clarity. This, however, was complicated by two facts: (1) virtually all of these variables allowed for multiple responses, and (2) different recording formats precluded an exact match between sites. In the end a qualitative analysis of the types of deviations from predetermined correct responses was employed as the best way of handling the data. Results were also compared between the three sites, concentrating on the relationship between the various recording formats and the accuracy of the recording.

RESULTS

With regard to deciding whether or not to open a file, 80% of the decisions recorded were correct, overall. However, when the correct answer was not to consider the patient a client, only 65% of the workers responded correctly. On the other hand, when the correct decision would have been to include the patient as a client, 88% of the respondents answered correctly. In other words, the social workers were more likely to err by including patients on whom reporting was unnecessary than to err by under-reporting.

Looking next at the variables with high face validity, the rate of correct answers ranged from 70% to 100% (Table 1). While for some variables, reporting was completely correct or almost so, there were a number of problems. In all cases of less than complete correctness, responses were examined in detail to try to determine the source of error. For instance, for the variable "living arrangements" 16% of the responses were wrong. This was attributed to lack of clarity in the definition of one of the categories. On the other hand, errors in determining "patient status" in the social work department (new, returning, or continuing) could be attributed to lack of clarity in the language of one of the case descriptions; hence no adjustment was required.

An example of a particularly problematic variable proved to be "sources of social care prior to the present contact with the social worker," which was answered correctly by only 69.7% of the respondents. Further examination showed that 83% of the errors were concentrated in two of the six case examples. Most errors reflected difficulty in understanding what was meant by "social care": Is it any care received for psychosocial needs, or only care provided by a social worker? Hence, the intent of the variable needed to be clarified.

For variables whose reporting requires some degree of judgment on the part of workers, reliability was somewhat lower than with the previous set of variables (Table 2). Levels of correct answers ranged from 43% to 81% for these variables. For example, in the categorization of psychosocial problems, several issues arose. First, while the intent was that only problems that had been worked on be reported, some of the social workers recorded a more comprehensive psychosocial assessment including all possible prob-

TABLE 1. Reliability testing, variables with high face validity (Selected examples).

Variable	% Correct	Notes for System Development
Source of income	93.1%	No change necessary
Living arrangement	76.2%	Clarify specific categories
Patient status	72.2%	Case description unclear No change necessary
Family status	100.0%	No change necessary
Religion	95.8%	If uncertain, refer worker to i.d. care (immigrants)
Ethnic origin	93.0%	Add examples regarding specific countries to guide
Type of medical insurance	100.0%	No change necessary
Referral source	87.7%	Create additional categories
Sources of prior social care	69.7%	Redefine variable
Prior home care arrangements	95.8%	No change necessary

lem areas. Furthermore, they often seemed to have difficulty making fine distinctions between related categories of problems. In particular, the issue of interpersonal problems between patients and their families required clarification. This included determining whose emotional reaction was at the focus, the patient's or the family's or both, and whether it was related to the illness or not. It is worth noting again that difficulties arose despite the fact that categories were rather gross, which had been expected to improve reliability.

Another problematic variable was that of worker activities. In addition to difficulties in determining and defining categories, we had, up to this point, experimented with two different recording formats–one problem-oriented in which up to four activities were recorded per problem; the other process-oriented in which up to four types of activities were re-

TABLE 2. Reliability testing, variables requiring discretion or judgment (Selected examples).

Variable	% Correct	Notes for System Development
Functional status	61.0%	Distinguish more clearly between categories reflecting temporary vs. fixed status
Services at discharge	63.3%	Distinguish more clearly between categories: (1) people discharged with no services arranged and (2) people not in need of services
Reasons for discharge delay	42.8%	Distinguish between categories attributing responsibility for different aspects of discharge planning and service provision
Types of psycho-social problems	77.6%	Stress reporting only on problems actually dealt with. Reporting must differentiate between "owners" of problems.
Unit of intervention	80.7%	Stress possibility of citing mixed client units (e.g., patient together with family)

corded per client per day. Reliability was considerably lower among the workers using the problem-oriented recording system than among the workers using the system based on activity-days. The reasons for this disparity are still not totally clear.

REVISING THE SYSTEM

Once the formal testing was completed, revisions were made in the system. In addition to test results, a large volume of comments about the reporting forms, the variables and the categories were gathered from individuals and groups of social workers, both in writing and in discussions. Project staff also analyzed together with workers a series of reports based on data gathered in the pilot tests. Inconsistencies and questions about the findings served to pinpoint additional reliability problems.

The final version of the information system reflects revisions based on feedback from all these sources. Social workers are provided with a detailed, user-friendly guide to filling out recording forms. It provides an overview of the system–its goals, operations and general instructions for filling out reporting forms. This is followed by a listing of all variables, clearly defined, as well as detailed definitions of all categories. Category definitions may include conceptual definitions, examples of items to be included and examples of items to be excluded, depending on the clarity and potential for misunderstanding.

TRAINING

Assuring reliability does not end with the implementation of recording tools and installation of the computer program. It is also a central focus of introductory and ongoing training in using the system. At each new site, project staff is available to meet with social workers, to explain and demonstrate the system and its components. This is followed by group sessions in which social workers practice coding and recording the material according to the information system criteria.

The process of learning to categorize data and use recording forms carries over beyond the technical demands of the information system. At one site the staff meets regularly in small groups to discuss actual cases and their recording. This has led to a more creative stage of thinking about the nature of social work practice and the way it should be reported and analyzed.

CONCLUSION

As noted at the outset, it is unrealistic to expect that all of the reliability problems in social work information systems can be foreseen, overcome or prevented. New problems continually arise, requiring system developers to work together with users to find acceptable solutions. It is clear that improving reliability is not a one-shot effort. Rather one must continually be on the look out for inconsistencies and incorporate retesting and retraining as a routine element in system maintenance.

REFERENCES

Benbenishty, R. (1993). *Clinical Information Systems for Human Services.* Jerusalem: Magnes Press. (Hebrew).

Bronson, D. E., Pelz, D. C., & Trzcinski, E. (1988). *Computerizing Your Agency's Information System.* Newbury Park, CA: Sage.

Cohen, J. (1960). A coefficient of agreement for nominal scales. *Education and Psychological Measurement,* XX, 37-46.

Cook, T. D. & Campbell, D. T. (1979). *Quasi-Experimentation: Design and Analysis Issues for Field Settings.* Boston: Houghton-Mifflin.

Epstein, J. (1988). Information systems and the consumer. In Bryan Glastonbury, Walter LaMendola & Stuart Toole (Eds.) *Information Technology and the Human Services.* Chichester, Great Britain: John Wiley.

Feine, R. J. (1988). Human services instrument based program monitoring and indicator setting. In Bryan Glastonbury, Walter LaMendola & Stuart Toole (Eds.) *Information Technology and the Human Services.* Chichester, Great Britain: John Wiley.

Finnegan, D. J. , Ivanoff, A., & Smyth, N. J. (1991). The computer applications explosion: What practitioners and clinical managers need to know. *Computers in Human Services,* 8 (2), 1-19.

Gripton, J., Licker, P. & deGroot, L. (1988). Microcomputers in clinical social work. In Bryan Glastonbury, Walter LaMendola & Stuart Toole (Eds.) *Information Technology and the Human Services.* Chichester, Great Britain: John Wiley.

Murphy, J. W. & Pardeck, J. T. (1992). Computerization and the dehumanization of social services. *Administration in Social Work,* 16, 61-72.

Mutschler, E. & Hoefer, R. (1990). Factors affecting the use of computer technology in human service organizations. *Administration in Social Work,* 31, 87-101.

Nurius, P. S. & Hudson, W. (1989). Computers and social diagnosis: The client's perspective. *Computers in Human Services,* 5 (1/2), 21-35.

O'Brien, N., McClellan, T. & Alfs, D. (1992). Data collection: Are social workers reliable? *Administration in Social Work,* 16, 89-99.

Raider, M. & Moxley, D. (1990). A computer-integrated approach to program evaluation: A practical application within residential services. *Computers in Human Services,* 6 (1/2/3), 133-148.

Selitz, Jahoda, Deutsch & Cook, *Research Methods in Social Relations (revised).* New York: Holt, Rinehart & Wilson, 1959.

Thomas, G. (1990). The making of COBRS 2.0: The competency-oriented behavior rating system for children and youth services. *Computers in Human Services,* 6 (1/2/3), 149-168.

Williams, S. & Forrest, J. (1988). Technology on trial. In Bryan Glastonbury, Walter LaMendola & Stuart Toole (Eds.) *Information Technology and the Human Services.* Chichester, Great Britain: John Wiley, 214-222.

Witkin, S. L. (1988). Guidelines for the development and assessment of human factors in software programs. In Bryan Glastonbury, Walter LaMendola & Stuart Toole (Eds.) *Information Technology and the Human Services.* Chichester, Great Britain: John Wiley.

The Quality of Information and Communication– Some Slow Remarks in a Rapid Age

Geert van der Laan

SUMMARY. The rapid developments in the field of software and hardware would lead one to expect an improvement in information processing in fields such as social work. However, that is only the case to a very limited extent. One of the most prominent problems with information systems is that they tend to apply bad classifications. Although an information system with broad categories is easy for employees to fill in, the problem is that they tend to paint the same picture year after year. A differentiated classification provides more and better information. A condition is, of course, that the classification is done carefully and contains logically exclusive categories. *[Article copies available from The Haworth Document Delivery Service: 1-800-342-9678.]*

Ours is a rapid age, an age of technological progress. Progress in fast times seem to forge ahead in a straight line. Computers are becoming ever smaller and more powerful, the software increasingly user-friendly, and expertise more and more rapidly obsolete. Our age of information technology however also witnesses the phenomenon of circular processes. Slow processes are often circular, rotating around or hobbling along on two ideas until they end up where they started. What often hampers progress in

---

Dr. Geert van der Laan is Social Psychologist at the Netherlands Institute of Care and Welfare, P.O. Box 19152, 3501 DD Utrecht, The Netherlands.

[Haworth co-indexing entry note]: "The Quality of Information and Communication–Some Slow Remarks in a Rapid Age." van der Laan, Geert. Co-published simultaneously in *Computers in Human Services* (The Haworth Press, Inc.) Vol. 12, No. 3/4, 1995, pp. 339-351; and: *Human Services in the Information Age* (ed: Jackie Rafferty, Jan Steyaert, and David Colombi) The Haworth Press, Inc., 1995, pp. 339-351. Single or multiple copies of this article are available from The Haworth Document Delivery Service [1-800-342-9678, 9:00 a.m. - 5:00 p.m. (EST)].

information technology are social impediments. Developing the contents of information systems and processing information in organisations are examples of such slow processes. By "content" here I do not mean the quality of the software or hardware, but rather the content, the substance of the information systems–the quality of the variables and classifications. These areas have seen little progress, which explains why information systems so often fall short of the mark. A system will feed back what has been fed into it. Inferior data will fail to yield useful information, without which an organisation cannot operate effectively. An ineffective organisation is unable to process information properly due to the obstructions to smooth communication–a vicious circle. On the surface, the organisation may even seem efficient and tightly run, but the internal wheels turn at a rusty, laborious pace.

QUALITY OF INFORMATION: SLOW PROCESSES IN FAST PROCESSORS

It is good to look back now and then, to assess progress carefully. I would like to turn now to Social work. The April 1981 edition of a social work review in the Netherlands commented: "This year, over 1500 social workers work will be filling in 100,000 client registration forms. The information obtained, however, will play little, if any, role in policy decisions" (De Tombe, 1981). How should we view this lament now, more than a decade later, in the light of the spectacular progress since made in the world of computers? Those years witnessed rapid progress in information processing. Initially, there were paper forms which were fed at the end of each year into a large computer at some central office in the country. Later, the forms became electronic as the rapidly advancing age of personal computers enabled institutions to process information by their own staff.

The rapid developments in the field of software and hardware would lead one to expect an improvement in information processing in fields such as social work. However, that is only the case to a very limited extent. The quality of information processing still leaves much to be desired. The slow processes determine quality, just as the weakest link determines the strength of the chain. In discussing this problem, I will describe one of these slow processes and make a few simple suggestions on how the quality could be improved. The main problem is the use of broad categories as "garbage cans," where information can be dumped.

CLASSIFICATION PROBLEMS

As noted earlier: what goes in comes back out. The notion that stream-lined equipment or fancy software will turn poor quality input into useful output is an illusion. One of the most prominent problems with informa-tion systems is that they tend to apply bad classifications. Traditionally, the so called "client registration forms" are comprised of different sections (variables) to identify the client's problems and the client characteristics. These sections, in turn, consist of categories which can be scored.

The variable "gender" thus consists of two categories, "male" and "female." Most other variables comprise a greater number of categories, though it would be interesting to mention as a side-note that in 1981 the former Ministry of Culture, Recreation and Social Affairs in The Nether-lands let it be known that as far as they were concerned, the variable, "source of income," need only consist of two categories. The Ministry expressed a desire to acquire the following official information from data-bases in social work: " . . . problems of clients, type of assistance pro-vided, age categories of clients, primary living situation and marital status, cultural minorities, people earning an income vs. people on benefits (fur-ther categorization of the latter category is unnecessary)." The last part of that sentence, the part between brackets, is especially interesting. Indeed, it certainly does not take thousands of registration forms to obtain that kind of information.

The variable "problems of clients," is seldom split into two categories, such as "material problems" and "non-material problems," but is usually divided into some ten categories. Typical examples of the categories which fall under this variable in the social work's nation-wide information system in The Netherlands are: problems with income, housing, employ-ment, education, leisure time, health, sexuality, relationships, social orga-nisations. Over the years, other problem areas have been added to the list: problems with divorce, loneliness, ability to cope, identity problems, ad-diction and multi-problem families.

What is the informative quality of general classifications? The time and trouble spent obtaining data has proven to be way out of proportion to the value of the information obtained. Although such classifications are very quick in providing a global view of the situation in some particular field, the problem is that they tend to paint the same picture year after year. The time and effort invested in the acquisition process, therefore, fails to ren-der any new, useful information. Although an information system with broad categories is easy for employees to fill in, it provides data which are hard to process. The employees, in turn, receive little serviceable feed-back. The process of acquiring information is too oversimplified to yield information intelligible to social workers who think inductively. They, in turn, lose their motivation to invest time in consistent information processing etc., and a vicious circle is set in motion.

ADDICTS IN ALL SHAPES AND SIZES

A simple example of a broad category as a garbage can is the category "addiction." An overview of social work's concern with this problem during the 1980s in the city of Groningen, in the northern part of The Netherlands, is shown in Figure 1. This clearly illustrates that the total actual number of clients with an addiction problem grew by leaps and bounds throughout the eighties, but levelled off after 1988. There is enough information on this category to print out. For one thing, 65% of the addicts appear to be female and 35% male. Furthermore, the information registered shows that a relatively large number of addicts have, at some earlier point in their lives, been in contact with social workers, that a significant number of clients are referred by GPs to social work and that a large group are referred by social workers to the Counselling Centre for Alcohol and Drug Addiction.

FIGURE 1. Total actual number of social work clients in Groningen with an addiction problem.

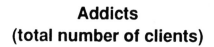

Addicts
(total number of clients)

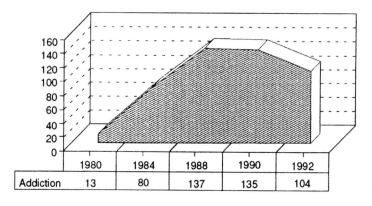

	1980	1984	1988	1990	1992
Addiction	13	80	137	135	104

▨ Addiction

Is this information useful to the institution? Let's test it on a typical practical example. Suppose that an experimental project has been set up in some particular district to identify alcohol addiction in the early stages and treat it in primary health care and social work. And suppose that a year later this same institution for social work is approached and asked to participate in a collaborative project on compulsive eating with the Regional Institute for Outpatient Mental Health Care and a psychiatric hospital. It is also easy to imagine how another year later, the police, in their new, growing concern about the rise of crime related to compulsive gambling, might inquire whether the institution for social work would consider setting up a new project to contact compulsive gamblers "on their own turf" to help "nip the problem in the bud."

These examples were not just made up helter skelter. Social work institutions are approached with such requests quite regularly. It is difficult to anticipate specific future requests. Therefore, the structure of an information system must lend itself to accommodating as many specific requests as possible. It should also be capable of providing an overview of the current situation and the developments leading up to it. It is important to know, for example, that it has not been until recently that an increase in the number of compulsive eaters has been registered. This trend may just as well be due to a population increase as to a growing "sensitivity" on the part of social workers to the problem. It may also be that over the last few years GPs have started recognizing the problem earlier on and consequently referring more cases.

The numerous collaborative projects the institution in our example would be involved in, make it necessary to chart the stream of clients and pattern of referrals to various other care providers and institutions, namely: GPs, primary health care teams, district agents, schools, the municipal social services department, welfare officers, the Alcohol and Drug Counselling Centre, the Regional Institute for Outpatient Mental Health Care, psychiatric and therapeutic services and the like.

It is also important to be familiar with the backgrounds of clients with an addiction problem–simple information, such as sex, age, source of income, primary living situation, as well as the inter-relationship between addiction and other problems of a material and non-material nature. Information about the nature and duration of the assistance provided is also necessary in order to obtain an idea of such aspects as the extent of the burden they place on care providers. Such questions cannot be answered without detailed information on the different kinds of addiction. A print-out on the category, "addiction" as a whole is insufficient. The extensive information

FIGURE 2. Subcategories of addiction problems and total number of addicts in social work in Groningen.

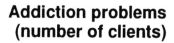

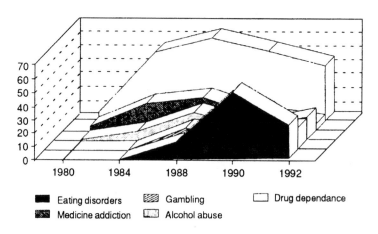

needed can only be provided by a system which distinguishes between different kinds of addiction.

Social work in Groningen has been working for years with an information system consisting of very detailed classifications and code lists. The figures registered paint the picture shown in Figure 2 of the developments in the field of social work among addicts during the eighties.

The graph illustrates that compulsive gambling, drug addiction and compulsive eating account primarily for the rise between 1984 and 1986. An exception to the falling trend among addicts between 1988 and 1990, is the sub-category of compulsive eaters. Although the other sub-categories of addicts showed a slow tendency to wane in the late 1980s, the same years witnessed a dramatic rise in the number of eating disorders. For the time being, we will not comment on the extent to which that indicates a real increase in the general population. The figures are the result of a research program on eating disorders of the University of Groningen, in which I took part. At the end of the program social workers and general practitioners in Groningen were advised how to handle eating disorders. Likewise we do not discuss the question whether eating disorders are correctly categorised under the classification of addiction. Before analysing this trend any further, however, one very striking finding should be pointed out, namely that 99% of the compulsive eaters are female. It was thought that most of those clients suffered from Anorexia Nervosa (Noordenbos, 1987).

We can conclude that the categories of addiction are comprised of important subcategories, the information from which could not be gleaned from broad categories and simple classifications. The significance of the sub-categories can be gathered from their combination with other variables. It appears that alcoholism and compulsive eating are the most prominent sub-categories. They have been placed side by side in Figure 3. The reader can get an idea from this information about the differences between these two subgroups of addicts.

FIGURE 3. Comparison of clients with alcoholism and compulsive eating.

ALCOHOLISM	COMPULSIVE EATING
Relatively more prominent among:	Relatively more prominent among:
Men:	Women;
The elderly;	Young people;
People on disablement benefits;	The employed:
Clients treated in the past by the Alcohol and Drug Counselling Centre	Clients treated in the past by therapists in private practice;
Clients referred to the Alcohol and Drugs Counselling Centre	Clients not referred by social services;
Clients with financial problems; Clients from broken marriages;	Clients with no financial problems; Clients given to anxiety and fits of crying;
Aggressive clients;	Clients with a poor ability to cope;
Is treated more frequently: in cooperation with GPs; in cooperation with welfare officers in consultation (information/advice)	Is seldom treated: in cooperation with GPs; in cooperation with welfare officers

FINANCIAL PROBLEMS

A comparable chart can be drawn up to trace the significance of financial problems. Suppose that during a discussion about debt problems of clients between an institution for social work, the municipal social services department and the municipal credit bank, the question arises as to the extent to which debts are related to an insufficient income. Could an institution for social work answer such a question on the basis of its information system? Is there only one type of financial problems, or should the problem be divided into various subcategories? Here again, one single category "financial problems" is not sufficient for a meaningful analysis. Let us begin by examining the different subcategories developed in the 1980s of financial problems as shown in Figure 4.

The graph shows that after 1988 the categories "insufficient income" and "problems acquiring an income" showed a sharper decrease than did "budgeting problems" and "debts." Research into the inter-connection between the financial problems recorded at Groningen's social work agencies (Span & Westerlaan, 1981; Van der Laan, 1990) shows that these two combinations of financial problems form significant sub-categories. On the one hand, requests are submitted for assistance with income acquisi-

FIGURE 4. Subcategories of financial problems at the Groningen Social work institute expressed in percentages of the total number of clients.

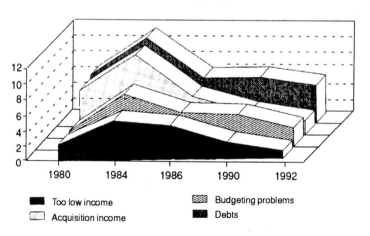

Financial problems
% of clients

tion, and on the other, for problems about budgeting. In the inter-connection between financial problems, these two aspects appear to form the two poles around which the other financial problems (costs of accommodation, bankruptcies, etc.) cluster. A study of the "carriers" (features of the clients) of these aspects of financial problems support this impression:

• Relatively speaking, problems with acquiring income occur more often among: women, single people, single-parent families, people on social security and "client systems" consisting of one person. This category of clients has relatively few debts. We call this configuration "type A."
• Problems with budgeting and debts occur more often among: men, complete families, clients in paid employment and "client systems" consisting of two or more people. This category appears to have debts relatively often. We call it "type B."

Figure 5 shows that financial problems consist of at least 2 subcategories. These subcategories become significant especially because of the "carriers" of these problems. Two different groups of clients appear to be involved here. Therefore, by combining the variable "problems" with other variables, such as source of income, age, sex, etc., we can reconstruct the meaning of the problem categories. Thus, on the one hand this is a question of definition a priori, and on the other, a reconstruction of meaning a

FIGURE 5. The interconnection between subcategories of financial problems in relation to other client characteristics. (The rectangles represent strong links, the circles weaker links, and the ellipse a weak link.)

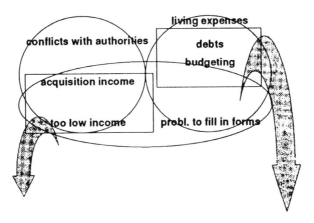

posteriori. This analysis of sub-categories of financial problems shows that the decision made in the beginning of the eighties to divide the broad category, "financial problems" into "income" and "budgeting/debts" in the national information system proved effective, as shown in Figure 6.

It is clear that the figures from Groningen reflect the figures from the nationwide information system. Further statistical analysis will be done in the future, to compare several sources of information about social work in The Netherlands. The analysis above also supports the recent decision to (give the option to) divide these two sub-categories in the 1992 social work information model into further sub-subcategories for internal use in the institutions, as in the social work information system in Groningen. We refer to the contributions of Potting and De Haas in this volume.

What about the interrelationship between material and non-material problems? It is striking that problems with acquiring income are very often accompanied by problems in raising children and that budgeting problems are least often involved. This gives type A a clear profile. The high number of single-parent families, in particular, contributes to this. It appears, therefore, that problems with acquiring income occur more often in combination with marital problems, while of all of the financial problems they are accompanied least by relationship problems (within existing relationships). All kinds of financial problems are often accompanied by anxiety, conflicts with government institutions, social isolation, alcohol abuse, suicidal behaviour and unemployment problems. In general we can say that

FIGURE 6. Financial problems in social work in the Netherlands.

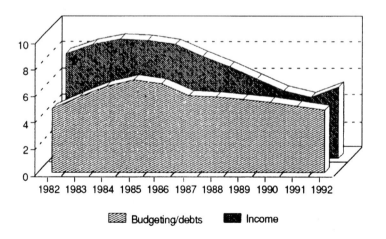

the inter-relationship between financial problems is no stronger than the inter-relationship between financial problems and other (particularly non-material) problems. Thus, poverty in the strict (financial) sense appears to be strongly linked to deprivation in other areas in the life of clients of social work.

It is interesting to see how the trends in social work are more or less a mirror image of the trends in society as a whole. At the start of the eighties unemployment in The Netherlands increased a lot. At the end of the eighties there was a considerable drop in the number of unemployed persons. That pattern is recognizable in the data from the social work information system in Groningen which reflect in more detail the trends in the nationwide information project in social work. Unemployment rates in The Netherlands showed a huge increase in 1993 so we can expect that the figures in social work, which are not yet available, will follow this trend. In that sense social work is a mirror of society.

NO GARBAGE CANS BUT SEPARATE COLLECTION AT SOURCE

Turning back to the hypothetical situation where a social work institution was invited to take part in collaborative projects on a local level, we can now evaluate the kind of data an institution can provide in order to obtain greater insight into the existing situation. It appears that implementing a policy at a local level requires detailed data. The institution must give a clear answer to clear questions. The (care provision) characteristics of compulsory eaters differ considerably from those of alcoholics. In the cooperation between the social services, it is also important to know that clients who have problems due to an insufficient income belong to a different category than clients with debts. A differentiated classification, therefore, provides more and better information. A condition is, of course, that the classification is done carefully and contains logically exclusive categories.

The lack of differentiation within broad classifications becomes clear when one has to choose between, for instance, "housing problems" and "financial problems." What to do with a client who has a problem with high costs of housing? Does that fall under "housing" or under "finances?" It would be better to include a separate category "housing costs" than to force workers to choose between "housing" and "finances." There is also a rule of thumb for analysing the streams of clients: make lists (code lists) with an exhaustive enumeration of all of the services available in the surroundings of the social work institution. This is the best way to answer concrete questions concerning the coordination and cooperation of the local welfare services.

STRAIGHT OR CIRCULAR

Figures from information systems do not lead automatically to unequivocal conclusions. Quality is a multi-dimensional phenomenon. An information system can provide no more than one of the many loops which are necessary to guide the organisation in the direction of quality improvement. These loops connect helping methods of practitioners to the policy of the institution. As in many institutions, there is a particular gap between staff and management. In most management information systems there is attention only to purposive rational activity: the instrumental way to assess the truth of facts in the objective world. There is a considerable discrepancy between the complexity with which social workers are faced and the simplicity of management discourse. It is important that information processing is embedded into careful procedures and adequate translations between the different user levels and between objective, normative and subjective aspects of human services. These "soft" communicative and cultural factors have an equally large influence on the quality of information processing as the information system itself.

Managers should be able to place themselves in the shoes of workers and be aware of the complexity of everyday practice. They should be able to identify the ethical and personal dilemmas of social workers. They are supposed to make a translation between the everyday predicaments of social workers and the demands of rationalized bureaucracies. The success of that translation is dependent on the quality of the communication between workers and managers. This communication should not be reduced to measurable facts in the objective world but should also cover normative and subjective issues (Habermas, 1984, 1987). Quality of information has to cover the quality of life of the clients.

Particularly in a sector in which a strong appeal is made to the moral and personal dedication of the people involved, the appropriateness of norms as well as the authenticity of subjective statements should not be neglected in worker-client relationships, supervision, team discussions, the development of professional theory and the interaction between social workers and managers (Van der Laan, 1990). Many managers think along rather straight lines. While, during some course or other, most have come across concepts from cybernetics, such as circular causality, equi-finality, feed-back loops, homeostasis and the like, they seem to go back, under the influence of the new business-like approach, to concepts from classical mechanics. In classical mechanics one actually does speak of linear causality, of predictability of effects and of measurable outcomes. However, the use of information in the social work sector for "measuring effects," "performance related pay" or "showing company profitability on the basis of hard figures" is, from a modern scientific point of view, highly dubious. In that sense progress does not move ahead in a straight line. The shortest way to the target is not always the best.

REFERENCES

De Tombe, E. (1981), *Zinloos registreren*. NOW-Nieuws 17 April 1981.

Habermas, J (1984, 1987), *The Theory of Communicative Action*, vol. 1 & 2, Boston: Beacon Press and Cambridge: Polity Press in association with Basil Blackwell, Oxford.

Noordenbos, G. (1987), *Onbegrensd lijnen*. Groningen/Leiden.

Van der Laan, G. (1990) *Legitimatieproblemen in het Maatschappelijk Werk*, Utrecht, SWP.

Westerlaan, L. & Span, J. (1981), *Classificatieproblemen in het maatschappelijk werk*, Groningen: Madi.

The Dutch Client Databank in Public Social Work

Jos Potting

SUMMARY. The history of the Dutch National Databank for Public Social Work began in 1960 in the province of Limburg. Social workers in that province met at a seminar and decided to set up a registration system concerning client characteristics and the counselling process which all the institutes of public social work in Limburg could be required to register in a uniform way. Thirty-three years later Dutch Public Social Work agencies are registering data according to a national system which was wanted, designed and developed by the united local authorities and all the institutes of Public Social Work. As a result, the National Databank for Public Social Work administers the data of all of the 166 institutes in the Netherlands and consequently is privileged to deal with the client characteristics and other specific data of the 250,000 client units that are involved every year with Public Social Work. *[Article copies available from The Haworth Document Delivery Service: 1-800-342-9678.]*

INTRODUCTION

In many ways 1993 was an important year for Dutch Public Social Work. From the beginning of January of that year, more than 2,900 people working in the sector of Public Social Work suddenly started to talk in the

---

Jos Potting, Drs, studied sociology and methods of social research at the University of Nijmegen in the Netherlands. After having worked for several years in higher education he is currently a staff member of the Limburg Institute for Social Service Support (FMDL) in Roermond, the Netherlands. This institute is the administrator of the National Databank for Public Social Work.

[Haworth co-indexing entry note]: "The Dutch Client Databank in Public Social Work." Potting, Jos. Co-published simultaneously in *Computers in Human Services* (The Haworth Press, Inc.) Vol. 12, No. 3/4, 1995, pp. 353-363; and: *Human Services in the Information Age* (ed: Jackie Rafferty, Jan Steyaert, and David Colombi) The Haworth Press, Inc., 1995, pp. 353-363. Single or multiple copies of this article are available from The Haworth Document Delivery Service [1-800-342-9678, 9:00 a.m. - 5:00 p.m. (EST)].

same way and using the same words about their clients and the counselling process. At the same time the "registration system war" that had been fought for too many years between the institutes in different Dutch regions came to an end. These institutes were the declared supporters of the registration system commonly used in their region and which they thought to be "simply the best." In the end the 175 employers of those 2,900 social workers agreed to send each year the registration data from their institutes to the National Databank for Public Social Work. The Netherlands finally have a uniform system of client registration, a system which for many years was sought by managers of the institutes and local and national administrators.

It almost seems too good to be true and actually it is not the whole truth. Although there is a national registration system that has been operational from 1 January 1993, not every institute was able to switch quickly to the new national system of client registration. By the beginning of 1994 most institutes for Public Social Work had joined the national system. Institutes who continue to register with their own conflicting systems are seen as real dissidents, frustrating the national system and excluding themselves from comparative analyses of neighbour institutes, regional data and national figures.

The social workers however did not have too many positive expectations about another way of registering their clients and their work, with consequently a new questionnaire. However they appeared to be very cooperative. The explanation for their compliance towards the new system can be found in the long tradition of registration in the Dutch Public Social Work sector; ever since 1982 data about clients and the counselling process were gathered by the social workers according to national rules and definitions and were collected for management purposes in the institutes and finally sent to a national databank. In certain regions of the country the tradition to register existed even longer–for example in the province of Limburg they had already decided to collect certain data about the institute and their clients in a uniform way in 1962.

IN THE BEGINNING

During a seminar for social workers in Limburg in 1960, the participators reached some important conclusions. They all worked in their own specific way and they all had their unique clients with unique problems, but there were also many similarities in the counselling methods used, in daily administrative actions, in the ways they characterized their clients and defined their methods of help. Therefore they decided that a registration system could be beneficial, a registration system that would be used in all the institutes for Public Social Work in Limburg. The developers of such a system would have to pay attention to several requirements that had been formulated. The registration system should be easy to handle and easy to interpret, it should not take too much time and the different parts of the system should be linked to each other. Also the system results had to be clear to the administrators in the institutes, and last but not least, the motivation of the social workers and the boards of the institutes had to be a matter of constant concern (CRM, 1973).

Only two years later this intention achieved the start of a system for all the institutes. One that was concerned with registration of client characteristics and problem definitions, but that also standardized administrative actions systematically. For instance a mailbook was developed, a financial form and a documentation card. On one form the contacts of a social worker had to be noted, on another form data about the family-situation; on the documentation card the most imported data for the central administration was collected. There was a list of all clients that had to be kept up to date, accompanied by data like the date of intake, the name, the address, the social environment and the problem the client had at intake. The financial status of the client was recorded on a financial form. A multitude of information and many forms to be filled in existed, but unfortunately it was not possible to relate the different types of data.

In 1966 there were arguments for reducing this comprehensive administrative system to a client registration system. Despite the disadvantages of the existing huge system, there was a growing interest in registration data in Limburg. In other Dutch institutes of public social work people also became aware of the potential use of a client registration system. However the most important reason for this change of view was that the social workers themselves, again united by a seminar, took the decision to evaluate the existing registration system. A research group started to select the data that had to be collected because of its relevance for administration. Special attention was given to the way this data had to be gathered. This study resulted in a system of registration per client, thus leaving out data that were only related to the social worker (for instance the contacts the social worker had in a day). For every client the following data had to be recorded;

1. serial number
2. dossier number
3. date of intake
4. client name
5. client address
6. parish, neighbourhood, local community

7. social worker
8. way of making contact
9. cooperation with
10. referred to
11. occupation
12. social environment
13. personal data, like age, sex, civil status
14. problem(s) at intake
15. treated problem(s)
16. date and reason for finishing counselling

In 1968 the new registration system became operational in Limburg. The Institute for Social Service Support Limburg (FMDL) in Roermond, which evaluated the previous system with the research group, now paid special attention to the motivation of the social workers to cooperate with the new registration system. In the former period it had become very clear that the social worker was the most important variable in getting valid and reliable figures. The social worker had to be convinced of the importance of seriously answering the questions asked about each client. The provincial service institute took the initiative to analyse the data of four Social Work Institutes within six months after the start of the new system. This analysis, meant as a stimulating action for the participation of the social workers, caused more requests for local figures. The staff member of the FMDL soon had trouble with meeting this large amount of requests and started to look for mechanical help.

As a result of analysing the potentialities of the computer, the logistic of the registration system had to be accommodated. Till 1969 the data about clients were written down on a collect form; from now on a registration form was filled in for each client and, with the help of a code book, these notes were transferred to a so-called "codeslip." Data on these codeslips were imported in a computer system which in 1969 was a mainframe with an internal memory of 64KB. This computer, owned by an agricultural organisation, was normally used for counting the beet harvest. The FMDL used it to produce tables and charts for the Limburg Institutes for Public Social Work.

THE FIRST NATIONAL
CLIENT REGISTRATION SYSTEM

After some years of studying, testing and discussing the pros and cons of the existing registration systems and testing some conceptual systems, the National Service Institute for Social Work (JOINT), started a national registration system. This so-called JOINT system made a distinction between two periods of registration; intake and the end of treatment. In the intake phase different questions were asked than at the end of the treatment. In fact the registration form consisted of two questionnaires each of which were sent to the central point, the JOINT, immediately after they had been completed to be processed.

An important innovative aspect of the national system was the possibility for extra, specific questions that could be formulated by the social work institute itself. Each team of workers could decide whether they wanted to register more than the national data simply because they themselves or the local government were interested in this specific data. This resulted in a more flexible registration system and it raised the motivation for management and workers to cooperate with the national registration project.

Another key issue was the incorporation of some data about the counselling process. Until then nobody, for instance in the Limburg registration system, had taken the risk to register the ways social workers worked. However from now on they were asked to define the way they worked using a pre-coded list of options. Despite these extensions the national registration system was not as national as it was meant to be. In the province of Limburg the institutes continued to work with their own registration system, but also in the rest of the country it was not easy to convince every institute to participate in the national system. In fact 80 of the 180 organisations joined the national JOINT system. Along with this there were the systems of Limburg, Groningen and Raalte, each proclaimed to be much better and more comprehensive than the others.

In 1985 the JOINT commissioned software for minicomputer systems, aiming to offer the institutes the option to process data locally instead of sending it to the JOINT. In practice this meant someone in the institute importing the data into a local database and producing output by choice. Soon this software was also made suitable for personal computers. With the introduction of software for personal computers by the national institute, other software made their entrée on the small market of Social Work to earn money. Within a short period there were software packages with mysterious names like MDS, V-Stat, Mirage, Regi, Roerstat, Crosstabs, Kernflex and ORKA. Nice names, good software but a uniform system for all Dutch social workers was not the goal of these software developers; several programs could not deliver databases that fully met the national requirements.

THE NATIONAL DATABANK FOR PUBLIC SOCIAL WORK

In fact from the moment the Social Work Institutes in Limburg began to collect registration data with the help of pre-coded questionnaires, a Databank for Public Social Work existed. This data was sent to the provincial institute where it was processed and on request figures were produced concerning the client population of the institute. Furthermore there was a growing agreement that it could be of great importance to present some figures to financers. The management of the organisation used the conclusions of these figures to emphasize the uniqueness and specialty of the work. In order to obtain more knowledge about the quantitative aspects of the clients, their problems and the region, the provincial databank received a growing number of requests for comparative figures which made use of the complete data of all institutes.

Shortly after the decision to register the client characteristics and counselling data according to a national system, the national databank was born. Not all institutes in the Netherlands however were willing or able to send their data to the national databank; they had different systems or no interest in national figures. Nevertheless 80 institutes of Public Social Work were willing to finance the development and organisation of this national databank. The logistics (from local data to databank data) had to be organised, an organisation for data processing had to be found, computer time had to be hired, computer programs developed for input of data and output of figures and finally a national helpdesk had to be organised.

Soon after the start of the national databank there were some changes in how data was delivered to the databank. At first the JOINT organisation received a great number of codeslips every three months, which were sent to a computer center for data to be entered into a computer system by data typists. The computer center then produced some standardized figures for every institute. At the end of a year all data of all institutes were amalgamated to produce national figures.

When several registration softwares offered options to process data in the institutes, there were two ways in which data was offered to the databank–on codeslips sent every three months or on floppy disks usually sent once a year as a ready-made database of the institute. As a result of these developments and the growing interest in the output of the national databank, the number of participating institutes increased from 80 to 125.

This introduction of other software packages into the market of client registration software at first had no influence on the number of participating institutes, although the JOINT software lost its monopoly status. The important effect was that the number of automated institutes grew rapidly, a process that began as soon as the FMDL took over administration of the national databank. This provincial institute produced the output the institutes used to get but it also organised the data input and wrote conversion programs with recoding options for newly-built databases. With a little help from the software houses that built the registration software, the FMDL succeeded in raising the number of participating institutes of Public Social Work.

THE INFORMATION MODEL OF PUBLIC SOCIAL WORK

Although there was a rise in participation in the national databank, it did not mean that the additional contributing institutes that were registering conformed to the national registration system. Several institutes continued using very different registration systems or software that could not produce a "databank-output" to the full requirements of the national system. For the sector of Public Social Work this was an annoying situation and often the sigh could be heard; *"There is so little we have in common; at least we should succeed in a common registration system!"*

In the Netherlands Public Social Work was decentralised from 1989. Since then, local authorities have had a bigger responsibility in administering and financing welfare. In fact local government paid for the help that Public Social Work offered to the citizen with problems. The quest for structured information was strongly felt by these local authorities.

That was one of the reasons for the start of the project "Information model public social work," the project was executed by the Cooperation of Local Communities (VNG) and the employers' organisation in the Public Social Work sector (VOG). A main goal from this project was to give the institutes for Public Social Work and the local authorities a better insight into their own information supply. The project also aimed at formulating a uniform data set, thereby stimulating a better exchange of information between the institutes, local authorities and other interested organisations. Finally the project should formulate the demands and wishes of the users of information and registration packages (VNG, 1992).

The most important result of this project is the data dictionary in which are entered the definitions of data which have to be registered by the institutes, and which are of major interest for local communities and the National Institute for Statistics (CBS). These are the so-called "central data" which not only concern client data but also organisational, personnel and financial data. This extra data had been collected until then by the CBS through an annual inquiry. Also in this data dictionary data was recorded on behalf of the Public Social Work sector, who proclaimed specific data to be important to them, mainly about the client and the counselling process. In this way a system arose with several registration levels. Nationwide the system consists of a central package and a sector package. The system can be extended with other data sets, under the strict condition that they do not violate the rules and definitions of the central and sector data.

Figure 1 is a schematic presentation of the registration system of Institute X. The circle and the oval represent the obligatory registration packages; all the institutes and all the social workers have to follow the rules, definitions and use codes in the same way. The outmost rectangle represents the local system of institute X. There is another rectangle in the scheme; institutes can make plans for collecting extra data. In the province of Limburg there is an LIO package, a set of data which all the institutes in this province will collect, with extra questions concerning for instance the status of the job (payed or voluntary) and the domicile of the clients. In this case the provincial service institute controls the use of this extra data and produces extra provincial figures and information based on this data.

The National Databank for Public Social Work and all the software developers were properly informed by the project leaders and got two messages: to plan for the new system and to be ready by 1 January 1993! The administration of the databank was prepared for anything with their

FIGURE 1

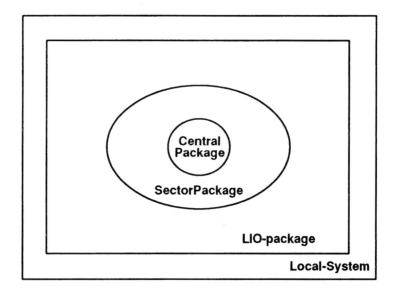

first test in 1994 when all national "new" registration data reaches the bank. There are five software packages which met the criteria and are able to work with the new registration system.

USE OF THE DATABANK FOR PUBLIC SOCIAL WORK

A scenario. On a particular day Mr. Qwerty telephoned the National Databank for Public Social Work and introduced himself as the director of the Institute for Social Welfare Faketown. This institute was a customer of the National Databank and every year receives a custom-built collection of tables produced from the client registration data. He said that he had called three months ago with some questions referring to the average number of contacts with clients in the first and last quarters of 1992. Mr. Qwerty asked politely if he could ask for some advice, but without waiting for an answer he dropped his cry of distress; *"The local authorities are 'phoning everyday, they want to know all sort of things concerning the social work target groups, the time spent on specific projects and when these projects finish? Moreover they also want to know how many social workers we have and how many we actually need?"*

There will be a meeting with officials of the local board the day after tomorrow, so yesterday he needed the answers on these questions! Using a software package at the institute, it was easy to provide answers to the questions at an institute level. Every contributor to the national databank receives each year three standardized reports with tables which present the figures about three different client populations–of the individual institute, of the institutes of the province and nationally. With the help of these reports, Mr. Qwerty was able to answer the following questions:

- What kinds of counselling are most often and less often offered by the institute? Does the local picture reflect the national client population? Is the average number of contacts per client in our institute high compared to the national figures?
- Is the impression correct that relatively more people of Faketown come with identity problems to Public Social Work then in the rest of the country? How much time does a counselling process take on average in our institute and is it a proper remark of an official of the municipality, that our clients remain for too long in the counselling or therapeutic process?

However the local authorities also asked for figures concerning problems of two specific groups of clients, namely young people and elderly people. Mr. Qwerty was not sure if it was possible with their own registration software package to produce a chart with both groups presented. Moreover he thought that it would be a good idea to make a comparison with the national figures, because he assumed that the Faketown situation was not typical. Another request from Mr. Qwerty was a table combining the frequencies of the problems of the clients of 1990, 1991 and 1992. He thought that with these figures he could demonstrate the effectiveness of the "Alcoholism" project that started three years ago.

All the questions could be answered by the national databank employees, it needed some operationalisation of the questions, some recoding to get the correct research populations and some attention to the layout in order to produce clear tables. However the tables that were sent to Mr. Qwerty were accompanied by a firm warning; if the national figures are used, be well aware of the fact that not all Dutch institutes participate in the national databank. It may become possible with the new registration system that 100% of the institutes for Public Social Work will deliver data to the national databank.

There are still questions that remain unanswered, simply because the dataset used in the national registration system does not have the right variables. That will always be a problem because the registration system and the resulting databank are a reduction of the complex world, or in this case a reduction of the complex client and the counselling process.

Besides directors, managers and social workers of the Dutch Institutes for Social Work, others showed great interest in the national figures. The VOG, the national organisation for employers in the Public Social Work sector, publishes reports about the sector and therefore uses data from the databank. The CBS uses data from the national databank to present demographic statistics about the sector and processes specific data in order to send them to the Ministry of Social Welfare, Health and Culture. Research institutes like the National Institute of Care and Welfare (NIZW) show a growing interest in the data of the National Databank for Public Social Work. Because of the new registration system, interest in the data of the bank will increase further, for instance local authorities will become interested in the figures produced with the "central data" of the national registration system. Hopefully social workers themselves will show a growing interest in the new registration data.

CONCLUSION

Public Social Work in the Netherlands knows a long tradition in registration of the client characteristics and some aspects of the counselling process. With the new national system, promises are made about the flexibility of the system and the increasing participation of the Institutes for Public Social Work in the National Databank. Whatever the future may bring, developments in this sector already serves in the Netherlands as a good example on how to set up a registration system. The history of the National Databank for Public Social Work is a bit shorter which is probably the reason that the potentialities of that data collection are not yet fully realised.

REFERENCES

CRM (1973). *Doelmatigheid in het maatschappelijk werk*, Ministerie van WVC, 's-Gravenhage.
VNG (1992). *Informatiemodel Algemeen Maatschappelijk Werk*, VNG, 's-Gravenhage.
VNG (1992b). *Eindrapport Landelijke Databank AMW*, VNG, 's-Gravenhage.
VOG (1992). *Landelijke AMW registratiesystematiek*, VOG sectie AMW, Rijswijk.

Information Technology
and Quality Management
in Public Social Work

Leon de Haas

SUMMARY. Managing a non-profit organization for public social work is primarily a matter of quality management which is the responsibility of the service manager. Because of (a) the actual state of quality assurance in the public social work branches, and (b) the professional character of the organizations, a Public Social Work Quality System asks for intensive involvement of professional workers in the development of the system. PS+QS is both a development method and a system model. It organizes the clients' routing through the institution. The major part of the workflow management concerns phasing of the service and counselling processes. PS+QS is a system of communication structured by information techniques. Professional counsellors and their service managers apply the professional standards and check on their application. *[Article copies available from The Haworth Document Delivery Service: 1-800-342-9678.]*

INTRODUCTION

Dutch society provides all its citizens with a specific kind of counselling facility called "public social work." The service is public in the sense

---

Leon de Haas, Drs, studied philosophy and the science of communication at the University of Amsterdam, and specialized in the application of information technology in the field of social facilities. He is currently a staff member of the Limburg Institute for Social Service Support (FMDL) in Roermond in the Netherlands.

[Haworth co-indexing entry note]: "Information Technology and Quality Management in Public Social Work." de Haas, Leon. Co-published simultaneously in *Computers in Human Services* (The Haworth Press, Inc.) Vol. 12, No. 3/4, 1995, pp. 365-376; and: *Human Services in the Information Age* (ed: Jackie Rafferty, Jan Steyaert, and David Colombi) The Haworth Press, Inc., 1995, pp. 365-376. Single or multiple copies of this article are available from The Haworth Document Delivery Service [1-800-342-9678, 9:00 a.m. - 5:00 p.m. (EST)].

that it is generally accessible and that its use is free of charge. It is also public in the sense that it is paid by the state, i.e., by the Dutch tax payer. The service is performed by professional counsellors, who are trained in special schools and have their own professional organization. The social worker has to meet the requirements of the profession as embedded in the code of social work.

Some years ago the task of subsidizing public social work in the Netherlands was transferred from the national government to local authorities. That is to say, public social work must be financially guaranteed by tight municipal budgets. Because of the lack of it, money has become a very important issue in matters of professional social work.

Local authorities and the board and managers of social work institutions are seduced by that structural shortage of money to think about public social work primarily as a budgetary question. In fact, however, public social work is still officially a public facility. The aim of public social work institutions is the realization of professional counselling of eminent quality. "*Social high tech*," freely available for everyone within Dutch borders, these institutions are not commercial organizations in which the quality of the products and services is just a function of making profits. In this kind of public facility financial management should be a function of the public services' high quality. Here, quality management is not just a commercial argument which can easily be over-ruled by the ever pressing financial arguments. Managing a professional, publicly available social work organisation is primarily a matter of quality management.

In the Dutch province of Limburg, several institutes for Public Social Work (PSW) are inventing and developing tools to regulate the quality assurance of the counsellors' work. Think of all kinds of *protocols* (e.g., for the Intake procedure and for special target or problem groups), *forms* with open questions, and *meetings* (like an Intake meeting or a Support meeting). The Limburg Institute for Social Service Support, the FMDL, is going to coordinate these local initiatives. So the project "Public Social Work Quality System" (PS+QS) is a complex project with several local workgroups, each with its own features, and a central point of coordination and tuning. This is possible thanks to the already existing networks of professionals and service managers in Limburg.

OUTPUT MANAGEMENT AND QUALITY ASSURANCE

The major impulse for developing PS+QS comes from the field workers and their service managers. They experience the inadequacy of the national Client Registration System in relation to their daily work. PS+QS is an enhancement of LIRS, the Limburg Information and Registration System, which has been developed since 1962 as a client registration system. It has been a major source for the development of the national Dutch Information Model Public Social Work in 1991 (VNG, 1992). The renewed LIRS is compatible with this Information Model and with the National Client Registration System, NCRS (VOG, 1992b), which started in 1993. The LIRS client registration system (LIRS-CRS) gathers data from *client systems* (counselling units consisting of one or more persons), *clients* (persons of the client system) and the *counselling process.* The data processing of this system delivers management information about the social service *output* of the organization. This information can be useful on the level of general policy concerning target groups, client problems, counselling functions, and the personnel/caseload rate. Neither the NCRS, nor the LIRS version of it are useful in the counselling process itself which is why the FMDL is developing the LIRS Public Social Work Quality System.

The NCRS is a quantifying system, in which the *object of knowledge* is an atomic fact, representing a specific reality. The system consists of related sets of related facts, the data, defined by a fixed range of permitted values. On NCRS forms the social worker describes the reality of a counselling practice by making his choice out of the prescribed pre-defined descriptions. The outcome of the description is a set of figures, some of which can be used by the service manager especially for logistical tasks. However for the quality assurance communication between the service manager and the professional social worker, qualifying propositions are needed.

In a qualifying information system, the possible descriptions of counselling practice cannot be pre-defined. As the counselling has to be effective, the diagnosis, prognosis and evaluation must be *creative,* touching the client's unique situation and possibilities. The art of counselling implies the art of describing which may not be among every counsellor's major skills. So it is one of the service manager's tasks to challenge the social worker to describe his case effectively. Steering tools are item lists and questionnaires that push the workers into the direction of professional standards.

There are identifiable objects–Client, Intake, Phase of the counselling process, Problem, etcetera–but the description of an object in a particular case cannot be the logical result of applying a pre-defined algorithm. The procedure of describing the object is an *open* procedure. Take, for instance, the object "Problem." Quality management can prescribe rules of communication for elaborating the client's problem, and rules of describing that problem. Those rules are of the kind of "point of attention" and "desirable approaches in case of . . . ;" they are not prescribed definitions of possible problems. That is the very essence of the quality approach of the VOG-section PSW, the employers' organization in the public social work sector (VOG, 1992a). Quality assurance is a matter of checking the application of those rules. That is the formal part of quality management and the service manager has to be strict on this point. The "open" part of quality management is a matter of discussion.

PS+QS: A MODEL AND A DEVELOPMENT TOOL

Being a communication system, PS+QS is a structured model of the communication settings needed for quality management of the counselling process. As an information system, it consists of tools like protocols, forms, check lists and reports. The integrated system is put into operation by its *actors,* who also *defined* the system. The actors are the social workers, their service manager, and to some degree the clients. The operation realizes the system's purpose, i.e., the quality assurance of the *object* of the system, which is the client's problem solving process as guided by the social worker's knowledge, understanding and skills.

So the PS+QS system is a material construction, which with a specific purpose is used by specific actors to control a specific object. The organization of the project is aimed at first, the process of defining the elements of the system, and second, at the construction of the material brickstones.

The social worker's professionality is supported by PS+QS. To some degree, the professional knowledge, understanding and skills are objectified in this system. The *problem researching communication* and the *process planning and evaluation* are directed by structured information. The workers should be challenged by the communication settings and information tools that form PS+QS, to get all the information needed and to take the best possible solutions. PS+QS does not afford the knowledge and the skills; it is not an expert system. It is a communication system aimed at *having the counsellor ask the right questions* and *having the team check some basic planning rules.*

PS+QS structures the *information* and *decision moments* of the counselling process. The counselling interaction between client and counsellor being a black box, i.e., principally uncontrollable by all those who are not participating in this interaction, it can be *discussed* by checking the application of protocols and forms. So, the institution's rule can be that all counselling interactions must be structured by official protocols and interrogation forms. The counselling interaction is structured by the communication between counsellor and client; communication techniques are among the counsellor's main technical means and can be structured by protocols and forms.

Figure 1 shows a schematic representation of a quality assuring system in an institute for Public Social Work. The three main stages of the service process are directed by **rules, protocols and structured forms.** The application of this steering information is checked in **structured meetings** between the service manager and the social workers. As a quality system cannot be developed and implemented without the creative involvement of the social workers, PS+QS is foremost a development tool for creating a working application of PS+QS in a Public Social Work institute. That is, by means of PS+QS the management and the workers organize their communication on the principles, structure and contents of their quality assuring system.

In this paper the PS+QS *twin model* is explained, i.e., both a model of the development tool and the *abstract* model yet to be made applicable in a Social Work Organization by the "actors" of that organization. The three main levels of the system are discussed–the workflow, the communication settings and the information tools. Finally, the framework of the development project is explained.

THE OBJECT: A WORKFLOW MODEL

What is public social work? It is a specific kind of counselling, delivered by professionals in a welfare enterprise. It is **part of the social**

FIGURE 1

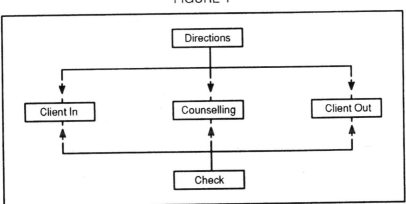

infrastructure of the local community paid for by local authorities. Citizens can use the social work facility as they can use the streets of the city. Economically speaking, the enterprise is a *non-profit* organization and, considering the primary process of the enterprise, it is a *professional* organization. The service delivered by the enterprise is professional. That means, first, that the counselling is to be performed according to the standards of the (inter)national community of social workers. From the organization's point of view it means also that the actual counselling interaction between client and counsellor is a *black box,* i.e., the "private enterprise" of counsellor and client.

Within the local social infrastructure, public social work functions as a social *safety net* for citizens, meeting problems they cannot afford by themselves, although they do not have refuge to "heavier" care facilities like psychotherapy. First of all, its public function is client oriented counselling (psychosocial counselling) and concrete and informative assistance. Its other functions are research and report service for third parties, and signalling (VNG, 1992). In the actual service the social worker applies the *paradigms* of his or her profession to these public functions. Those paradigms concern the following items (PBM, 1987):

1. *Knowledge* of problems and available problem solving methods, and knowledge of laws, juridical rules and available social facilities
2. *Vision,* that is, ethical and philosophical propositions on people and society and their relation
3. *Attitude* towards (his/her relation to) the client
4. *Skills* in the art of understanding and changing the client's behaviour; actually, the main skill is the art of challenging and supporting the client's own understanding and behavioral change.

The *aimed effects* of public social work are the improvement of the client's personal and social functioning; the improvement of the client's relations; and the realization of abilities. The aimed *users* of public social work are all those who have material and non-material problems. Mostly the clients are people who are involved in a complex cluster of problems, but are considered to be able to handle them by themselves when supported to do so. As the client's problem is usually complex, the counselling is an integration of different techniques and skills. A quality assurance system must reflect the professional paradigms and check their application.

PS+QS distinguishes three organizational levels concerning quality assurance in a public social work institution. The basic level is the workflow, which is the client's route through the institution. The implied conditional levels are the management flow and the information flow. The workflow is a problem analyzing and solving process that develops through seven phases:

1. *Entrance* in which the client asks for help by giving personal data and formulating problem(s)
2. *Intake* in which the counsellor and the client communicate on the client's problem(s) and the aimed solution
3. *Research* in which the counsellor analyzes the information from the Intake (Problem Research) and identifies the client's problem(s) and personal and social context, and defines problem solving goals and means (Diagnosis)
4. *Strategy* in which the counsellor translates the Diagnosis into a problem solving strategy (the Counselling Plan), and counsellor and client agree upon this Plan (Contract)
5. *Counselling phase* in which the actual counselling takes place
6. *Evaluation*, in which counsellor and client check the past counselling phase on the Counselling Plan; the Evaluation can result in either the last phase, the Conclusion, or a new Strategy and a new Counselling phase (repetition of step 5)
7. *Conclusion*, in which counsellor and client agree upon the fact and the way of ending the counselling process.

COMMUNICATION SETTINGS

The management of a public social work organization has the duty to guarantee the realization of the mentioned *social safety net* for all those who seek the organization's help. At first sight, and in the daily practice, there is the **paradox** between the "separate reality" of the management and the autonomous authority of the professional.

Professional social workers are not just employees who merely perform the activities the employer wants them to do. Actually, the very act of counselling is, in terms of controlling the organisation, a black box. The actual counselling is the responsibility of the counsellor. Afterwards, the service can be checked and evaluated, given the professional rules of good counselling, but at the end only the social worker can fully judge the counselling situation. Others can only check whether the proper procedures have been followed. So, the professional social worker is his own manager as far as he or she has to manage the planning and quality of the counselling. He or she manages his or her counselling by applying criteria of quality, as set by the professional community. This setting should be the client's guarantee of quality. Meanwhile, the institute's management has, for the organization's board and for the authorities outside the institution, the main responsibility for the enterprise's activities.

The service manager should play a **key role** in this management paradox. His main task is assuring the institute's interest in high quality service and counselling. The service manager incorporates the institute's quality by directing and checking the professional counsellor's planning and evaluation. Actually, quality assurance in this kind of professional organization is a matter of communication and information structure, which challenges the professional worker to fit to high standards of quality. The organization, in the function of the service manager, is able to set and check those standards.

As it is a profession, the standards of quality are (inter)national standards, which cannot be the result of individual arbitrariness. As social work is a profession, its performance must be checked by (or at least related to) those (inter)national standards. The service manager represents those standards within the organization. The organization's *quality system* reassures the application and checking of the standards. The medium of quality management is live communication; its tools are standard procedures and *free text* descriptions following structured questions. Various different means of communication are actually being practised in public social work institutions. There is not (yet) a standardized way of managing counselling processes.

The information needed here is just partly quantifiable, such as some of the clients' personal data, the number of each social worker's clients, and the problem that is treated in the actual phase of the counselling process. Most information consists of propositions which cannot be reduced to pre-defined categories. They are the professional counsellor's *qualifications* of the client's problem(s), of the actual and planned approach, and of the progress made in the counselling process. These *open text* qualifications are structured by pre-formulated item lists and questions, but not pre-defined as to the categories allowed.

Two-Way Communication

The NCRS is exactly what it is, a *registration* system. It is a matter of one-way communication, from the workers to the management and the national databank. The counsellors register data about the client systems; management and all kind of policy makers use those data as a source of information. Those who "know" by means of the data are the managers and the policy makers, not the workers.

A Quality Information System has to be a two-way communication system. The quality system is a *communication system* in the first place and, in the second place the communication uses information tools. The partners in the *counselling management system* need to communicate. All partners, i.e., the counsellors and the service manager, need to get information from each other and to provide the others with information. That is because the standards of quality and the quality control are matters of collective discussion and decision-making, not just a matter of the manager checking items on a list. The standards themselves must be the result of collective decision making, because the professional has to be convinced the standards are right. The professional counsellor must be able to use the standards as if they are his or her own standards. Therefore he or she must be enabled to reason out the *why* and *how* of the standards of quality and the quality control.

The professional community of social workers has already developed some standards. The national organization of social workers set up the professional code of the social worker (LVMW, 1990). The co-operation of different organisations in the field of social work resulted in the professional profile of the social worker (PBM, 1987a; PBM, 1987b). The above mentioned VOG is developing criteria of quality (Dym, 1993), to be used by all members of the VOG. So there are national standards of quality, or they are being developed. The development of instruments for improving and evaluating the quality of counselling within the institutions is still *work in progress*. It is partly a matter of national standards; for the most part the service manager and the social workers of a particular institution have to develop their own quality system. Communication between institutions about the local initiatives would improve the quality of the local systems. That communication should be stimulated by regional and national support and research institutions.

The report of the Project Quality Care Public Social Work (Dym, 1993, p. 18-19) distinguishes the following quality instruments: the counselling system and procedure; the system and methods of the support meeting; an evaluation system; systems of structuring the work; and policy-development.

At the management level, the workflow is directed by communication in a standardized set of meetings. The *Intake meeting* is the setting in which the counsellor and the service manager communicate on the diagnosis and the counselling plan. The second workflow step, Intake, and step 4, Strategy, are linked (see the seven workflow phases above). The *Support meeting* is the setting in which the counsellor and the service manager communicate on a particular case in which the counsellor wants the support and advice of the service manager and/or his colleagues. Such a meeting can take place sometime during phase 5, a counselling phase. The *Evaluation meeting* is the setting in which the counsellor and the service manager communicate on the evaluation of a completed counselling phase. The counselling process is either ended or continued by another Counselling phase.

INFORMATION TOOLS

At the information flow level the management is supplied with structuring and guiding tools. Each of the workflow steps is directed by procedures and protocols, the total set of which is called the Service Guide. The gathering of information is guided by prestructured forms. During the service process the forms are filled in, and the Client Dossier is built up. Protocols and forms direct the Entrance and the Intake. The protocols tell the counsellor how to act in case of specific kinds of questions. For example, the intake protocol can prescribe that in case of evident *female* problems the specific Intake form for *female* counselling must be used. The entrance and intake communications between counsellor and client are structured by the forms, i.e., by the questions that must be asked. Protocol and form are the techniques by means of which the counsellor organizes the professional quality of the entrance and intake communications.

At the service managing meetings the completed forms are used to check the quality of the actual workflow steps. In the Intake meeting the service manager, possibly in consultation with the team of counsellors, checks upon the actual application of the prescribed protocols and forms, and upon the application of professional knowledge and techniques in the diagnosis and the plan. At the Evaluation meeting the case discussion is directed by the Case discussion form and protocol. At the Evaluation meeting the Counselling Plan is checked (Have the phase's aims been reached? How is the service process to be continued; by a new counselling phase, by referring to another social service, or by ending the service?). The Evaluation is directed by the Evaluation form; the Evaluation meeting is directed by the Evaluation protocol and report.

Automation

It is clear, that PS+QS is not just computer software, but first and foremost a communication system that sets and controls standards of professional quality. Parts of the system might be automated. Think of the word processing in the dossiers, and of the data processing in forms and reports. It is one of the project's aims to integrate the registration of the NCRS-data into the PS+QS form handling. The quantitative NCRS-data must be automatically retrieved from the qualitative form information made and used in PS+QS. Conversely, data from the NCRS can be used in this quality system, e.g., data about a counsellor's caseload. Such integration is necessary to avoid double registration and data storage. It supposes both systems tune to each other.

The PS+QS development tool is a computer aided scenario for designing a PS+QS system. Both the planning and the system building is supported by a computer program. The development tool is basically the information designer's concern. The project plan actually is a prototype of the tool that is to be one of the project's products. It is a scenario with building and implementation guidelines for developers, and with a *model* of the PS+QS system as material.

THE DEVELOPING ACTORS

The definition of the system is performed by the system partners, who constitute the quality circle of the organization. They define and shape the system, with the help of professionals in the fields of social work methodology and information technology. In the Netherlands, PS+QS is being developed by two *workgroups* that consist of representatives of the professional social workers of the organizations involved, the service managers of the organizations involved, an expert in the field of Theory and Methods of Public Social Work, and an expert in the field of information system design. The project manager plans the project and controls the progress of the project. The members of the workgroup must agree upon the target of the project.

The workgroups define and shape the building bricks of the system as outlined in the previous paragraphs. The basic modules are the communication structuring tools; i.e., the meeting structures and the responsibility structures. The second group of modules are the information structuring tools, i.e., the protocols, forms, and reports. The third group are the standardizing rules, structured in item lists and check list, and partly derived from (inter)national quality standards.

The two workgroups are developing different groups of modules. One workgroup aims at elaborate intake procedures and counselling protocols specifically for female clients with female problems. Preliminaries have been done by the Dutch project Female Counselling in Public Social Work (VHV, 1992). The other workgroup is developing a total frame of communication and information tools. So, the PS+QS will, at the end of 1994, deliver four products; i.e., a Development scenario, a Workflow model, a Service guide with a set of protocols, and a Dossier model with a set of structured forms.

Not all Limburg social work institutions with their own quality assurance protocols are represented in the workgroups. Nevertheless, it is of importance to use those concepts and material in the project. Besides, the findings and results of the project will have to be distributed to all Limburg social work organizations. Therefore the Quality Circle PSW Limburg is created, a communication network of possibly all social work managers in the region. The quality circle is supposed to survive the project as an institutionalized network.

CONCLUSION

The features of public social work institutions determine the characteristics of the information technology those institutions need. The Dutch quality management project PS+QS coordinates several local quality assurance initiatives, and aims at bringing the locally scattered expertise to a more generally accessible level. In the workgroups field workers, quality managers and system designers are developing a flexible, modular system for quality assurance of counselling processes in public social work. In the future the diagnosis and evaluation parts of the system might grow into a regionally and nationally administered knowledge bank and system.

REFERENCES

Dym, S. (1993). *Actuele en potentiële kwaliteit van het Algemeen Maatschappelijk Werk, Tweede voortgangsrapportage Project kwaliteitszorg*, VOG sectie AMW, Rijswijk.

LVMW (1990). *Code voor de maatschappelijk werker*, Landelijke Vereniging van Maatschappelijk Werkers LVMW, Utrecht.

PBM (1987a). *Beroepsprofiel van de maatschappelijk werker*, Projectgroep Beroeps-vraagstukken Maatschappelijk Werk (PBM).

PBM (1987b). *Professional Profile of the social worker*, Committee on Professional Questions regarding Social Work, 's-Hertogenbosch.

VHV (1992). *Handleiding VIVA-model*, Landelijk Integratieproject Vrouwenhulpverlening in het algemeen maatschappelijk werk.

VNG (1992). *Informatiemodel Algemeen Maatschappelijk Werk*, VNG, 's-Gravenhage.

VOG (1992a). *Identiteit en Kwaliteit. Definitieve Strategie-en Beleidsnota van de VOG-sectie AMW voor de jaren 1993 tot en met 1996*, VOG sectie AMW, Rijswijk.

VOG (1992b). *Landelijke AMW registratiesystematiek*, VOG sectie AMW, Rijswijk.

A National Registration System
for Youth Assistance

Anja Smorenburg
Jules Prickarts

SUMMARY. The SRJV (Registration Foundation of Youth Facilities) is a national Dutch organisation that is responsible for setting up a national registration system for youth services. The main objective of the foundation is to generate information for government policy and management information for the involved organisations. To gain better insight into this territory, it is essential to have knowledge of a number of developments within youth assistance in the Netherlands. This will be in line with the new law on youth assistance, which has been effective since the middle of 1989.

The previous history and the development of the registration system will be discussed. Attention will also be given to the actual structure of the system. A look into the future will conclude this article. *[Article copies available from The Haworth Document Delivery Service: 1-800-342-9678.]*

YOUTH ASSISTANCE IN THE NETHERLANDS

Doing more with less money and increasing effectiveness calls for a business-like approach, and a business-like approach calls for figures. In the Netherlands youth assistance has for quite some time suffered from shortcomings in the structure and equipment of its services. The need for

Anja Smorenburg and Jules Prickarts are Consultants at the Foundation for the Registration of Youth Services, Utrecht, The Netherlands.

[Haworth co-indexing entry note]: "A National Registration System for Youth Assistance." Smorenburg, Anja and Jules Prickarts. Co-published simultaneously in *Computers in Human Services* (The Haworth Press, Inc.) Vol. 12, No. 3/4, 1995, pp. 377-390; and: *Human Services in the Information Age* (ed: Jackie Rafferty, Jan Steyaert, and David Colombi) The Haworth Press, Inc., 1995, pp. 377-390. Single or multiple copies of this article are available from The Haworth Document Delivery Service [1-800-342-9678, 9:00 a.m. - 5:00 p.m. (EST)].

377

cuts in combination with a growing demand for help necessitates effectiveness and optimum results from the invested resources.

To meet this need for improvement in the quality and efficiency of the help, a great number of changes have been introduced, such as restructuring, cooperation and a reorganization of institutions at a regional level, norm harmonization, differentiation, and expansion. For the coming years youth policies will focus on increasing the efficiency and the quality of youth assistance. Where necessary, customized assistance should be provided. The Dutch Ministry of Social Welfare says this calls for a flexible adjustment of the supply to the client's demand and a smooth shift between the various forms of help. If prevention and efficient help prove inadequate, the policies should pay more attention to specific categories of youths with serious problems. A new emphasis in this so-called catch-up policy is needed during the coming years because of new problem groups with which society is faced.

The 1989 law on youth assistance regulates some of these aspects. One of the means available to the government for generating policy information is the creation of a national registration system. In chapter XI of the law, "control and information," clauses 54 through 56 stipulate that: "A national registration system will be set up to ensure optimal administration of the data issued to the ministers. Policy-makers will be able to make use of the data collected and processed here and so be in touch with youth assistance in practice" (Rijpma and Brand-Koolen, 1989, p. 15).

This development of a national registration system is an extensive (organizational) operation, which may provide new insights into the developments and trends in youth assistance. It will, in any case, bring quite a number of changes for the roughly 700 services involved. The next section will go into youth assistance in more detail from the perspective of the law on youth assistance.

A NEW FRAMEWORK FOR POLITICIANS, INSTITUTIONAL POLICY-MAKERS AND MANAGERS: THE LAW ON YOUTH ASSISTANCE

In 1984 it was announced that the organization and control of youth assistance would come under a law on youth assistance. Five years later, on 1 July 1989, the law (partly) came into effect.

The government's starting points are that youth assistance should be as temporary as possible, as light in form as possible and as close to the home as possible. Youth assistance offers many forms of help, ranging from light to intensive. It is important to assess at which stage, which kind of help is best for which young person, i.e., customized help.

Important characteristics of the law on youth assistance are:

1. decentralization and planning;
2. budgeting and norm harmonization;
3. redistribution;
4. monitoring and improving quality;
5. registration.

Decentralization and Planning

The law on youth assistance includes provisions to transfer a number of tasks in the field of regulating, planning and financing of regional services from the state to the provinces. After 1 January 1992 the provinces plan and finance their own regional services and cooperative clusters, for which they receive a target subsidy from the state. Even after that date the national services and experiments will remain a national responsibility. The four major cities and their suburbs have a special role within the decentralization, because according to the legal conditions, they can be put on a par with provinces.

Each year the Ministers of WVC and Justice set up a 4-year plan, indicating which national services and regional centres will be financed and to what level. The Provincial States make plans for four-year periods on regional services and cooperative clusters.

Budgeting and Norm Harmonization

A budgetary system has now been set up for the greater part of the services. Up to now this has been done on the basis of the way budgets developed in the past, but this is no longer desirable. The objective is "to reallocate the available resources, which are currently being apportioned in a way which has developed historically, in such a way that, considering the actual targeted performance, a more justified and efficient allocation of resources is achieved" (Ministry of WVC/Justice, 1989, p.30). This is the task of the Committee for Norm Harmonization, set up in 1988, which presented its final report in January 1991. The committee uses a functional approach, i.e., they depart from a number of elementary functions which characterize youth assistance.

Redistribution

Regional distribution across the country is important, because the law dictates that each region should offer sufficient services to meet the demand. In order to achieve a coherent network of services at a regional level, a Study Group for Redistribution was set up in 1989 in which the State, the provinces/major cities, and private enterprise are represented. According to the law, regional services should be organized in regional cooperative clusters. These clusters direct the activities in the region and their task is to coordinate and support activities. They also oversee exchanges of information and advise the provinces on developments in youth assistance. One of the main tasks cooperative clusters have is to guarantee the existence and functioning of a JHAT (Youth Assistance Advisory Team). At the request of aid-workers, placing institutions, or the magistrate of a juvenile court, this team gives advice on complicated problems or on which method of treatment should be chosen. In addition, the JHAT takes care of the registration of placements and investigates the policies of placing institutions in the region.

Quality Control and Improvement

The government is responsible for quality control and improvement and will adopt a monitoring policy through the registration and evaluation of the performance put up by the institutions providing youth assistance. Services will have to determine the requirements of skilled and reliable assistance on the basis of a framework of general rules. There is a joint obligation to set up a working plan each year and to draw up a youth assistance plan for every young person. Children's helplines, medical examiners' centres, and information services on child play and education are ambulant services exempt from this obligation. With the introduction of the law the existence of an independent inspection authority has also been settled. Its main task is to monitor voluntary assistance, partly on the basis of the given quality standards.

Registration

A national registration institute will be established to ensure that the data issued to the ministers is administered as well as possible. One of its tasks is to develop a uniform system of registering data on institutions and clients. "Policy-makers will be able to make use of the data collected and processed here and so be in touch with the practical aspects of youth assistance" (Rijpma and Brand-Koolen, 1989, p. 15).

The schedule of the law mentions all categories of services which form part of youth assistance and to which the given rules apply. The law also relates to the institutions for family guardianship and guardianship, which are not officially youth assistance services. In addition, the law regulates the involvement of the RIAGG's (State Institutions for Ambulant Mental Health Care) and the Child Welfare Council in youth assistance.

Under this law, all institutions falling within the scope of the law are obliged to supply data to the national registration institute for use as policy information by providers of subsidies and as management information for the institutions. In this way attempts are made to link up with youth assistance in practice.

A NATIONAL REGISTRATION SYSTEM FOR YOUTH ASSISTANCE

Previous History: Contending Parties Opt for a Pragmatic Solution

Discussions among policy-makers on the setting up of a registration system date from years back. After some earlier attempts, the Interprovincial Consultative Body (IPO) worked out a proposal for registration in the residential and day-care treatment sectors. However, the parties involved could not reach agreement on the actual details of the proposal, so that the plan seemed to get stuck in endless consultations.

While ministries, provinces, employers' organizations, cooperative clusters, and youth assistance institutions were locked in a conflict of interest, the following questions seemed unanswerable:

- Which items exactly should be collected?
- Who should be collecting the data?
- Who should administer the data?
- Who should have access to the results?

Most important, however, was that there was no clear policy framework within which a registration system could function as a useful aid, if people do not agree on which policy to adopt, collecting data on that policy area is certain to meet with distrust from all quarters. People will of course be worried that the other party will be given the means to implement a controversial policy. In other words, if you cannot say what you will be collecting data for, you do not have a legitimate reason for doing it (Prickarts and Smorenburg, 1992).

After the attempt at registration through the IPO had failed, the consultation partners put the matter before a steering committee. In the early part of 1988 this steering committee for the Registration of Youth Assistance advised the ministers concerned to strive towards the establishment of a single (national) coordination centre for the registration of youth assistance. The steering committee held the view that, following the new law on youth assistance, it would be logical to develop a national system which would offer insight into the facilities available for and the use made of youth assistance. Such a system would be able to generate relevant policy information for a large number of interested parties. This counsel has been adopted by the ministers. The steering committee, for its part, consulted a management consultancy agency, viz. Kleynveld, Bosboom and Hegener (KBH). This agency carried out an extensive survey, using a pragmatic argumentation.

Despite the fact that a joint registration system within youth assistance has not yet come about, registration is taking place within the various sectors and work areas. If a set of items is formulated similar to those used at most subregistrations, it could be the pragmatic beginning of a common registration model.

By the end of 1988 the model was ready. However, it was hardly more than a list of items to be registered. Only a few general remarks were made on the desired implementation.

During the next two years a few things were done towards the realization of this idea. For instance, it was decided to leave the implementation of the registration in the hands of the institutions for youth assistance themselves, represented by the employers' organizations. They actually make up the board of the Foundation for the Registration of Youth Services (SRJV), which started setting up the registration system in mid-February 1991.

In preparation for the operation, the Registration Foundation of the day had already undertaken two activities during the course of 1990; firstly they had asked the SAG (Foundation for Supplying Health Care Information) for advice and subsequently they requested an independent adviser (H.J. van de Linde, Director of the Groningen Academic Computing Centre) to write a Plan of Approach. This report was ready in September 1990. One of its conclusions with respect to the previous period was that in one crucial area no progress whatsoever had been made; "The question as to which policy information is actually needed and for whom, and how frequently it should be generated, has remained totally unanswered" (p. 5). The same conclusion had been reached before in the "Exploratory final report on youth assistance," published by SAG Services for the board of the Registration Foundation.

Secondly, at the invitation of the board of the SRJV, a project group has been engaged on highlighting and putting into operation the list of items for the national registration of youth assistance. As a basis they used the list of items and the corresponding table of codes as designed by the consultancy agency Bosboom and Hegener. The following questions were asked repeatedly:

- Is the definition clear and unambiguous?
- Can the requested data be collected reasonably and reliably?
- Do the items meet the probable information need of the various clients at management level?
- If the answer to 1, 2 or 3 is no, can the items be changed or replaced by other items?

In comparison with the list of the project group and that of Bosboom and Hegener it appears that the project group has abandoned a large number of items as "not unambiguously definable" or "not collectable." For instance: the nature of the problems, the indication for placement, the kind of help offered, the reason for terminating the help, the reason for leaving the service. The project group states that it realizes a number of clients would regard exactly this kind of information as relevant to policy. They suggest that if there is a need for information on these subjects on a national level, tools for collecting such data could be developed with the help of scientific research (Project Group for the Standard Definitions of the List of Items Youth Aid, 1990).

Eventually, the last agency produced three lists of items. These have been laid down in the protocol for the transfer of data, on which subject it has been agreed that no alterations should be made in the data set before 1 January 1993:

1. ambulant, excluding information/advice function;
2. day care, fostering and residential youth assistance;
3. information and advice list, the so-called tally list.

The registration system deals with data both on the institution itself and on the young people who have been admitted to the institution concerned, are treated by or receive counselling from it. The registration model consists of two parts, namely "institution registration" and "client registration."

As far as *institution registration* is concerned, the data will be collected at the institutions by the SRJV and be kept up-to-date. This has to do with factual information, such as address, kinds of services and capacity.

As far as *client registration* is concerned, a reasonably extensive set of forms had been developed, in which a number of questions on the young person had to be filled in at the beginning and at the end of the help provided. These mainly dealt with factual information, such as age, sex and place of residence. But some more profound questions were also included, for instance on the nature of the required help and the diagnosis at the time of placement in a residential service.

For the output of information, a thematic approach has been chosen so that the various items can be related to each other in a logical way. Standard output, which will be generated each quarter, will consist of basic reports with figures on the capacity utilization of the institution. In addition, reports will be issued for each service area on the basis of four subjects. These subjects have developed from the starting points of youth assistance, namely that youth assistance should be as short as possible, should be as light in form as possible, and should take place as close to the home as possible. The subjects are:

- *Duration:* figures on the length of treatment, stay, or counselling offered by assistance services.
- *Distance:* surveys on the background of the young people, on the institutions which carry out placements and those which provide the treatment. It is the relation between these data which is important.
- *Course:* data on the assistance provided to the young people before and after the assistance they currently receive.
- *Demographical data:* surveys of, for instance, the distribution by sex and age.

Shortly before, the law on youth assistance had come into effect. This law also includes obligations with regard to registration on the part of the institutions for youth assistance. This means that it has now become mandatory to take part in the registration of youth assistance. The Order in Council (AMvB on the registration of youth assistance) would then stipulate which data should be produced and which institution should be responsible for administration. The coming about of this AMvB has now passed the Council of State stage and will probably come into effect shortly. It stipulates, among other things, that the registration is to be introduced as of 1 January 1994, with a transitional period lasting until 1 January 1996 at the latest.

ACTUAL APPROACH: REGISTRATION AS AN ACTIVITY OF THE INSTITUTIONS THEMSELVES

The original registration system was clearly set up from a traditional approach to data processing. For instance, it was primarily geared towards forms which institutions would send to a central point to be key-punched. On the basis of this processing of data they had put in themselves, the SRJV would send periodic summaries to the subsidizing government authorities. From the start the SRJV has adopted a completely different starting point, one geared towards electronic service to the institutions taking part in the system. Such a starting point offers scope for more functionality than just supplying summaries to authorities on the basis of reports by institutions. The SRJV's starting point differs in three crucial aspects:

1. The attention has shifted from data on institutions and youths towards information in the area of youth assistance. This shift in attention offers the opportunity to gain an overview of youth assistance in its totality and to continually search for new information entities. This has created the possibility to pay attention, to matters like waiting lists, vacancy bulletins, capacity measuring tools, and advice to institutions in the area of information supply without encountering fundamental problems.
2. The focal point has shifted from the subsidizing authorities towards the institution providing the help. The consequence of shifting the attention in the direction of the institutions providing the help has been that the SRJV has come to function primarily as an instrument for these institutions. In addition to the execution of the statutory task on behalf of these institutions, this left scope for attending to other matters which institutions themselves consider important. This meant that client administration programmes could now be taken over or developed in-house without too many problems. Also, it was now fitting to the new SRJV image to establish a commercial branch (the SOAJ), which can occupy itself with the sale of hardware and software as well as the supply of computer services.
3. The basic method has been changed from manual processing to electronic data processing. The disappearance of manual processing in favour of electronic data administration has improved the reliability of the system considerably: checking the information on a particular institution is now done completely by the institution itself. This has also made the system cheaper, although on the other hand a large part of the savings have subsequently been spent on the expansion and improvement of the electronic service system.

The Electronic Infrastructure

The electronic infrastructure set up by the SRJV allows the whole process of input, throughput and output of data to be run electronically. It is now possible for each institution to collect and check the necessary data within their own client administration system on their own computers. From there, data are sent via a modem to SRJV's Bulletin Board System (BBS) after which summarized lists are produced by a flexible processor. These can then be downloaded by users for further use within their own systems.

Linking Up with Practice

During the process of setting up the national registration system for youth assistance, a number of rules and conditions were drawn up with the aim of linking up with practice aspects as closely as possible. As the first starting point it was decided to take as a basis the administrative procedures in use at the time the project was started by the institution providing the help. In the second place, the organization of the input and administration of the registration data was set up in such a way that the various institutions were and remained themselves responsible for the correctness of the data and for checking their input. In the third place, discussions on changing the actual data that are to be input are avoided as much as possible, in favour of discussions on changes and additions to the summaries and surveys that are produced from the data. In the fourth place, the system offers extensive possibilities for the SRJV to provide electronic services to the various institutions, but functionalities will only be added if several institutions request their addition.

An Example of a Policy Relevant Summary

A method of checked output was chosen for the production of summaries (OUTPUT), output can only be generated to authorized users of the system and only with the knowledge and consent of the institutions that are involved in that particular survey. Authorized users of the system are of course the institutions themselves and also the subsidizing authorities, the cooperative clusters in which the institutions operate, their employers' organizations and the youth assistance inspectorate. Standard summaries are used, i.e., summaries drawn up according to a predetermined list of possible surveys. The summaries are sent to all those involved. Additional summaries will only be made on written demand, with due regard for privacy (no numbers that are too low in the case of multiple selections) and all institutions involved will receive the summaries. In general, a minimal supply of information is what is strived for, only the necessary summaries and no other. This is to prevent users from being swamped by too much information.

The standard summary programme includes the so-called MACRO surveys, which, for each youth assistance region, show the realized supply (what was the pattern of use made of the services in the region concerned) and the apparent demand (to what extent did the youth in the region make use of the services). This survey gives an interesting impetus to policy development, taking into account both the number of services in the region and the number of youths from the region.

A LOOK INTO THE FUTURE

For the near future plans are being prepared to further increase service in the field of registration. The most important plans are the Results Flow-Chart (RSD) and the Regional Registration Point (RAP).

RSD, Results Flow-Chart

During the development and implementation of the national registration system for youth assistance, the SRJV regularly consulted the institutions. Until recently, for instance, such consultations would take place through weekly presentation meetings. During these meetings, the institutions could have a look at the summaries that were produced for them each quarter, and comment on them. A frequently uttered complaint was the lack of historical overviews with too little insight into client flows, while it is essential from a point of view of management and policy to have some insight into the "careers" of young people in and around youth assistance.

In 1992 the SRJV began thinking of a facility which could provide insight into these matters on a statistical basis. It was important to find a method with which, on the one hand, groups of clients, "flows," could be followed over a long period of time, but which, on the other hand, would not infringe upon the privacy of individual clients. For reasons of privacy it is not possible to work with unique numbers. In collaboration with the academic computing centre of the University of Utrecht (ACCU) a statistical model was produced which seems to offer some solutions. A "statistical fingerprint" of the client is used on the basis of a number of data which should be included in the national data set (the data sent to the SRJV by the institutions). However, the method still needs to be tested and refined.

The method is based on the assumption that entries from different institutions on the same youth can be recognized by the system, with an uncertainty margin of five percent. In this way, it is never absolutely certain that two entries concern the same child, but that is not what the system is intended for. Such an uncertainty margin is small enough to be able to provide the policy-makers and management of institutions with surveys in the form of a RESULTS FLOW-CHART (RSD). In this way, different institutions can, in the course of time, acquire information on different dimensions of their service provision. These include e.g., how large a percentage of youths has previously had any form of help, at what type of institution, for how long. Subsequently, information can also be obtained about what has become of the youths, to whom they have given counselling or treatment themselves, whether they received subsequent forms of help, and if so, in what form and for how long.

Further research into the reliability of the selected calculating model is needed if this project is to be realized for 1994.

RAP, Regional Registration Point

Another functionality frequently mentioned by institutions is the possibility to gain insight into vacancies in homes, day care and fostering. In combination, insight could be provided into "compacted waiting lists" (waiting lists from which double entries have been removed) and current information on the supply of services in a particular region. To achieve this, one region (Amsterdam) started a Regional Registration Point (RAP), in which the intended information is input and kept up-to-date by the institutions themselves through SRJV's BBS. A method has been devised to track down double entries without infringing upon the client's privacy. If it proves successful, it is the intention to introduce this RAP in more regions. There is plenty of interest in the system.

CONCLUSION

With the enactment of the law on youth assistance, the setting up of a national registration institute has now become a fact. It has been decreed that mandatory registration is to be introduced at all institutions for youth assistance falling within the scope of the law. The aim of the registration is to generate policy information for the various authorities. Through an AMvB (an Order in Council), the Foundation for the Registration of Youth Services (SRJV) will be appointed as the institute in charge of the organization and introduction of a national registration system for the institutions falling under the law. The system is intended to be operational by January 1994 at the latest. The data to be collected are factual data. Data on matters such as the nature of problems and indications for placement will not be collected. These items proved difficult to define unambiguously or impossible to collect at all.

The board of the SRJV consists of representatives of the four employers' organizations involved and an independent chairman. In addition, there is a users' council, which monitors the protection of privacy and gives advice, either on request or voluntarily, to the board of the SRJV. Members of the users' council are: the government authorities (WVC, Justice), the provinces/major cities, and the employers' organizations. The registration system deals with data both on the institution itself and on the young people who have been admitted to the institution concerned, are treated by or receive counselling from it.

The institutions for youth assistance themselves were given major responsibility for the implementation of the registration system. They are the ones who will take care of the supply of full and reliable data. In addition, a great deal of attention has been paid to developing an input method using computers and electronic data transfer. This has led to new points of departure for further developments in electronic services for the benefit of all those involved in youth assistance: institutions, authorities, cooperative clusters, and the youth assistance inspectorate.

REFERENCES

Commissie Harmonisatie van Normen, Harmonisatie van Normen op het terrein van de jeugdhulpverlening, deel 3: einadvies. Distributiecentrum DOP, 's-Gravenhage.

Commissie Jeugdonderzoek (1989). *Programma Interdepartementaal Jeugdonderzoek.* Ministerie van WVC, Rijswijk.

Hovingh M., & Lucas, P. (1990). *Verkennend Eindrapport Jeugdhulpverlening.* SIG Services BV, Utrecht.

Kapteyn, B. (1987). *Organisatie voor non-profit.* Nijmegen.

Kleynveld, Bosboom en Hegener (1989). *Eindrapport adhoc-werkgroep structuur en organisatie om te komen tot een landelijk registratie systeem t.b.v. de jeugdhulpverlening en tot oprichting van een landelijk registratie instituut.*

Linde, H.J. van de (1990). *Registreren is vooruitzien, Plan van aanpak voor de landelijke registratie van de jeugdhulpverlening.* Haren.

Prickarts, J.D.W., Smorenburg, D.J. (1992). *De bouw van een registratiesysteem voor de jeugdhulpverlening,* in: *Registreren in Zorg en Welzijn.* SWP, Utrecht.

Smorenburg, D.J. (1991). *Van registratie tot beleidsinformatie.* Doctoraal scriptie Sociale Pedagogiek, Faculteit der Psychologische en Pedagogische Wetenschappen, Vakgroep Pedagogiek, Vrije Universiteit Amsterdam

Van Bennekom D. & Elling, M. (Eds) (1989). *Vernieuwing in de jeugdhulpverlening.* Utrecht.

Verslag van (1990). *Projectgroep Standaarddefinities Itemlijst jhv.* Utrecht.

Wet van 8 augustus 1989 (1989). houdende regelen ten aanzien van de jeugdhulpverlening (Wet op de jeugdhulpverlening), Staatsblad van het Koninkrijk der Nederlanden, nr. 385

WVC, Ministerie van (1990). *Manifestatie Jeugdbeleid.*

WVC, Ministerie van (1988). *Meerjarenprogramma jeugdbeleid.* Sdu uitgeverij, Rijswijk.

WVC, Ministerie van (1990). *Vernieuwing in het jeugdbeleid.*

WVC, Ministerie van, Justitie, Ministerie van, Onderwijs en Wetenschappen, Ministerie van (1984). *Tussen droom en daad.* Eindrapport van de IWAPV, Rijswijk.

WVC, Minister van, Justitie, Staatssecretaris van (1991). *Concept Besluit gegevensverstrekking jeugdhulpverlening.* 's-Gravenhage.

Solving the Problems of Computer Use in Social Work

Peter G. M. Roosenboom

SUMMARY. The problems encountered when introducing information technology in social work are commonly considered as caused by computer fear among social workers. A distinction is introduced between automation and "informatisation." Introduction of IT applications in social work is an informatisation process most of the time, which means that new information is produced whose role in the organisation is not yet defined nor accepted. Organisational as well as technical suggestions are made to solve this problem. *[Article copies available from The Haworth Document Delivery Service: 1-800-342-9678.]*

AUTOMATION AND INFORMATISATION IN SOCIAL WORK

It is considered as common knowledge that social work lags behind in adopting information technology as a tool for improvement of social work practice and social work management (Cnaan, 1989, and Phillips 1990). Implicitly it is taken for granted that there is much more progress made in mathematically based sciences, in the medical sector and in industry and commercial services. Cnaan (1989) gives as reasons that knowledge of social work is not systematic and social work is not prepared for quantification and strict regulation; that social work is a small market with a lack

---

Peter G. M. Roosenboom is affiliated with CAUSA, Hogeschool Eindhoven, The Netherlands.

[Haworth co-indexing entry note]: "Solving the Problems of Computer Use in Social Work." Roosenboom, Peter G.M. Co-published simultaneously in *Computers in Human Services* (The Haworth Press, Inc.) Vol. 12, No. 3/4, 1995, pp. 391-401; and: *Human Services in the Information Age* (ed: Jackie Rafferty, Jan Steyaert, and David Colombi) The Haworth Press, Inc., 1995, pp. 391-401. Single or multiple copies of this article are available from The Haworth Document Delivery Service [1-800-342-9678, 9:00 a.m. - 5:00 p.m. (EST)].

391

of financial resources. Apart from these reasons Cnaan lays stress upon more psychological and cultural factors. Social workers are considered professionals who are reluctant to use new technology in general and who are feeling anxious and fearful about computers. Social workers fear over-bureaucratisation of social work. Cnaan argues that a clash exists between the culture of social work, its values and norms and the world of computers. This clash is partly real and partly a myth, but nevertheless a lot of social workers are to be considered as antagonistic to the new information technology. Some of them are even quite simply cyberphobic. In the schools of social work developing software or specialising in the field of information technology is considered as unrewarding which leads to a lack of leadership and of role models.

The position of Cnaan reflects the position which is generally taken when observing the problems of computerisation in social work. The problems are for the greater part explained from a psychological point of view. Social workers are presented as persons full of fear of technical, quantitative and managerial approaches. This at least partially irrational and emotional reluctance to accept information technology becomes stronger when the implementation of information technology applications takes place outside the domain of financial and wages administration and logistics. As soon as data of clients or the position of the workers themselves are involved, or new management information is introduced, trouble starts.

In the observations to follow I will restrict myself to registration systems which are the most commonly used information systems in social work that are specific for social work. Of course word processing and financial bookkeeping are more commonly used, but they are not typical for social work and the development and implementation causes no particular trouble. In social work, registration systems are comparable with management information systems as used in for-profit companies.

In the early nineties, information technology industry got into a deep crisis. Hardware prices fell in an unknown and unexpected way. It became more and more clear that newly developed software tends to fail. They are full of bugs and lack functionality, it simply did not provide what was paid for. IT budgets are increasingly spent to maintain existing IT applications, which are technically obsolete, but produce at least reliable information. Big corporations and their organisations in the Netherlands confronted the IT business overtly with the question: "What is information technology good for?" And the painful question was raised as to why the promised gain in productivity in the commercial services never occurred. The IT crisis makes organisations reluctant to invest in IT, it forces software developers to look for new methods of programming (like object oriented programming), for new methods of analysing information needs and describing processes in organisations (like Infomod and Aktimod). Polytechnics and universities are looking for new profiles for software engineers educated by them.

What is going on? Decision makers being suspicious of information technology, being reluctant to invest in it, are now no longer only to be found in human services and related kinds of human activities, but there exists a widespread distrust in the profits of information technology all over society in the developed countries.

Introducing a distinction between two general kinds of IT applications: informatisation and automation leads to an explanation.

AUTOMATION

Automation consists in principle of the copying of existing information producing processes in automated processes. The processed data (the input) remains the same, the algorithm used to process the data remains the same, the output (which is considered as information) remains the same. In fact the whole process remains the same, only the instrument changes. Paper, pencil, typewriter and calculator are replaced by functions of the computer. Once automated the process is supposed to be faster and more accurate, to need less staff at lower wages, to produce more beautifully printed output and, very importantly, state of the art. But still, the product is the same information. The final test of IT applications in the case of automation is an accurate comparison, over quite a long period, under different circumstances, between the output of the old information producing process and the new automated one. Only when the new system produces the same information as the old one or when the differences are caused by the new system being more accurate, and the new system proves to be more reliable and cost efficient, the old system is stopped and the new system is implemented. Typical examples of automation are to be found in the domain of administrative processes like computerising bookkeeping systems, scheduling systems, keeping records of stored goods, order processing. These processes, entirely done by hand not long ago, are mostly processed by computers nowadays. Especially where financial data are concerned, IT applications are very successful and rather easy to develop and implement. Even in social work nobody cares that wages are calculated by computers as long as the amount of the monthly wage is correct and arrives in due time.

INFORMATISATION

In informatisation completely new information generating processes are built. Newly gathered data are processed by a new algorithm to produce new output. This output is new to the user and the user has to take new decisions based on this new information. In informatisation the power of the computer is used to explore new resources of information, information that without computers cannot be obtained, because gathering and processing of the data is too time consuming and costly.

An example of informatisation is the management information system. Management information systems provide decision makers in organisations (top management, middle management, staff services) with information about production processes, developments in the markets of raw materials, developments in the consumer markets and so on. The information is quantitative such as: productivity per employee. The aim is to provide the management with more information to gain more control over the organisation in order to have an advantage over the organisation's competitors. Management information systems give information supplementary to the financial system which remains the main information source in a commercial enterprise. Management information systems produce information that is less abstract than the financial information. They produce information connected to the real processes in the organisation. These include the number of defective products related to the total number of products and the average number of illness related absence per employee.

Management information systems are until now not very successful. Most management information systems fail to produce useful information at the right time at the right place. There seem to be two major problems.

The First Problem: Unpredictable Information Needs

The management information need of an organisation is very specific, varies in time and is by consequence unpredictable. As a not very satisfactory solution computer departments tend to produce growing amounts of statistics, probably thinking: we do not know the questions, but by producing as many possible answers as we can, we have the greatest chance to cover the questions. As a result managers then have to select the information they need from a growing pile of unstructured data. Only the computer department considers the output as information. In fact management information systems produce, in this way, not information but just processed data. When management information systems do not produce output which is concise and easily interpretable, management information systems are practically useless.

The Second Problem: Social Implementation

Software engineers generally assume that when raw data are processed to computer output, information is produced. This is true in automation, but not in informatisation. Two examples. Firstly, using the same data and the same algorithm to calculate the profit of a corporation, and the computer program not containing any errors, the produced output of the computer, i.e., the profit rate, is the same as in the non-computerised situation. In order to verify this, administration by hand is continued for some time while the computerised administration is already installed. The output of the computer system is verified by the output of the administration done by hand. The output can, when it is verified to be correct, be considered as information. It is the good old profit rate, calculated only in a new way by the computer. The profit rate, calculated correctly, is information which the management of a corporation is perfectly well able to handle. And not only the management of the corporation, but also for corporation employees, stockholders, stock market analysts and tax authorities the profit rate is a meaningful figure and they know how to use it in the debate about wages, value of shares, or the amount of taxes to be paid by the corporation. Automation produces information as an unchanged element of an unchanged debate in a technically new way.

Informatisation produces information as a new element in often a new debate. An example of informatisation. In two large organisations a personnel management system is introduced. Among other figures in both organisations a figure is produced about the employment rate of women. In one of the organisations the employment rate is 50%, in the other 60%. What do these figures mean? Is this computer output information? Information on what question? When organisations are supposed to contribute to equal opportunities for women in our society, is it then true that we have the right information? Supposing that the contribution of an organisation to women's equal rights is correctly measured by the mere percentage of employed women, the organisation that employs 60% women, contributes most. The situation changes by providing some additional information. The first organisation is a social work organisation, employing 50% women. The director, vice-director and administrator are women, the social workers are men and women and the doorperson is a man.

The second organisation employing 60% women is a health care organisation in which nearly all management and medical personnel are male and where the nurses are nearly all female. Now not only feminists will agree that it will take more information than the mere percentage to decide whether or not an organisation contributes sufficiently to the equal opportunities of women. So in this case the information system did not produce the right information, in fact it only produced a new element into the discussion about how to decide whether an organisation fulfills one of its duties or not. The most important problem of management information systems is that real information is produced in a two step flow. The first step is that the computer calculates a result from data according to the strict rules of the algorithm. The second step is defining the meaning of the output of the computer. This second step is a social process consisting of discussion and learning. The discussion is needed to define the meaning of the output of the computer. The learning process is needed to distribute the knowledge of this definition to all relevant persons inside and outside the organisation.

To evaluate the contribution of both organisations to equal opportunities for women a discussion is needed about the figure that reflects correctly the success of the organisation in attaining this target. In the aforementioned case, the outcome of the discussion between general management, personnel management, trade unions, and a feminist action committee could be that the algorithm is changed in such a way that the percentage of female employment is corrected by the proportion of the total wages formed by the wages paid to the female employees.

Assuming that the discussion produces consensus that the last figure, percentage of employees corrected for wages, gives adequate information about the organisation's effort to contribute to the equal opportunities for women, this definition has to be formalised in a decision of the general management or maybe even in a contract with the trade unions. After that the employees of the organisation and all relevant persons and institutions outside the organisation have to be informed. The personnel information system produces every year from then on information on this subject. It produces a figure that reflects the position of the organisation and the evolution of this position. This figure contains the same information for everybody concerned. In fact this is a simple example because there is no problem on the input side. The gender of employees in an organisation is in all cases easy and unambiguous, determinable as are the wages. In most cases management information relies upon new data, which are not always easy to obtain in a reliable way.

Informatisation needs two implementation efforts. First there is the technical one: implementation of computers and software including training on how to operate them. Secondly, there is the social effort: implementation of the newly produced information. Or otherwise put: automation has the advantage that it restricts itself to the production of information of which the social implementation has already taken place.

In general the IT industry has been successful in automation. This needs to be understood as: in computerising existing information processes. In general IT applications tend to fail when engaged in informatisation processes. In reality pure automation and pure informatisation processes are scarce. In most cases automation processes contain some new elements and so informatisation is mostly only a part of an automation project.

IMPLEMENTATION OF IT APPLICATIONS IN SOCIAL WORK

The attitudes of social workers, which are supposed to be negative towards the use of computers, are not the main problem. The main problem is that in social work the processes to be automated are less in number and of less importance then in profit oriented business.

Use of IT in social work is to a much greater extent exploring the difficult new domain of informatisation. Two arguments support this hypothesis. The first argument is that the automation of the financial administration and the administration of wages in social work in the Netherlands has been computerised since the late seventies and early eighties without great problems or heavy discussion. The second argument is the following: profit business is legitimated in its existence and in its functioning when it is profitable. A profit oriented organisation pays two tributes to society. Firstly it produces goods, which are legitimated by the fact that people buy them. Secondly, it pays taxes based on the financial administration. In principle there is no public control on the continuity of the organisation. It goes on as long as it is profitable. Profit is the proof of success. Which means that the financial administration is the most important source of information. Centuries of development have gone into it to produce consensus about how financial administration is done and how to interpret its output.

In the case of nonprofit organisations like social work which are state financed, financial administration only shows that the money is spent. Financial profits and losses both pose a serious problem for an agency manager but they give no information on the continuity of the agency nor on the effectiveness of the social work done by the agencies nor on the appreciation by the clients of the care given to them.

Social work in our culture can not conclude it is successful on the basis of the financial administration. This means that the easiest form of IT applications, automation, does not provide the vital information for social work. But social work is put under growing social and political pressure to prove that it is successful in solving individual and collective problems. And not only social work has to prove that it is successful, it has to grow more productive: social work is forced by lowering of budgets to be more cost-effective.

In the Netherlands, both on a national and on a local level, social work has to compete with other institutions depending on diminishing public funds. So social work has to develop information systems that provide information about the care providing processes in the agencies just to prove that the production targets have been met, exactly the kind of systems that in profit business are so difficult to develop.

Social work has to provide information on the number of clients, their age, their family relations, their income, their jobs and so on depending on the actual government programme. Production of these kinds of figures is already quite a task, but the most important question of whether the clients well-being has been raised by social work intervention and whether it was worth the cost of it, cannot be answered by these figures.

Van der Laan (van der Laan, 1992) observes an underestimation of the methodological problems when determining effects of social work. The fact that the registration is based on data produced by the social workers themselves adds to the problem.

Van Ewijk (van Ewijk, 1992) sees output financing as an aspect of professionalisation in the near future. State and local authorities see themselves more and more as buyers of care on behalf of the clients. They want annual reports with clear figures of what is produced and with what means. They want to pay only for clearly defined products (output). Van Ewijk writes that these changes demand registration as a fundamental change in the practice of social work. The conclusion is that social work is under pressure to legitimate its contribution to society and is involved in a process of informatisation. It has to produce information which is as vital to the continuity of social work agencies as it is difficult to produce.

The nature of the information generating process, being an informatisation process, is more responsible for the lag behind in use of IT applications in social work than the attitudes of the social workers. Maybe their attitude is a result of the problem, more than the cause of it. When IT implementation results in management information being produced without a consensus existing regarding the meaning and purpose of this information, people tend to get suspicious about the purposes of implementing IT applications. In fact social work faces the challenge, as all publicly financed services, to use IT applications in a field where profit oriented businesses often fail. Then the position of social work on IT is not one of lagging behind but of slowly proceeding under difficult circumstances.

SOLUTIONS

Is there a way out of the problem? Some suggestions for solutions on two levels. The level of implemented information and the level of technical progress. Implemented information is, for example, the aforementioned employment rates of women and the profit rate. These are quantitative bits of information or figures. They are meaningful for the people concerned. When they are implemented well in the process of social implementation, they have the same meaning for all the people concerned, they are accepted as trustable information, and there is consensus about the way the figure has to change in the future. Well developed information consists of figures. These describe the current situation correctly and formulate a target in the future and are known and accepted by the relevant actors in decision making.

The key issue in informatisation is then the development of new concepts of information and the social implementation of them. Politicians finance social work without clearly defining quantitative criteria for success or failure. New concepts of quantitative information can regulate the relationship between agencies and financing authorities and provide a basis to legitimate social work. The same goes for the processes inside the agencies. They can be better managed and supported by well implemented quantitative information.

In the Netherlands GFO's have been developed. GFO stands for local authority functional design. In GFO's minimum sets of data are defined. Agencies have to register at least these data. In fact the data are prescribed so that it is predictable that they will be needed to produce information on the number of clients and type of treatment. In GFO's no new concepts of information are presented. I consider however GFO's as an important step towards new concepts of information because a minimum set of data gathered for a whole branch of social work, like it is done for Social Casework and Community Organisation, will favour the development of new concepts of information based on and restricted to the minimum set of data. In fact politicians can now formulate measurable targets for social work using the minimum set of data in dialogue with the agencies.

As Crooijmans (1992) states, GFO's change when essential changes in legislation or otherwise occur. This suggests that GFO's are implicitly based on vague new concepts of information. In informatisation the development of new concepts of information and the social implementation of them is the key issue. The process of informatisation has to start there. Classic automation procedures however are not interested in new concepts of information. They just look for information needs. Information needs are the output of the computer and the input in existing decision making processes. From the point of view of the classical software engineer that's what he/she needs.

Informatisation processes are often started as if they were automation processes, with software engineers just looking for information needs. When no clearly defined information needs are found, a guess is made at what could be important information needs. These information needs become the output of the computer and then by using the output of the information system maybe some useful new concepts of information are found and each single information need turns out to be useful or not. The production of an information system functions, in the case of informatisation, often as a catalyst for the assessment of new concepts of information. This is one solution on the level of implementation of new information. It may not be the best one, but it works, especially when the process is iterative. By trial and error new concepts of information are tested. Not only the technical system is prototyped but also the criteria for decision making.

The best solution seems to be in developing criteria for decision making, implementing them to produce consensus on their validity, defining information needs, and finally then defining the data model and the algorithm. But it is a long process as discussions of this kind and the building of information systems both take a long time. Because management information often changes, this may after all not be such a good solution. Further research on this subject is needed to decide which method produces in practice the best and the quickest results.

On the technical level there is a solution to be found by building systems without predefined output. Systems of this kind are open to users to use their own algorithm to produce output. In fact, this comes down to a large database with a kind of SQL-interface. The SQL-interface gives easy access to the data and enables flexible change of output. It is important that the database contains a large quantity of data, because it is unpredictable beforehand what data have to be processed to obtain new information.

I see two major bottlenecks in this solution. Users have to learn to use SQL-interfaces and the process of social implementation has to take place in order to make the produced output function in the decision making process. Both requirements are not easy to meet. SQL-interfaces are less user friendly than programs with menu driven predefined output. The conceptualisation of new information, the operationalisation of it in terms of data and algorithm requires sociological imagination and sociological abilities. The process of social implementation requires negotiating abilities. These abilities go beyond the scope of technically trained automation staff. Neither social workers nor social work management, however, are trained to participate in the informatisation process.

Schools of social work have an important mission in this field. They have to educate students for social work professions, who are not only able to use computers technically, but are able to participate in developing new concepts of information and implementing them in order to maintain or raise the level of care given to their clients. The Dutch "national" curriculum social informatics is designed to educate social workers to play their part in the informatisation of social work (Roosenboom,1993; Grebel, 1993; van Lieshout, 1993).

CONCLUSION

The problems of computer use in social work to produce management information are not only due to the reluctance of social workers. Vital information generating systems are the subject of informatisation processes, which are far more difficult than automation processes. Technological means cannot solve the problem alone. New concepts of information have to be developed, implemented in the decision making processes, and operationalised. Social workers in general do not have the skills required for the informatisation processes. Schools of social work have to lay stress on the training of these skills.

REFERENCES

Cnaan, R. (1989), *Social work practice and information technology-an unestablished link.* in: Cnaan, R. and Parsloe, P. (eds.), *The impact of information technology on social work practice.* Binghamton.

Crooijmans, J. (1992), *Het belang van gemeentelijke functionele ontwerpen voor zorg en welzijn.* in: Van Ewijk, H. (ed.), *Registratie in zorg en welzijn.* Utrecht.

Van Ewijk, H. (1992), *Inleiding, registratie in perspectief.* in: Ewijk, H. van, (ed.), *Registratie in zorg en welzijn,* Utrecht, 1992.

Grebel, H. (1993), *Information technology in the care of the mentally handicapped: an educational approach.* in: Leiderman, M., Guzetta, C., Struminger, L., Monnickendam, M. (Eds.), *Technology in peoples services, research, theory and applications.* New York.

Van der Laan, G. (1992), *Kwaliteit van registratie: langzame processen in een snelle tijd.* in: Van Ewijk, H. (ed.), *Registratie in zorg en welzijn.* Utrecht.

Van Lieshout, H. (1993), *More than computers,* in Glastonbury, B. (Ed.), *Human welfare and technology,* Assen.

Phillips, D. (1990), *The underdevelopment of computing in social work practice.* in D. Macarov (ed.), *Computers in the social services: papers from a consultation.* International journal of sociology and social policy, Vol. 10, nrs. 4/5/6.

Roosenboom, P.(1993), *The Dutch "national" curriculum computer applications for schools of social work.* in: Leiderman, M., Guzetta, C., Struminger, L., Monnickendam, M. (Eds.), *Technology in peoples services, research, theory and applications.* New York.

REFLECTIONS

Introduction

Jan Steyaert

The three papers in this final section of this book discuss some of the broader, underlying dimensions of the HUSITA 3 conference. These include Yitzhak Berman and David Phillips' account of the tense relationship between social work and new information technology, and Robert MacFadden's paper on expected changes in information technology in the coming years and its effect on knowledge development within the profession of social work. We conclude this section and this volume with Bryan Glastonbury returning to ethical themes and dilemmas that particularly shaped the first section on the book and which are at the heart of the HUSITA movement.

Whilst other sections of the book have marked out new projects and developments that show real progress in the task of "building the future," these papers bring us back to a more reflective assessment of the present state of progress. These commentators, bring out once again the tension between optimism and pessimism that runs through all of this work. This

Jan Steyaert is Consultant at Causa, the innovation centre of the Institute of Higher Education, Faculty of Health Care and Social Work, Eindhoven, The Netherlands.

[Haworth co-indexing entry note]: "Introduction." Steyaert, Jan. Co-published simultaneously in *Computers in Human Services* (The Haworth Press, Inc.) Vol. 12, No. 3/4, 1995, pp. 403-406; and: *Human Services in the Information Age* (ed: Jackie Rafferty, Jan Steyaert, and David Colombi) The Haworth Press, Inc., 1995, pp. 403-406. Single or multiple copies of this article are available from The Haworth Document Delivery Service [1-800-342-9678, 9:00 a.m. - 5:00 p.m. (EST)].

403

tension stretches back not just to the first HUSITA but into the very nature of our civilisation and culture. For every exciting new project that enhances the quality of the services we can provide, the shadow of unemployment threatens with many projects driven by economic forces rather than human needs. Notwithstanding earlier contributions by Hanclova and others on helping the unemployed, the impact of IT on employment is perhaps the issue which receives least attention, even though service sections of most economies, such as banking, have seen a massive hemorrhaging of jobs through information technology.

Berman and Phillips reflect on the relations between social work and information technology by describing the nature of IT, the nature of social work and making a comparison between the two. They introduce a distinction between what information technology is and what it does. This resembles the distinction Roosenboom introduced in the previous section between automation and informatisation. Rather than consider information technology to be a deterministic (and usually pessimistic) actor within an organisation, as many commentators have done, or adopt the other extreme of a utility-centred approach that empowers the individual, the authors consider the nature of information technology to be socially constructed. In this model human services can shape how it is or can be used to reinforce human values and purposes. This view sees IT as reinforcing prevailing tendencies within organisations. However, it is arguable that their account does not sufficiently take into account the interaction between the arrival of IT and the combined impact of new economic constraints and managerial theories which emphasise control in the name of accountability.

The nature of social work is more difficult to describe, and the authors build on the work of David Howe to shed some light on the issue. They describe four main orientations or paradigms within social work. These are labelled "fixers," "seekers after meaning," "raisers of consciousness" and "revolutionaries." They acknowledge the difficulties inherent in any taxonomy of social work which as a discipline can be described as having "a rich diversity" or being "hopelessly fragmented" according to choice. However they see individual/community and stasis/social change as key dimensions of analysis.

In the relation of social work to information technology, they see the art-science continuum within these distinctions as relevant. By describing the case study of behaviourism and its use of information technology, Berman and Phillips invite us to their conclusion that information or "working knowledge" is a vital ingredient of the service delivery in social work with clear common ground between social work and the use of information technology.

MacFadden takes up the theme of computers contributing not just to "working knowledge" in day-to-day practice, but looks into the effect of information technology on professional knowledge development as a whole. He identifies the contribution of information technology both as a useful tool and a cause of shifting paradigms. As a tool "without precedence" he identifies its contribution and potential for knowledge acquisition. These contributions include its analytical powers, the accessing that networking provides, as well as its capacity to handle huge amounts of data on CD-ROMs and its ability to present information in new ways through multimedia.

From this perspective he then analyses the impact on knowledge use and development within human services. He notes the intrinsic bias towards "hard facts," evaluation and accountability at the expense of the subtleties and complexities intrinsic to social work. He picks up on Berman and Phillip's themes about the intertwining of art and science in social work but sees information technology significantly tipping the scales towards the measurable. However MacFadden sees the emphasis on information "permeating into all facets of human service work" and he presents an optimistic perspective about the robustness and pluralism of social work itself. This is matched by optimism that computers will "reflect the range of creativity. . . . . .in (social work) knowledge development." The final section of MacFadden's paper examines some of the promise of IT taking up Kay's conception of the computer as meta-medium rather than just a tool. Here he looks at research into the computer not just within an empirical, rational framework but in approaching intuitive thought, naturalistic knowledge and as a means towards qualitative as well as quantitative analysis. Apart from these directions, it will be most interesting to see whether the introduction of neural networks and fuzzy logic, now so popular in the area of artificial intelligence, has anything to offer to human services. Except from one presentation that worked from a neural network approach to social work assessment, they were largely absent from this conference, but may be the more present at the next HUSITA.

Whilst MacFadden's approach is perhaps one of guiding and shaping the potential of IT towards the needs of practice, the closing paper by Bryan Glastonbury presents a more urgent and partisan viewpoint that demands attention. His paper on "The Ethics and Economics of IT" takes up themes that he has elaborated elsewhere (Glastonbury, 1993) that the development of information technology, as well as its obvious benefits, presents us with major ethical dilemmas about its use and its effect on our lives. These are identified as important issues that not only frame the environment within which human services operate but go to the core of human service values and work. His theme is elucidated through consideration of themes of personal privacy, empowerment, unemployment, criminal and delinquent behaviour, smart weapons and citizenship. As such it has clear echoes of papers in the first section such as Varghese's work on technology transfer to the developing world, Busby's work on facilitating citizenship, Bhatti-Sinclair's work on immigration controls and van Hove's work on privacy legislation, although Glastonbury seems to regard this as virtually a lost cause.

His conclusion that the human services need to not just see themselves as a casualty of service but to be in the vanguard of developing an ethical framework for IT is a fitting point of conclusion for this book. It started, as did the conference, from a concern with ethical values which underpinned the conference theme of "the quality of life and services." This theme is not unique to this conference only. It was also present at the first HUSITA conference in Birmingham and was passionately and powerfully expressed from a developing world perspective from South America at HUSITA 2 in New Jersey. Whatever else the future may bring in terms of achievement, challenges, disappointment and fulfillment, these themes will continue to be at the core of the HUSITA movement, and will no doubt continue to be so at HUSITA 4 in Lapland in 1996.

REFERENCE

Glastonbury, B. and LaMendola, W., (1993). *The Integrity of Intelligence.* Macmillan, UK and St. Martin's Press, USA.

Two Faces of Information Technology: What Does the Social Worker See in the Mirror?

Yitzhak Berman
David Phillips

SUMMARY. The relationship between social work and information technology (IT) is explored and conclusions are drawn about using IT effectively within a social work value framework. Conceptions of the nature of IT within social work are reviewed, followed by a discussion of different paradigms of social work. Behavioural social work is used as an example of effective interaction between IT and social work. It is argued that IT can enhance professional practice across the whole spectrum of social work approaches without compromising their humanistic value base. *[Article copies available from The Haworth Document Delivery Service: 1-800-342-9678.]*

In this paper we bring face-to-face the nature of information technology and the nature of social work and then look at the relationship between the two.

THE NATURE OF IT

LaMendola (1987) in an article entitled "Teaching Information Technology to Social Workers" makes one of the rare attempts in the human

---

Yitzhak Berman is Director of the Department of Planning and Social Analysis at the Ministry of Labour and Social Affairs, Jerusalem, Israel. He is also associated with the School of Social Work, Bar Ilan University, Israel.

David Phillips is Senior Lecturer in Social Administration at the Department of Sociological Studies, University of Sheffield, U.K.

[Haworth co-indexing entry note]: "Two Faces of Information Technology: What Does the Social Worker See in the Mirror?" Berman, Yitzhak, and David Phillips. Co-published simultaneously in *Computers in Human Services* (The Haworth Press, Inc.) Vol. 12, No. 3/4, 1995, pp. 407-418; and: *Human Services in the Information Age* (ed: Jackie Rafferty, Jan Steyaert, and David Colombi) The Haworth Press, Inc., 1995, pp. 407-418. Single or multiple copies of this article are available from The Haworth Document Delivery Serivce [1-800-342-9678, 9:00 a.m. - 5:00 p.m. (EST)].

service literature to give an appropriate definition of information technology. He does not find it an easy task. "It would possibly be most accurate to define information technology as the codification of the human way of doing things with data in order to derive meaning" (p. 55). In using this formulation he is attempting to find a definition which is as user friendly as possible to the human services. His motives are noble: he is trying to make the important point that IT did not commence with computers. For example, the use of video in human services education is well established and acceptable. He is on to the right track because he is trying to find a way to conceptualise IT in a way which is relevant to the human services and can be taken on board within the context of its value system.

It is important at this stage to make a distinction. There is a difference between what IT does and what IT is–between its utility and its structure. If we concentrate our attention on structural technicalities–on what IT actually "is"–then we are likely to get bogged down either in metaphysical speculation or become overwhelmed by technical details. On the other hand, if we concentrate on utility–and ask what it is that IT can do for us–we will get a clearer and more useful idea of its possibilities.

An extreme example of metaphysical reductionism is given by Wilson (1989; emphasis in original):

> Technology demands characteristic ways of thinking . . . Technology sets its own objectives, and would have us evaluate progress towards those objectives in terms of its own criteria and logic. These demands and criteria are quite independent of the "content" of the technology. Technology is more than an expression of culture–technology drives culture. In a real sense technology is culture.

Fortunately, this sort of approach is rare, even in human services literature.

Concentrating on the structural technicalities–which is what many observers have done–can be dangerous too, particularly as it runs the risk of us coming under the spell of "techno-value systems" (even if they are subtler than Wilson's). This leads to IT taking a central place in the organisational framework and with the technology itself–instead of the purposes for which it was introduced–playing a dominant role in organisational activities: "Computers create a unique presence in an organization, which requires that life be altered in many significant ways" (Murphy and Pardeck, 1990). This overly-deterministic and rigid perception of the nature of IT means that IT will impact on the value system of the organisation, the organisational framework, the roles of the personnel of the organisation and the organisation's normative behaviour. By viewing the nature of IT in this manner the social service organisation ends up with the tail wagging the dog and changes its activities for the sole purpose of fitting in with the technology instead of doing what it should be doing and using the technology to enhance its activities.

Kling (1980) criticizes this approach to the nature of IT stating that "Only the most ardent technical determinist would claim that the consequences of computer use depend exclusively on the technical characteristics of the mode of computing adopted" (p. 62). Yet when we look at the literature on IT in human service organisations we often find such a deterministic approach. Let us see what phrases, processes and ideas are found in the literature about the requirements for an organisation in the context where IT is a focal point in the organisation's framework. "Service work has to be restructured and adapted to the requirements of the hard and software offered on the market" (Brinckmann, 1988, p. 22).

"A computer system is structured, standardised and explicit." (Glastonbury, 1986, p.11)

"Technological innovation shifts more control over to management by incorporating some worker skill and knowledge directly into the technology itself." (Kraut, Dumais and Koch, 1989, p. 220)

"Automation increases the interdependence between the data processing units of an organisation and those divisions relying on information generated by these units." (Meyer, 1968, p. 258)

"The pace of the job, the type of data that can be collected, and even the questions that can be raised, appear to be dictated by what is believed to be technically feasible." (Murphy and Pardeck, 1990, p. 2)

"A client's record begins to determine his and her identity." (Murphy, Pardeck, Nolden and Pilotta, 1987, p. 68)

"Decision making becomes more structured and less flexible." (Schoech, 1982, p. 217)

"Technical expertise will be necessary to aid in the interpretation and summarizations of the knowledge produced by the system." (Wodarski, 1988, p. 47)

An alternative perspective of IT based upon its utility is to view IT as a technological means in achieving organisational or professional goals. In this approach IT does not have any intrinsic value in itself but rather is a mirror of its user. How IT is used depends on the user. This may be called a utility-centred approach to IT. Isaksson (1991) writes "Computerization reinforces the prevailing structure–this means that an undemocratic system becomes more undemocratic with computerized routines and a democratic system becomes–or has the necessary requirements for becoming–more democratic" (p. 3). He presents data indicating that computing should not be viewed as a technology with inevitable, fixed patterns of use and consequences. Kling states that "computing is selectively exploited as one strategy among many for organizing work and information. The patterns of computer use appear to fit the workplace politics of the computer-using organization" (1980. p. 78). The utility-centred perspective of the nature of IT places the individual at the hub of the organisation framework. The individual is not a "servant" to IT rather IT empowers the individual. IT is viewed as a flexible process. Kling's findings indicate that the technology does not necessarily lead to a dramatic change in the character of work; rather it can have a benign and minor influence on the work of the computer user. Its role of IT within the organisation is determined by the needs, norms and values of the organisation. He goes on to say that computer-based information systems reinforce the structure of power in an organization. "Automated information systems should be viewed as social resources that are absorbed into ongoing organizational games but do not materially influence the structure of the game being played." He then concludes: "computers by themselves "do" nothing to anybody. Computer use is purposive and varies between social settings; little causal power can be attributed to computers themselves" (Kling, 1980, p. 100). This is in stark contrast to Wilson's doomsday scenario, reported above.

Let us see what phrases, processes and ideas are found in the literature about the requirements for an organisation where the individual is a focal point in the organisation's framework and where IT is used as a functional process to achieve organisational goals.

> "The use of computer technology in the area of professional decision making involves professional standards and ethics." (Boyd Jr., Hylton and Price, 1978, p. 370)

> "Carefully designed information systems for social work could provide individual social workers or decentralized teams with the expert knowledge they need while leaving decision-making authority at the local level." (Brauns and Kramer, 1981, p. 147)

> "Involve your staff" (Bronson, Pelz and Trzcinski, 1988, p. 20)

"Expert systems technology offers the possibility of designing systems to aid nonexperts in dealing with large complex bureaucratic organisations. This brings about a redefinition of the power relationship between claimants and social welfare bureaucrats." (Dawson, Buckland and Gilbert, 1987, p. 17)

"The impact of technology is dependent on the organisational context in which it is employed." (Karger and Kreuger, 1988, p. 115)

"If an organization collects information, someone decided which data are necessary." (Keen and Morton, 1978, p. 56)

What then is the nature of IT? It is obvious from the differing perspectives above that its nature–or its identity–is socially constructed. If it is seen in terms of what it can do then obviously it can do good or it can do harm. If it is seen as a thing then it can work properly or it can malfunction. Malfunctions are no good to anybody. But this isn't the end of the story. Things which work properly can still be harmful as well as useful. But these are only the minor issues. The major problems occur when the IT is in good working order but is taking the wrong direction. This is a real danger with IT; that the user becomes mesmerised by its power and forgets that the whole idea of using it is to be of assistance to the organisation. So the socially constructed nature of IT can be seen to have two different identities. It can be seen as a service facility–a process in achieving goals. Or it can be seen as having a will of its own–it can help you but only on its terms.

Or perhaps it is the social service agency which can have an identity problem? The humanistic, socially sensitive, participatory, interactive value system of the social services ought to prevent IT from becoming the dominant factor in the organisational framework of the social service agency. At the same time there is a danger of lack of knowledge, fear, distrust and a general negative bias to IT which might prevent the social service worker from developing a process perspective of IT thereby enabling a positive impact of IT within the social services.

Therefore, the nature that IT takes within a social service agency is related to the perspectives of social service personnel. It is not just a question of social service workers knowing IT. Rather it is social service workers integrating IT within a social service (value) framework.

In an Israeli Decision Support System for juvenile offenders (Shapira, 1990) the probation officer inputs the offenders characteristics (demographic, family, crime, etc.) then the computer delivers its recommendation regarding the disposition of the offender. But first the probation officer must key in a disposition recommendation. A disagreement between the computer and probation officer is discussed in a case conference. Here IT is used within the social service process and does not dominate the organisational setting.

When IT is embedded in a complex social setting, it becomes a social object, and the development and use of IT based services a social act. Consequently IT demonstrates social characteristics. It is not only a "problem solver" as is often portrayed but also a "problem generator." On the technical side this includes the proper design of a computer application, IT responding to new work conditions, getting and using adequate and timely data, finding skilled computer experts, correcting errors in data and systems, etc. On the human side this includes management-worker relations, changes in the power structure, impact on informal communication networks, worker isolation, etc. Part of this IT-worker "social relationship" mimics human relationships. When the worker is forced to interact with IT the reaction is usually negative on the part of the worker. When people have substantial discretion in their decisions about whether, when, and how to use computing and can use it as a relatively flexible resource to fit many social agendas (Kling, 1980), they are therefore "happier" with the relationship to IT.

THE NATURE OF SOCIAL WORK

Social Work has an even more complex nature than does IT. There is much common ground on its purpose and even–at least on a high level of abstraction–on its value base. But it has a diversity of theoretical paradigms, problem-solving strategies, and perspectives on interactions between service user and social worker. This can be seen either as a healthy diversity or as hopeless fragmentation–or a mixture of the two.

Things were not always this complex. Social work has gone through a variety of stages in its development and growth–each of which has left its mark (Howe, 1987). The initial impetus in the nineteenth century was directed towards action, based upon empiricist social investigation not upon the great normative theories of laissez faire or Marxism. Then in the 1920s the (in)famous psychoanalytical deluge commenced. Social work, once and for all, lost its innocence. This was followed by the development of the insight-oriented diagnostic school which was heavily influenced by Freud.

After this a wide range of new theories and approaches blossomed in the post-war era of rapidly expanding welfare provision. The functionalist school (which had been around before the war) was joined by a range of theories drawing on the disciplines of psychology and sociology, which themselves were expanding rapidly and thus spawned even more social work theories. At least four main strands had developed by that time, each based on a different tradition–empiricism, drawing upon natural science; "insight" based on deep self-knowledge; "scientific psychology" of learning theories and behaviourism; and sociological theories of symbolic interaction and structural inequality. The natural science paradigm was pretty straightforward and homogeneous, but each of the others spawned a range of differing theories.

It is not surprising, therefore, that attempts were made to consolidate and unify social theory (and, along with it, the social work profession) via the unitary "system theories" of the 1970s. System theory of course led to a false dawn–just as did the initial mainframe-dominated onslaught of computerisation in the 1970s. "In spite of the widespread fashion for systems theory throughout the 1970s, the unification of social work theories was premature, incomplete and illusory. It was the product of epistemological myopia" (Howe 1987, p. 21).

Running parallel with these developments within social work were larger social movements throughout the developed world. Social work was not immune to the political radicalisation of the 1960s. The rise of the New Left made its mark. Radical Social Work and political polarisation ensued. This was not so much "social work theory in practice" but "social work practice as applied social theory."

So much for the "case history" of the growth of social work. What about assessment/diagnosis/insight/appreciation (take your pick!) of the situation it finds itself in?

Howe uses a taxonomy of social work theories based on the work of Burrell and Morgan (1979) which brings together two dimensions–order/conflict and subjective/objective–and produces four paradigms: radical humanists; radical structuralists; interpretivists; and functionalists. His taxonomy of social work theories fits thus:

- functionalists   "the fixers"
- interpretivists   "the seekers after meaning"
- radical humanists   "the raisers of consciousness"
- radical structuralists   "the revolutionaries"

He sees *the fixers* as empiricists operating within the functionalist paradigm and having an objective view of social reality. He sees system theorists, behaviourism, task-centred and even psychodynamic theories as coming within this group (or at least the psychodynamically influenced psychosocial approaches of e.g., Hollis). Loosely, we can call these approaches "scientific social work."

The seekers after meaning are best exemplified by client-centred (Rogerian) approaches, "loving" (Halmos), interactionalist and labelling approaches. Humanism, love, art, intuition, understanding, and appreciation are all used in this paradigm–social work as art.

The raisers of consciousness include adherents to: radical social work, empowerment, feminist and anti-racist practice. Based in a political analysis; their aims are to raise awareness and take control. Their methods are: consciousness raising, collective action and organising for power.

The revolutionaries aim for the redistribution of wealth and power. Its methods are those of aggressive welfare rights work and collective action via socialist and Marxist social work (unfortunately Howe does not tell us what the latter entails–and we have not been able to find any other source which does either).

These latter paradigms have two similarities which are of interest to us. First, they both take group and community perspectives–they deal with neighbourhoods, communities or groups which share a common interest. Secondly, they are concerned about change in society.

The difficulty with Howe's classification lies in the very fuzzy border between his "fixers" and "seekers after meaning," particularly in relation to psychosocial theories. Their very nature leaves them with a foot in both camps. For heuristic purposes he is postulating a split at the art-science border where in reality the shading between them is more akin to that of a continuum. Markus (1990) makes a helpful contribution to this area:

> "One of the most pervasive themes underlying social work practice and education is the confusing and complex interface between art and science in therapeutic counselling. These two approaches seem at times to blend together in near-perfect harmony and at others to lock horns in unresolvable conflict. The helping professions have developed and learned to live with these apparent incongruities: art is art and science is science and apparently the two are forever entangled and intertwined and never the twain shall part." (p. 31)

SOCIAL WORK AND IT–THE NATURE OF THE RELATIONSHIP

So, where does this leave us? If we take a utility-based perspective on IT we can define its nature for our purposes as *"a technological means for achieving organisational or professional goals."* The nature of social work is more problematic but we can at least identify a "mainstream" art-science continuum, along with two more peripheral strands of community orientation and concern over societal change as relevant features.

It is clear from Howe's list of approaches within his "fixers" and "seekers after meaning" paradigms that most of our time will be taken up with the mainstream of the art-science continuum but the "fringes" occupied by the "consciousness raisers" and "revolutionaries" need to be touched on here. Their community and group orientation of is indicative of a commonality of interest with community activists and pressure groups in general over the use of new technology (Phillips, 1989). Concern over social change, which is by no means their monopoly–it is shared by some elements in the mainstream paradigms too–is a large issue which transcends the day-to-day problems of social workers grappling with technology in their working environment. Rather, it leads to the expansion of the human services to take on board issues of social justice and empowerment (Phillips, 1991). We will give an example of perfect harmony between IT and an approach to social work. The nature of this approach will come as no surprise!

Case Study–Behaviourism

There are some areas where the nature of IT and the nature of a social work paradigm are inextricably intertwined. As we mentioned above, the development of case management (particularly as related to community care in the United Kingdom) is dependent upon sophisticated and up-to-date data bases and financial packages.

But there is also one area of social work practice where the philosophical paradigm itself has extensive commonalities with the underlying logic of IT systems analysis and programming. This is behavioural social work.

Terry Holbrook in a seminal article explicates these commonalities and makes a strong case for behaviourism per se. He advocates a "marriage between behaviour therapy and computer technology given that the principles and practices of behaviourism dovetail effectively with the programming and monitoring capabilities of computers." This leads him to predict "that behaviourism or some variant of it will be utilised increasingly and promoted as the ideal therapeutic approach to complement the computer revolution." (Holbrook, 1988, pp. 89-90)

The basis of his claim is not just the chance coalescing of a social work paradigm and new technology. He sees both as being in the vanguard of the advance of science: "Because of behaviourism's identification with ideas, values and patterns of thought associated with modernisation, e.g., progress, faith in science, the quest for mathematical certitude, and prediction and control in decision-making, this theory will continue to shape the future for a long time to come" (ibid.)

His detailed exposition of this position is worth quoting in full:

> . . . Computer technology has also been heralded as providing solutions to the difficulties involved in information processing, production and control. There are a great many theoretical and practical similarities between behaviourism and computerisation that lead logically to their effective combination. Computer programming, for instance, assumes that most decision-making is routine, repetitive and follows rational rules. Information processing requires that data (behavioural or otherwise) be objectified, decision-making criteria be clearly outlined (process), and service units assume a measurable form (output). Behaviour therapy, on the other hand, assumes that all the therapist has to do is target a specific behaviour, introduce a stimulus (input), and modify the stimulus until the desired behavioural change occurs (feedback). Both technologies are based on the premise that complex human behaviours can be reduced to their simplest parts, manipulated, and altered to attain some predetermined goal. Since both technologies are goal-oriented and stress measurement, as a result of establishing clearly defined objectives and specified frames for change, the capability for judging success or failure is built into each system. . . . (Holbrook, 1988, pp. 91-92)

THE SEARCH FOR COMMON GROUND– A PRAGMATIC APPROACH

Let us now look at this issue from a practical perspective. We will investigate the processes associated with good social work practice and good IT practice in systems analysis and programming.

This approach redirects the debate which normally takes place over the implementation of IT. Instead of it being viewed as either the take-over or absorption of a caring, flexible and humanistic profession by an impersonal, rigid and mechanistic juggernaut–or replacement of disorganised, inconsistent arbitrary processes by clearly thought-through, consistent and naturally just procedures (depending on one's prejudices)–we can start off from a clear understanding of the extent to which there is common ground in approaching day-to-day work in the two fields.

Social work practice is a process which involves the interaction between social worker and client in order to deal with defined problems. Geiss (1983) points out that the practice of social work is an amalgam of humanistic values, practice experience and science-based knowledge.

Information in social work as in any other profession is a key in the delivery of services. Information technology in a social service framework can be used in the application of social service knowledge. It is a facilitator of the information mechanism used by social workers in transferring the science-based knowledge, of the profession, "knowing," to working knowledge, "doing." The value of information technology within the social services is that it can be used to relate to and adopt social service knowledge to a human end (Layton, 1974). Information technology accesses social service knowledge while social work practice applies that knowledge. Therefore, one may see a continuum between social service knowledge, information technology and social service practice.

Information technology can provide the social service worker with the "working knowledge" needed to practice. Social work practice is therefore not the scientific application of a technological decision. Social work practice is the "artistic" application of social work values based on a working knowledge of a social service knowledge base.

REFERENCES

Boyd, H., & Kramer, D. (1981). "Social Work in an Information Society: New Challenges and Opportunities," in H. Nowotny, (ed.) *The Information Society: Its Impact on the Home, Local Community and Marginal Groups*, Vienna, European Centre for Social Training and Research, 143-151.

Brinckmann, H. (1988). "Rise or Fall of the Expert: The Position of the Service Worker in an High Tech Environment," *New Technology in the Human Services*, 4/2: 19-24.

Bronson, D. E., Donald C. P. & Trzcinski, E. (1988). Computerizing Your Agency's Information System, Sage Human Services Guide, 54, Newbury Park, Sage.

Burrell, G. & Morgan, G. (1979). Sociological Paradigms and Organisational Analysis, London, Heinemann.

Dawson, P., Buckland, S., & Gilbert, N. (1987). "Expert Systems and the Public Provision of Welfare Benefit Advice," Paper presented to the British Sociological Association Annual Conference at the University of Leeds.

Geiss, G. (1983). "Some Thoughts about the Future: Information Technology and Social Work Practice," *Practice Digest*, 6: 33-35.

Glastonbury, B. (1986). "Managing the Social Services Computer System Some Problems and Pitfalls," *Computer Applications in Social Work and Allied Professions*, 3/1: 10-13.

Holbrook, T. (1988). "Computer Technology and Behavior Therapy: a Modern Marriage," *Computers in Human Services*, 3/1-2: 89-109.

Howe, D. (1987). *An Introduction to Social Work Theory*, Aldershot, Wildwood House.

Isaksson, T. (1991). *The BITS-Project: Child Care in the Admass Society*, University College of Falun/Borlange, Sweden.

Karger, H. J., & Kreuger, L. W. (1988). "Technology and the 'Not Always So Human' Services," *Computers in Human Services,* 3/1-2: 111-126.

Keen, P.G., & Scott-Morton, M. S. (1978). *Decision Support Systems: An Organizational Perspective,* Reading, MA, Addison-Wesley.

Kling, R. (1980). "Social Analysis of Computing: Theoretical Perspectives in Recent Empirical Research," *Computing Surveys,* 12: 61-110.

Kraut, R., Dumais, S., & Koch, S. (1989). "Computerization, Productivity and Quality of Work Life," *Communications of the ACM,* 32: 220.

LaMendola, W., (1987). "Teaching Information Technology to Social Workers," *Journal of Teaching in Social Work,* 1/1: 53- 69.

Layton, E. T. Jr. (1974). "Technology as Knowledge," *Technology and Culture,* 15/1: 31-41.

Markus, E. J. (1990). "Computerisation: a Precondition for, or a Product of, Responsible Social Work Practice," *International Journal of Sociology and Social Policy,* 10/4-6: 30-53.

Meyer, M. W. (1968). "Automation and Bureaucratic Structure," *American Journal of Sociology,* 74: 254-264.

Murphy, J. W., & Pardeck, J. T. (1990). "Introduction" in Pardeck, J. T., & Murphy, J. W. (eds.) (1990). *Computers in Human Services: An Overview for Clinical and Welfare Services,* Harwood Academic Publishers: Chur. 1-8.

Murphy, J. W., Pardeck, J. T., Nolan, W. L., & Pilotta, J. J. (1987). "Conceptual Issues Related to the use of Computers in Social Work Practice," *Journal of independent Social Work,* 1/4: 67-73.

Phillips, D. (1989). "Human Services Computing: The State of the Art," New *Technology in the Human Services,* 4/4: 23-32.

Phillips, D. (1.991) "Information Technology and the Human Services: Implications for Social Justice," *Computer Use in Social Services Network,* 11/1-2: 34-35.

Schoech, D. J. (1982). *Computer Use in Social Services,* New York, Human Sciences Press.

Shapira, M. (1990). "Computerised Decision Technology in Social Service: Decision Support System Improves Decision Practice in Youth Probation Service," *International Journal of Sociology and Social Policy,* 10, 4-6: 138-153.

Wilson, J. (1989). "High Technology and Social Services," in Spence, W. R. (ed.) *New Technologies and Social Intervention,* Jordanstown (Northern Ireland), University of Ulster, 48-69.

Wodarski, J. S. (1988). "Development of Management Information Systems for Human Services: A Practical Guide," *Computers in Human Services,* 3/1-2: 37-49.

IT and Knowledge Development in Human Services: Tool, Paradigm and Promise

Robert J. MacFadden

SUMMARY. The role of computers in knowledge developments is explored from two perspectives: the computer as a tool to enhance knowledge development and the computer as a major influence or paradigm affecting the nature and structure of knowledge development. As a tool, the computer is without precedence, continually transforming to meet current and future knowledge needs. Examples of this are provided. As a paradigm, the computer will support the positivistic development of knowledge, emphasizing structure, taxonomies and operational definitions. Computers, however, also offer the potential to develop knowledge through other, more exploratory, creative and intuitive ways. In summary, computers will respond to meet the challenge of pluralism in knowledge development and our *many ways of knowing*. *[Article copies available from The Haworth Document Delivery Service: 1-800-342-9678.]*

Robert J. MacFadden, PhD, is Associate Professor at the Faculty of Social Work, University of Toronto, Canada. He has written extensively in the area of information technology in human services and has a particular interest in computer-assisted instruction and information system development as it relates to assessing and monitoring service effectiveness. Professor MacFadden has been active internationally in Information Technology and Human Services through the HUSITA conferences as Canadian Co-ordinator.

Address correspondence to: Robert J. MacFadden, Faculty of Social Work, University of Toronto, 246 Bloor Street West, Toronto, Ontario, Canada M5S 1A1.

[Haworth co-indexing entry note]: "IT and Knowledge Development in Human Services: Tool, Paradigm and Promise." MacFadden, Robert J. Co-published simultaneously in *Computers in Human Services* (The Haworth Press, Inc.) Vol. 12, No. 3/4, 1995, pp. 419-430; and: *Human Services in the Information Age* (ed: Jackie Rafferty, Jan Steyaert, and David Colombi) The Haworth Press, Inc., 1995, pp. 419-430. Single or multiple copies of this article are available from The Haworth Document Delivery Service [1-800-342-9678, 9:00 a.m. - 5:00 p.m. (EST)].

INTRODUCTION

This article will explore the role of computers in knowledge development in human services. Computers can be viewed from two perspectives: basically as tools to improve knowledge development and more fundamentally, as representing a significant influence or paradigm which affects the nature and structure of knowledge development. Both viewpoints will be elaborated on within this paper.

THE COMPUTER AS A TOOL

Upon some reflection, one comes to believe that the computer is but a tool . . . a remarkable tool, a versatile and immensely powerful tool, but a tool nonetheless (Geiss and Viswanathan, 1986, p. 22)

A tool can be defined as . . . *anything used to accomplish a definite purpose* (Random House, 1980). Certain tools like the wheel and plough have revolutionized work and society. The computer, however, is a tool without precedence. Unlike most tools which retain their shape and function, computers are highly metamorphic in nature. Similar to a child's transformer toy, the computer's shape and particularly functions are constantly changing and elaborating. As a programmable tool, the computer alters its functions and purposes based on instructions provided by the software. Thus a computer can be used to play a child's game like *Pong* or chart the unique DNA structure reflected within a single cell.

Given this high malleability, it is certain that the computer will function as a tool for tasks we have not yet identified and to meet needs which have not yet arisen. As a tool, computers are strong contributors to knowledge development in several ways and are impacting on how this knowledge is created and disseminated.

Data and Data Storage

Computers process and analyze certain types of data exceptionally well. While humans have always been able to perform this function, computers have been designed for this specific purpose. This ability has increased exponentially in terms of capacity and speed. Desktop units now have the capability of supercomputers. In terms of knowledge development, this means that researchers and practitioners have the ability to perform extensive analysis and exploration of data looking for patterns and connections. Apart from the initial costs, no other expense is involved and the time needed for these operations has been reduced significantly. This increased processing ability alone should have considerable ramifications on the volume, systematic nature and extensiveness of the knowledge produced. It is important to acknowledge that increased power and capacity does not necessarily mean an increase in knowledge development. Clearly more information is generated but it still requires human creativity and imagination to develop knowledge.

Conceptually, data are discrete elements without any inherent meaning. When patterns are identified, data become information. When meaning is attributed to this information, this becomes knowledge. One is reminded of the plea . . . "Data, data everywhere, but not a thought to think" (Shera, 1983, p.649). Of course more information and greater analytical capability can also lead to increased *fishing expeditions* where patterns are sought and identified but the meaning of the information is unclear. It is reasonable to assume, however, that given more analytical power and extensive information sources in the hands of more people that knowledge development will increase.

Advances in statistical software permits users with only a rudimentary knowledge of statistics to conduct sophisticated analyses. Again, however, appropriateness and interpretation of this analysis must be made by the consumer. User friendly interfaces (e.g., Windows-based statistical programs) encourage use by a wider range of professionals. The movement towards integrated programs has meant that basic spreadsheets now contain the ability to perform sophisticated statistical operations and then immediately display the results in complex and full featured graphics. This data can then be sent via modem to other sources for further analysis.

The ability to process and store large amounts of data locally represents another important feature to aid in knowledge development. One half gigabyte drives are becoming standard on desktop units. Combined with rapid processing, this capacity permits the researcher to examine all but the largest of data sets. Additionally, increased storage and processing capacity is fostering the growth of large and small databases. Social agencies are computerizing their manual databases and collecting significant amounts of data in electronic form. Increasing sophistication of agency information systems will permit the analysis of data that up to this point was not possible. Such information represents a wealth of information to increase our knowledge about a range of factors, including services, resources, clients, and outcomes. In this sense our knowledge about a range of our *selves*–organizational, professional and community, as examples, should be enhanced.

Other types of storage and databases are also improving our knowledge acquisition. The increasing popularity of CD-ROM citation databases like *PsychLit,* and *Sociofile* is placing extensive information directly in the hands of researchers and practitioners. These easily searched formats, in combination with bibliographic managers permit quick retrieval and production of information. Literature reviews, using electronic abstracts, can be performed rapidly and conveniently and is resulting in more dissemination of knowledge.

Linking Computer Data

Telecommunication is another function of computers that has emerged which has implications for knowledge development. This involves linking two sources (e.g., people) via computers. It permits the reliable transfer of data at great speeds and over large distances. Networks have developed at several levels and for many purposes. Many social agencies are operating local area networks which link people via computer within their immediate organizations. Wide area networks have been developed to expand this link across sites and individuals. International networks like Internet link researchers worldwide. These networks permit the sharing of information and the development of knowledge via this medium. Networks of experts can be formed to consult and share knowledge on specific topics. Special interest groups also exist to share information. Such networks can be attached to databases, as described above, to access large amounts of information. Large information services such as CompuServe are like information highways which route and match people and information.

The trend towards using computers as a networking tool may also have additional impacts on knowledge development. The earlier stand-alone personal computer fostered more individual work and local storage. Although data could be and was shared, it was not as simple as it is now with networks. Networks are constructed on the principle of maximizing the ability to integrate and share information and communications. Groupware, as a new software trend, capitalizes on this orientation and allows multiple users to work jointly on projects, documents, collectively schedule activities and other collaborative features. This collaboration is essential in knowledge development and is designed to be convenient and economical.

Data Presentation

The increased ability of computers to present information has improved knowledge development and dissemination. Desktop publishing, computer-assisted instruction, graphical presentation software all permit the display and use of information in a manner that adds clarity and impact. The trend towards multimedia offers an opportunity to retrieve, explore and display information in a multi-sensory fashion. Portable CD readers are now available to play various types of books and materials. CD technology offers collections of materials available to be scanned for more specific information in quick targeted ways. The power of these search engines should permit more extensive use of these materials than ever before.

Information is no longer solely textually based but can also contain sound, colour, graphics and animation. The modern textbook is becoming a dynamic type of medium that presents information in an array of engaging forms. It is becoming more routine for some books to be sold with computer disks enclosed. One recent book (Nurius and Hudson, 1993) comes complete with software for making case recordings, rapid assessment instruments to evaluate client progress and computational and graphics capabilities for single system analysis of practice. The content of the book has been made dynamic through the use of the accompanying software program. Thus the learning potential of this text moves far beyond the impact and message of the printed words to include a computer software system that offers additional learning opportunities and experimentation.

A recent music industry innovation offers customers the opportunity to select an album and have it produced on-the-spot, onto a CD. New software vending machines store shareware titles on CD-ROM and purchasers pay to have the software copied onto their own disk (*PC Magazine,* September 14, 1993, Vol.12, No. 15, p.30). Such instant publication opportunities should also be possible for books and other materials. This could broaden the range of texts, journals, reports, and other material available and perhaps reduce the price of this material (overhead in the form of inventory would be reduced). Given the high cost of published materials in many countries, combined with shrinking educational dollars available, this innovation could improve our access to significant information and promote knowledge development.

Apart from expanded functions, the lower prices of computer technology has led to a form of knowledge empowerment through making it more available to non-traditional sources. Historically large organizations and scientists had access to this computing power and computers were a tool for the privileged. More recently the reduced cost has meant that a range of groups and individuals have more access to the technology. Small interest groups and variously challenged individuals are utilizing computers to analyze and present information. No longer completely dependent on the information produced by other sources, these groups are becoming skilled and knowledgeable at how to collect, identify, analyze, extract, interpret and present information that supports their causes.

One of the claims of the futurists (Naisbett, 1984) is that computer technology will flatten organizational hierarchies and put information (i.e., power) into the hands of more people. While these organizational changes are not clearly evident, some trends suggest that computers are being shared more widely across a range of agency personnel. Information systems, as examples, are being constructed to not only serve management, but to incorporate features that front-line workers can use to inform their practice.

THE COMPUTER AND THE IT PARADIGM

While computers are unique tools, the technology they represent and the characteristics and requirements of their operations exert a significant influence on knowledge development and dissemination. Computers are more than a tool. Information technology represents a major societal force which impacts on the way we think, feel and act. Information has been termed the new GodWord (Roszak, 1986) and knowledge developed via computers takes on an added level of validity and importance for many people. Use of computer technology, to some extent, reflects a paradigm or influence on knowledge development.

The requirements of technology itself exert some impact on the way information is structured and knowledge developed. As an example, computers, in many respects, support the scientific and empirical perspectives related to knowledge development. With increasing computerization, much of the data used by human service professionals will require modification. Data will be made more hard, clearly defined, mutually exclusive and operationalized. Concepts which are loose, abstract, or *soft* are more problematic in terms of use by computer. In order to maximize use of this hard, computerized technology our characteristically soft, professional technology will be tempered to meet these requirements.

The very act of refining our professional knowledge base to meet these criteria may produce fundamental change. Many of our current formulations, theories, and practice models will not survive this conversion. Other theories and concepts will be modified and operationalized. New theories, concepts and models will arise. The process of refining our professional technology may provide new perspectives on the nature of practice itself—the scientific dimension and the artistic, creative dimension and the consequent blend of these two realities.

The process of preparing our knowledge base for computerization and the increasing use of data-based practice requires specification and standardization. Data dictionaries are being developed to define and operationalize concepts, constructs and interventions (Gripton et al., 1988). This process frequently reveals an array of theories and practice models utilized in most human service organizations and the lack of a consensus as to the precise meaning and referents of many of these fundamental concepts. This lack of consensus can occur across and within professions. Creating data dictionaries, while increasing the reliability of definitions, may also promote considerable dissent and conflict and engender power struggles among groups wishing to establish and promote favourite frameworks and models.

Computer technology, influenced by empirical practice, will increasingly function as a sieve to screen out ambiguous formulations, loose definitions and concepts and force more clarification and specificity.

> Users of software systems designed to improve clinical practice will be obliged to engage in conceptual clarification of the nature of their practice. Computer representations of the therapy process do not yet capture its subtleties and complexities. Nor can they resolve ambiguities or correct faulty logic (Gripton et al., 1988, p. 94).

As our adoption of these technologies proceeds, future practice promises to be more defined, refined, precise and measurable. This has implications for evaluation and accountability of service, and the development and transmission of our professional knowledge bases. As an additional result of computerization and trends towards empirical practice, practice may be conceived of more discretely and atomistically and in more digital/scientific terms than analogic/artistic terms (Gripton et al., 1988, p. 94). With this focus on components, it may be more difficult to assess the contribution of the parts to the whole–the emergent quality of practice.

With the shift towards empirically-based practice and information technology, human service organizations will increasingly be viewed as joint human-computer knowledge processing systems (Holsaple and Whinston, 1987) and human service professionals characterized as *knowledge workers*. The development of comprehensive, dependable information systems is becoming a priority as human service managers track a broader range and depth of information about their organizations. Similar to developments clinically, managers are experiencing pressures to codify and standardize dimensions of the organization to enable use of information technology. Agencies are increasingly using computers for program evaluation and to report to funding sources on a variety of dimensions.

Computer technology promises to structure and refine professional decision-making in other ways. The database emphasis not only applies to the increasing empiricism of clinical practice but also the use of information technologies to support decision-making. Databases, or collections of information will become ubiquitous. The agency information systems will emerge as a major database for all levels of practitioners, enabling them to assess outcomes, identify patterns and obtain complex service information. Similarly, these information systems will eventually be made available to various agency stakeholders, including board members, funders and other community organizations, increasing the knowledge level of these stakeholders of the agency, its resources, services and impact.

Specialized databases relevant to agencies and field will proliferate within and across agencies and include major external databases, private and public. Specialized human service databases, for instance, could be programmed into a ROM cartridge and slotted into handheld computers. These ROM cartridges could be updated regularly and users could carry this unit in a pocket or purse and retrieve information quickly and reliably. Information could also be uploaded or downloaded between this unit and a full-sized computer. These specialized, hand-held computers have already entered the market as electronic thesauruses, language dictionaries and spelling checkers. New hardware innovations like an optical monocle worn on one eye which presents a computer screen output in a heads-up display (HUD) promises to popularize and further miniaturize computer technology.

Professionals will become major information brokers, linking clients with appropriate information based on need. Practice will become increasingly monitored and evaluated with the results utilized to refine treatment models. The emphasis on information will permeate all facets of human service work, from intake through termination, from direct service to board work. Professional decision-making will require reference to data and databases.

The trends identified above are significant and promise to influence how we conceive of and develop knowledge. Critics will continue to decry this movement towards empiricism (Cooper, 1980) and computerization (Abels, 1972) as threatening our humanistic approach to knowledge development. Feminists have critiqued our current knowledge base and scientific methods as being seriously biased with patriarchal values. Such knowledge and development represents faulty, dichotomous thinking, infused with a binary world view (e.g., the convenient separation of public and private lives). Thus science, traditional knowledge, and computers are interwoven into the same fabric by these critics.

Concern is also expressed about our movement from the art to the science elements of practice, reducing practice to a series of abstract concepts and interaction with a machine thereby increasing the distance between practitioner and client. What is lost when so called *fuzzy* concepts are eliminated? Is there a danger that we may begin to reify the definitions created during these process or perhaps deify the technology? Human service professionals, in this scenario, will become technicians constantly feeding the technology that functions as another wall between those who need help and those who provide it. Knowledge developed will be biased towards an incomplete, atomistic understanding of phenomena.

In one sense, applying computer technology to our professional knowledge reveals some of the structure and qualities of our knowledge base. As Fischer (1978) points out, much of our professional knowledge is theoretical, foundation knowledge at a high to medium level of abstraction. Many concepts are pre-operational. Some empirical and intervention knowledge exists but these are smaller in scale. As such, social workers use many types of knowledge, including personal, intuitive, and artistic ways of knowing.

Computers have been most associated with supporting the empirical, positivistic model of knowing. One of the challenges is whether computer technology can address the needs of these other types of knowledge and what role these other types of knowledge have within our profession. It is tempting to assume that the computer will only serve to promote more definition and structure in knowledge development, fuelled by the trend towards data-based, empirical practice. Given, however, our limited yet dynamic history with computers and pluralism within human services, it is more likely that computers will be expanded and used to reflect a range of creativity and less structured methods involved in knowledge development.

In summary, a computer is a tool but represents something more than a tool. The malleability of the machine, combined with the growing influence of factors like feminism, multiculturalism, qualitative and ethnographic approaches to knowledge development, promises an interesting and productive future.

THE COMPUTER AND THE PROMISE

It is not a tool, although it can act like many tools. It is the first metamedium, and as such has degrees of freedom for representation and expression never before encountered and as yet barely investigated. (Kay, 1984, p. 59)

The progress of the computer in our professional knowledge development is dependent, in part, on its ability to meet the needs of a range of sources. Given that the history of computers has been one of constant elaboration and change there is no reason to believe it will not be adapted by various sources to promote knowledge development. While it may foster more definition and structure, it will also be employed to assist with more intuitive processes and creative ways of knowing.

Part of the difficulty with this is that these other ways of knowing are not well defined. Intuition, as an example, has been viewed as an innate gift that is part of our human species. Some feminists suggest that women particularly, are imbued with this gift. Other intuition theorists view this process simply as preconscious logic made below human awareness. In the latter case of pre-conscious logic, computers might be helpful in assisting the expression of such intuition. In the former case, it is difficult to imagine the role of computers in developing intuitive knowledge. The question remains, can computers assist in knowledge development in processes other than the empirical, positivistic models?

As one example, Besher (1985) reports that the *Japanese Science and Technology Agency* announced a plan to harness various forms of parapsychological and extrasensory perception. It is thought that the human body possesses sensors that can act as electrical transmitters and be connected to computers. Thus the computer is being viewed as being able to assist us with non-traditional ways of knowing, blending the psyche and computer.

Similarly, the hypertext approach to knowledge development has been termed . . . *a means of democratizing knowledge* (Larson, 1990) and avoids directing the research and provides non-linear avenues to pursue research paths (King, 1993). The user moves around various databases in non-structured ways that have personal meaning and utility and the computer acts as a knowledge navigator directed by the researcher. This is a naturalistic approach to knowledge development that permits individualized use of the technology.

A major component of our professional knowledge base is experiential knowledge. Yet this type of knowledge is difficult to articulate and analyze. Historically, experiential knowledge has been transmitted through supervision and apprenticeship. Such practical knowledge frequently does not emerge beyond the network of the individuals involved. The development of computerized expert systems represents an attempt to codify and systematize experiential knowledge in specific domains to provide a wider range of professionals with a decision-support tool. Knowledge in the form of decision rules is utilized to assist in problem-solving. More recent directions suggest that effective expertise may be based more on memory than on analysis and logic and computer systems are being designed to capture such memory-based expertise (Carlson, 1993, p. 339). The evolution of expert systems, although slow, reflects an attempt to capture this important experiential component of our knowledge base and through its successes and failures is serving to illuminate facets of how we think and know professionally.

Although computers have largely been applied for quantitative analysis, development of computerized, qualitative applications is also occurring (Tesch, 1990). Software exists which screens textual material and identifies frequency and occurrence of words and manages this textual content like a database. This permits the researcher to identify and label themes, search, order, track and produce outputs of this thematic analysis. The increased use of computers in this area has empowered qualitative researchers and provides a powerful tool for systematic review of textual material. Ironically, the use of computers in this area may add more legitimacy to qualitative approaches by associating the method with the power and status of computer technology. Given that it has frequently been difficult to secure research grants using a qualitative methodology, the use of computer analysis may be an increasingly significant advantage and result in more studies and knowledge development using this approach.

Additionally, the computer as a tool is elaborating in other ways to meet the demands of qualitative approaches to knowledge development. As an example, recent technological advances in transforming verbal input directly into digital/text data would permit qualitative interviewing to be instantly and reliably recorded into digital and text formats in several languages. Once costs come down, this process in combination with more refined text-based analytical software promises to greatly enhance the quality and quantity of ethnographic types of research. Thus the technology may assist in empowering more *voices* to be heard and inform knowledge through the participation of a wider range of persons.

In summary, computers are unique knowledge development tools with chameleon-like qualities, adapting to the needs and orientations of users. Additionally, this information technology emphasizes and reflects certain orientations and features. The continuing influence of computers on knowledge development promises to be varied and exciting, offering new opportunities for approaches to knowledge development that have not traditionally employed the technology.

As Turkle (1984) asserts, computers are highly evocative objects which force us to consider the difference between mind and machine. It is in the reflection of this machine that we see aspects of what it means to be human, how we think, and importantly, how we develop our knowledge. This is both the challenge and opportunity that computers present.

REFERENCES

Abels, P. (1972). Can computers do Social Work? *Social Work* 17, 5-11.

Besher, A. (1985). Pacific Rim column. *San Francisco Chronicle,* July 15, p. 31.

Carlson, R. (1993). From rules to prototypes. *Computers in Human Services* 9(3/4), 339-350.

Cooper, S. (1980). *The master's and beyond.* In J. Mishne, *Psychotherapy and training in clinical social work.* NY: Gardner Press.

Fischer, J. (1978). *Effective casework practice.* NY: McGraw-Hill.

Geiss, G. & Viswanathan, N. (Eds.) (1986). *The human edge.* NY: Haworth Press.

Gripton, J., Licker, P., & de Groot, L. (1988). *Microcomputers in clinical social work.* In Glastonbury, B., LaMendola, W., & Toole, S. (Eds.) *Information technology and the human services.* ENG: John Wiley & Sons.

Holsapple, C., & Whinston, A. (1987). Knowledge-based organizations. *Information Society* 5, 77-90.

Kay, A. (1984). Computer software. *Scientific American* 251 (3), 53-59.

King, M. (1993). Using hypertext in human services. *Computers in Human Services* 9, 3/4, 293-299.

Larson, N. (1990). *Hypertext Newsletter.*

Naisbitt, J. (1984). *Megatrends.* NY: Warner Books, Inc.

Nurius, P. & Hudson, W. (1993). *Human services practice, evaluation and computers.* CA: Brooks/Cole Publishing Company.

Roszak, T. (1986). *The cult of information.* NY: Pantheon.

Shera, J. (1983). Quoted in Machlup, F., & Mansfield, U. (Eds.), *The study of information.* NY: Wiley, p. 649.

Tesch, R. (1990). *Qualitative research: Analysis types and software tools.* PA: Fallner Press.

Turkle, S. (1984). *The second self.* NY: Simon and Schuster.

The Ethics and Economics of IT

Bryan Glastonbury

SUMMARY. This paper argues for the recognition of the ethical dimension in the use of IT to promote economic development. It analyzes four areas in which the spread of new technologies are having an impact on individual and community life–unemployment, delinquent and criminal behaviour, smart weapons, and citizenship–in an attempt to establish that IT is too important to be left to politicians and business people. Instead it should be treated as a matter of great relevance and decision for the whole of society. *[Article copies available from The Haworth Document Delivery Service: 1-800-342-9678.]*

INTRODUCTION

The aim of this paper is to look at the relationship between IT, the standards by which we conduct community life (that is, our ethical framework), and approaches to the maintenance of economic development. The intention is to argue not only that there is a close relationship between these three, but also that the outcome is of vital importance for all of us in the human services.

We take for granted many of the great range of benefits of IT, and it is important to keep these benefits in clear focus during any debate about the problems IT has thrown up. Most of us would find our lives severely impoverished if the technology advances of recent decades were taken away. Nevertheless, we need also to recognise that these very advances

Bryan Glastonbury is Research Professor and a member of the Centre for Human Service Technology at the University of Southampton, UK.

[Haworth co-indexing entry note]: "The Ethics and Economics of IT." Glastonbury, Bryan. Co-published simultaneously in *Computers in Human Services* (The Haworth Press, Inc.) Vol. 12, No. 3/4, 1995, pp. 431-437; and: *Human Services in the Information Age* (ed: Jackie Rafferty, Jan Steyaert, and David Colombi) The Haworth Press, Inc., 1995, pp. 431-437. Single or multiple copies of this article are available from The Haworth Document Delivery Service [1-800-342-9678, 9:00 a.m. - 5:00 p.m. (EST)].

431

have provoked an ethical dilemma for our society and it is just as important that this too is fully recognised. The ethical agenda which has most directly impinged on our professional work as human service workers has been about the role of IT in weakening the ability of individual citizens to keep their private lives private. The political decision of a majority of western nations to abandon the protection of personal privacy in the face of arguments about the potential beneficial uses of information systems based on personal data, not to mention the profitability of the information industry, has demolished one of the core theoretical tenets of the caring professions. Personal information is no longer personal property, perhaps to be shared within the confidential framework of a relationship with a therapist; personal information is now a tradable commodity in many societies, while in others the element of control we can exercise over the recording of our personal histories is severely limited.

On a wider level there are other ethical concerns. Having or not having the benefits of IT has pointed up the growing gap in technology resources between rich and poor communities, and impediments to free and smooth technology transfer. Ownership of advanced technology, and even more the ability to undertake developmental work, has carried with it enormous political power across a wide spectrum, ranging from control over global communications to access to new forms of warfare using "smart weapons." The technical ability to use IT, especially when so many do not possess that ability and are forced into trusting others, has opened up wide scope for economic manipulation, some of it falling over clearly into the arena of illegality, into computer crime.

More could be said to justify the argument that we are going through an ethical crisis related to IT, but it may be of greater use to move forward in search of explanations, perhaps to go back to some of the ideas of the pioneers of technology planning. Yoneji Masuda, who oversaw the planning process leading to vital political decisions which have underpinned Japan's technological progress, initiated discussion around the idea that a major scientific advancement will always stimulate the formation of an ethical watchdog, but with a delay before it becomes operational (1981). Hence we can expect the IT industry to be shadowed by an "ethics industry," of which, incidentally, human service workers are seen as a part, but those whose preoccupation is ethical will always be running to try to catch up with the technology.

This argument, that ethical development and integration will always lag behind technological progress, has been further refined by Walter LaMendola (Glastonbury and LaMendola, 1992) in his theory relating to the technological/cultural/biological three speed. In essence his argument is that in order for a new development to become fully integrated into society it has to go through three phases of development. Technological development shows us what the new science can offer; cultural development seeks to integrate this new science into our lifestyles and value systems; while biological development takes account of any evolutionary changes which are necessary to adapt ourselves to the new situation. The time scale needed for each of these adjustments is very different. A major technological change can occur, as has happened with IT, is two or three decades. The corresponding cultural adjustment can take most of a century–it will after all take from 70 to 80 years from the first introduction of computer teaching in schools to the point where everyone in a community has received such education. Biological change is measured in hundreds, if not thousands of years.

The inevitable conclusion from Walter LaMendola's work is that any major scientific change, and IT is a massive one, will bring forward a list of cultural, ethical and economic questions. Some of the answers will be happy ones–such as that IT offers a much less polluted and despoiling environment than traditional heavy industry. Other questions will have less happy answers, or seem, at least for the present, to be unanswerable. Only experience will tell us what is happening to our lives, but four disadvantages have already emerged to present the main challenges for the human services for the coming decades. IT may not be the sole cause of these problems, but it is a significant factor.

UNEMPLOYMENT

Keynesian economic theory postulates a close dependent relationship between economic welfare and levels of employment. An economically healthy society has full employment: an economy falling into recession sheds jobs: a government wishing to pull out of recession creates employment, thereby encouraging increased economic activity. After little more than two decades of IT the position has changed radically. An economy falling into recession makes savings by cutting levels of employment and replacing the work force with new technologies, from word processors to robots. An economy coming out of recession does much the same thing, putting an increasing proportion of investment into technology rather than labour. The reason is clear–that new technologies are often more productive than human labour, and therefore, from the point of view of an employer, more profitable. The outcome for people is devastating. As we emerge from the current global recession it will become apparent to everyone that national economies can thrive at a macro level while maintaining, at the same time, very high levels of unemployment. For the first time the comforting association of fuller employment and general economic good health is no longer dependably present.

Chronically high unemployment is a major challenge for the caring professions, not only for the direct impact of having so many people without work, but more importantly for the spread of social problems it engenders, ranging from increased suicide and crime to all the impact on family and community life of poverty.

DELINQUENT AND CRIMINAL BEHAVIOUR

Links are argued between unemployment and the levels of criminal behaviour within a society, with unemployment viewed as a causal factor. Patterns of criminal activity are enormously complex, and many explanations have been given as to why people commit crimes, ranging from psychological and physiological theories about "criminal types" to the deterrent impact of forms of punishment. In a context where there is limited consensus one of the more durable beliefs has been in the view that well distributed economic welfare reduces the need or incentive to commit crimes (particularly those such as theft and burglary). In contrast increased poverty and unemployment works in the opposite direction, providing the opportunity of unoccupied time, the need to help maintain acceptable living standards, and a motivation born of despair to try any path to a better future. These trends are, perhaps, exacerbated by a prevailing political philosophy of individualism rather than collectivism, in the way that John Mortimer suggests, only half in jest–"Criminals are, by and large, of an extraordinary Conservative disposition. They believe passionately in free enterprise and strict monetarist policies. They are against state interference of any kind" (1988, p. 74).

Another relationship is conjectured between criminal behaviour and the impact of the media. The possibility that violence on TV promotes violence in the family and on the streets is a topic of endless discussion. What is less frequently considered is that such a debate can only occur if we take for granted the trivialisation of the media, the acceptance that the standard diet of the media contains large portions of violence. While the IT industry may not be responsible for the output of television companies, it is responsible for trivialising the domestic use of information technology, of ensuring, because the profits are greater, that the home computer is a games machine not a serious contribution to the quality of domestic life. The failure of IT to do for the home something as important as it has done for the office has both helped undermine the family as a viable social unit, and ensured that many children will spend hours playing computer games of uncensored brutality.

In the longer term we must be anxious about the gradual coming together and resultant confusion between "reality" and "virtual reality," with many members of society finding it increasingly difficult to modify their behaviour and attitudes according to whether they are in the real world or an artificial world, or to understand differences between real world values and those which prevail in computer games.

SMART WEAPONS

Nowhere is the ethical confusion of real and artificial worlds more apparent than in the development of the tools of war, with computer guided missiles and star wars programmes mimicking video games creations (or is it the other way round?). There has been a startling change in people's attitudes towards warfare in recent decades. The development of the nuclear bomb sparked off a wave of revulsion, a feeling that warfare was getting out of hand and would have to be banned in some way. In contrast the development of smart weapons, characterized by a supposedly much more precise and selective targeting, has lulled anti-militarist sentiment, and almost made us feel that war can be acceptable because we can ensure that very few innocent people suffer.

Leaving aside the validity of such claims for the technology, it is a matter of observations that the market in IT based armaments is almost out of control, and the end of superpower confrontation has not brought an end to war. For the caring professions the task remains, as it has always been, to help innocent victims. Across the world there are, now, as many displaced persons, refugees following military action, as there ever were during the second world war.

CITIZENS AND NON-CITIZENS

Most refugees have lost all effective rights of citizenship and join with another major population group, economic migrants, for whom a sense of belonging and a secure home in a supportive community is a highest priority. In its moves towards greater cohesion the EU has rightly recognised the issue of citizenship and the importance of ensuring the welfare of people who live within Europe, whether they are ethnic or religious minorities, or face additional challenges such as a handicap. IT is a mixed blessing in this context. On the one hand it enables us to identify, track and direct help towards people who need it. On the other hand IT exercises a strong pull towards standardization, and in that sense it can be used to support and promote both gentle moves towards weakening diversity and making us all more homogeneous, and the vicious opposition to diversity which continues to be a feature of racial attacks. Here is yet another area where one of the basic theoretical tenets of the caring professions is being challenged, and it is important for the challenge to be resisted. From their inception the caring professions have recognised, cherished, and fought for the uniqueness of each individual and the right which we all have within the framework of the law to "do our own thing." The caring professions are the upholders of tolerance and diversity, at a time when intolerance is widespread, and the information systems which increasingly order our lives would prefer us all to conform to a stereotype.

CONCLUSION

Drawing these arguments together, we can see that IT has developed with hugely significant positives and negatives for all our lives. Therein lies the dilemma. The particular feature of the dilemma presented in this paper arises from the dynamic interchange of economic and ethical pressures, and the fall-out which has to be tackled by the caring professions. Masuda saw a future possibility in which the economics and ethics of IT stayed in alignment when he wrote "information technology is both public and international in character, a point that must receive special emphasis. . . information is by nature a public property; it is non-expendable, non-transferable and has a cumulative effect" (1981, p. 124). Instead of Masuda's vision we have information and its technology both drawn into the circle of governmental secrecy to spawn tools of destruction and control, and privatized as a market commodity to displace the human labour force. Information technology is far too important in our lives to be left to politicians and business people. The nature and economics of the technology need to be moderated by a strongly represented ethical framework. It is vital for all our futures that the caring professions do not see themselves solely as a casualty service when facing up to the challenges outlined above, but maintain broader and more far-sighted horizons as part of the vanguard of a thrust towards a better IT.

REFERENCES

Glastonbury, B. and LaMendola, W., (1992) *The Integrity of Intelligence.* Macmillan, UK and St. Martin's Press, USA.

Masuda, Y., (1981) *The Information Society as Post-Industrial Society.* World Future Society, USA.

Mortimer, J., (1988) *Rumpole for the Defence.* Penguin Books, UK.

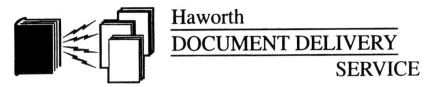

Haworth
DOCUMENT DELIVERY
SERVICE

This valuable service provides a single-article order form for any article from a Haworth journal.

- *Time Saving:* No running around from library to library to find a specific article.
- *Cost Effective:* All costs are kept down to a minimum.
- *Fast Delivery:* Choose from several options, including same-day FAX.
- *No Copyright Hassles:* You will be supplied by the original publisher.
- *Easy Payment:* Choose from several easy payment methods.

Open Accounts Welcome for . . .
- Library Interlibrary Loan Departments
- Library Network/Consortia Wishing to Provide Single-Article Services
- Indexing/Abstracting Services with Single Article Provision Services
- Document Provision Brokers and Freelance Information Service Providers

---

MAIL or *FAX* THIS ENTIRE ORDER FORM TO:

Haworth Document Delivery Service
The Haworth Press, Inc.
10 Alice Street
Binghamton, NY 13904-1580

or FAX: 1-800-895-0582
or CALL: 1-800-342-9678
9am-5pm EST

PLEASE SEND ME PHOTOCOPIES OF THE FOLLOWING SINGLE ARTICLES:

1) Journal Title: _____
   Vol/Issue/Year:_____Starting & Ending Pages:_____
   Article Title:_____
   _____

2) Journal Title: _____
   Vol/Issue/Year:_____Starting & Ending Pages:_____
   Article Title:_____
   _____

3) Journal Title: _____
   Vol/Issue/Year:_____Starting & Ending Pages:_____
   Article Title:_____
   _____

4) Journal Title: _____
   Vol/Issue/Year:_____Starting & Ending Pages:_____
   Article Title:_____
   _____

(See other side for Costs and Payment Information)

COSTS: Please figure your cost to order quality copies of an article.

1. Set-up charge per article: $8.00
   ($8.00 × number of separate articles) _____

2. Photocopying charge for each article:

   1-10 pages: $1.00 _____

   11-19 pages: $3.00 _____

   20-29 pages: $5.00 _____

   30+ pages: $2.00/10 pages _____

3. Flexicover (optional): $2.00/article _____

4. Postage & Handling: US: $1.00 for the first article/
   $.50 each additional article _____

   Federal Express: $25.00 _____

   Outside US: $2.00 for first article/
   $.50 each additional article _____

5. Same-day FAX service: $.35 per page _____

   GRAND TOTAL: _____

_____

METHOD OF PAYMENT: (please check one)

❏ Check enclosed ❏ Please ship and bill. PO # _____
   (sorry we can ship and bill to bookstores only! All others must pre-pay)

❏ Charge to my credit card: ❏ Visa; ❏ MasterCard; ❏ Discover;
   ❏ American Express;

Account Number: _____ Expiration date: _____

Signature: ✗ _____

Name: _____ Institution: _____

Address: _____

_____

City: _____ State: _____ Zip: _____

Phone Number: _____ FAX Number: _____

_____

MAIL or *FAX* THIS ENTIRE ORDER FORM TO:

Haworth Document Delivery Service	**or FAX:** 1-800-895-0582
The Haworth Press, Inc.	**or CALL:** 1-800-342-9678
10 Alice Street	9am-5pm EST)
Binghamton, NY 13904-1580	